A. Munro Neville · Michael J. O'Hare

The Human Adrenal Cortex

Pathology and Biology – An Integrated Approach

With 173 Figures

Springer-Verlag
Berlin Heidelberg New York 1982

A. Munro Neville, PhD, MD, MRCPath,
Director, Ludwig Institute for Cancer Research (London Branch),
Royal Marsden Hospital,
Sutton, Surrey SM2 5PX, England

Michael J. O'Hare, MA, PhD,
Ludwig Institute for Cancer Research (London Branch),
Royal Marsden Hospital,
Sutton, Surrey SM2 5PX, England

ISBN 3-540-11085-2 Springer-Verlag Berlin Heidelberg New York
ISBN 0-387-11085-2 Springer-Verlag New York Heidelberg Berlin

Filmset and printed by BAS Printers Limited,
Over Wallop, Hampshire

2128/3916-543210

All these things here collected are not mine,
But divers grapes make one kind of wine,
So I from many learned authors took
The various matters written in this book;
What's not mine own shall not by me be father'd,
The most part I in many years have gather'd.

John Taylor, the Water-Poet, 1580–1654

Preface

We would like to take this opportunity of expressing our sincerest thanks to the many persons who have made adrenal tissue and related materials available to us for our work. Our especial gratitude is extended to Drs. J. J. Brown, A. Lever and J. I. S. Robertson of the M.R.C. Blood Pressure Unit, Glasgow, Dr. J. K. Grant, Royal Infirmary, Glasgow, Professor R. B. Welbourn and Dr. W. Kelly, Royal Postgraduate Medical School, Drs. D. B. Grant of Great Ormond Street, J. Ginsberg, Royal Free Hospital, D. C. Anderson, Hope Hospital, Salford, C. R. Edwards, St. Bartholomew's Hospital and Professor I. Doniach (formerly of the London Hospital) and Messrs. J.-C. Gazet, A. McKinna and P. Greening, Royal Marsden Hospital, London.

The preparation and presentation of the material and the results would not have been possible without the help of Dr. P. Monaghan and his Electron Microscopy Unit, Ludwig Institute for Cancer Research (London Branch), Sutton, Mrs. Mitchell and her Histology Team, Royal Marsden Hospital, Sutton, Mr. K. Moreman of the Photographic Department of the Royal Marsden Hospital and Institute of Cancer Research, London and Mr. M. Hughes for graphics. Particular thanks are due for the untiring efforts and assistance of Mr. J. Ellis and Mrs. D. Corney of the Ludwig Institute for Cancer Research (London Branch), Sutton, for most of the photographic and secretarial work respectively.

Professors G. Dhöm and E. Mäusle kindly provided material for Figs. 6.7, 6.8 and 6.9, 6.10 respectively. Professor J. R. Anderson for Figs. 18.1B and 18.2, Dr. J. Powers for Figs. 18.4 and 18.5 and Dr. B. Fox for Fig. 21.1 for which we are most grateful.

Finally, we would like to extend our appreciation to Sir Thomas Symington, our former mentor, who initially stimulated our interest in the adrenal gland, and our many previous co-workers including Drs. A. M. MacKay, K. Grigor, P. Hornsby and E. Nice.

Sutton, September 1981
A. Munro Neville
Michael J. O'Hare

Contents

Chapter 1
Introduction

We have been interested over the past two decades in aspects of both the functional biology and pathology of the human adrenal cortex. During this period, a substantial number of papers and monographs have been published by many investigators on various topics relevant to the animal and human adrenal glands and knowledge has been advanced in many respects.

Our purpose in compiling this book has been threefold. First, we have attempted to present an integrated approach to the pathology of the human adrenal gland, based in part on our personal experience, but also incorporating and summarising much of the recent data thereby providing the working pathologist with a single up-to-date volume.

During the past two decades several books have dealt with the adrenal cortex and its diseases from clinical (Soffer et al. 1961a; Mills 1964; Nelson 1980), multidisciplinary (Currie et al. 1962; Eisenstein 1967; Chester Jones and Henderson 1976, 1978, 1980) and comparative anatomical (Chester Jones 1957) viewpoints. However, only two books have been primarily directed towards aspects of diagnostic histopathology (Dhöm 1965; Symington 1969) and both are now well over a decade old. Consequently, as a second objective, we have attempted to produce a well-illustrated reference together with a comprehensive description of the underlying biology of the human cortex derived partly from our own experience. This should, we hope, enable the accurate pathological classification of adrenocortical disorders to be made on a rational basis.

Finally, we have endeavoured to provide a book where the biology, pathology, biochemistry and salient clinical features have been integrated in such a way as to interest the scientist as well as the clinician in the problems that remain to be solved, as we believe that such an integrated multidisciplinary approach will continue to prove of value in the future.

Chapter 2
Historical Aspects

Although the human adrenal gland was illustrated by Eustachius in 1563, the descriptions of Caspar Bartholinus the Elder (1611) were the first to receive significant attention because Eustachius' illustrations were immured in the Papal library and remained unknown until the early eighteenth century when they were republished by Lancisi.

For two centuries, debate took place as to whether the adrenal or suprarenal glands, as they were called by Riolan (1629), possessed excretory ducts and a central cavity. These imagined attributes, considered evidence for a supposed function of processing 'atrabilia' or black bile, gradually fell from favour and, by the beginning of the 19th century, their ductless nature and the probability that they formed some secretion which was returned to the blood stream was generally accepted (Sorkin 1957).

The gross distinction between the cortex and medulla was noted by Cuvier in 1805 although Huschke (1845) was the first to apply these terms to the adrenal. Ecker (1846) gave the first detailed histological description of the human adrenal gland and Arnold (1831) was the first to study their embryology but erroneously believed that they were derived from the Wolffian bodies. A relationship between the gonads and adrenals was also suggested on comparative grounds by Meckel (1806). Thomas Addison (1855) provided the first concrete evidence of the vital nature of the adrenal gland describing accurately the symptoms of adrenal insufficiency and their association with destruction of the gland by a variety of infective diseases and neoplastic lesions. In his own words, he 'stumbled upon' these symptoms, which he believed usually included idiopathic anaemia, while searching for the cause of pernicious anaemia, although, in fact, the two diseases (i.e. Addison's disease and Addison's anaemia) are seen together only in a minority of cases.

Early experimental adrenal research was subject to misinterpretation and controversy. In a much quoted study, Brown-Séquard (1856) demonstrated by extirpation that the adrenals were essential to life. His experiments were prompted specifically by Addison's pathophysiological observations; they were, however, poorly controlled and the death of his animals was probably due as much to shock and sepsis as to true adrenal insufficiency. The failure of many subsequent experiments by other workers to give a consistent picture led to many decades of fruitless debate. The root of the problem lay not only in a failure to distinguish between medullary and cortical functions, but also in the widely varying frequencies with which accessory cortical tissues occur in various animals (noted in man by Marchand in 1883). Final proof that the cortex and not the medulla was the vital tissue was not obtained until the studies of Wheeler and Vincent (1917) and Houssay and Lewis (1923).

The second half of the nineteenth century had, therefore, seen little further progress in adrenocortical physiology; nevertheless, the structural relationships in the tissue and its development were further defined. Thus, the zonation of the cortex was recognised by Harley (1858) and Arnold (1866) coined the terms zona glomerulosa, zona fasciculata and zona reticularis (Fig. 2.1). The independent origin of the medulla and its homology with ganglionic elements was described by Balfour (1878) and

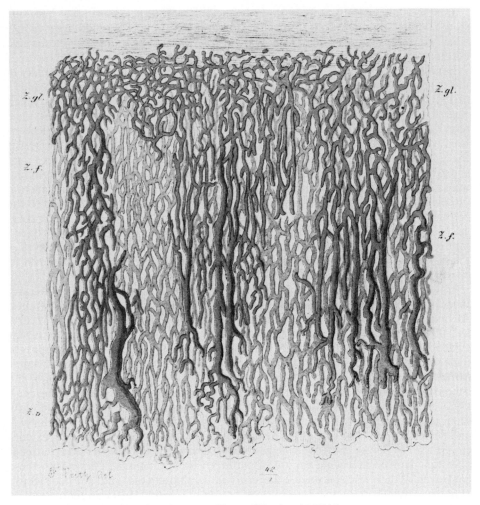

Fig. 2.1. The zonation of the adrenal cortex as illustrated by Arnold (1866).

Mitsukuri (1882), although these observations had been pre-empted to some extent by
Leydig (1852) and Köllicker (1854) with their descriptions of the gland in the German
literature. Balfour was, however, the first to describe correctly the development of the
cortex from coelomic mesothelium dorsal to and separate from the Wolffian body, and
dynamic relationships between the constituent cells were first suggested by Gottschau
(1883) who originated the concept of centripetal adrenal cell migration.

   Experimental interest in the adrenal cortex during the years 1890–1920 was largely
overshadowed by the medulla, its relation to the sympathetic nervous system and the
general concepts of reflex nervous action that were then fashionable. Thus the
endocrine secretions of the gland were by and large identified with adrenaline, which
had been isolated and characterised in 1901. Many attempts to prepare adrenal
extracts active in Addison's disease had been made during this period, but most met
with little objective success (Adams 1903). Reasons for the 80-year gap between
Addison's description of adrenal insufficiency and the success of Swingle and Pfiffner
(1930) in preparing active cortical extracts are not, however, hard to find.
Contemporary studies of other endocrine tissues had been facilitated by factors such as

the water-soluble nature of their products, the relatively large quantities of hormone stored within the tissue, and in several cases identification of specific target tissues which served as assay systems. None of these criteria could be fulfilled by the adrenal cortex.

Early studies of adrenal pathology (e.g. Woolley 1903) did not assist materially in the identification of cortical hormones and their effects although Bulloch and Sequeira (1905) subsequently described a series of adrenal tumours and hyperplasias which elicited precocious or inappropriate development of secondary sex characteristics. The term 'suprarenal virilism' or 'adrenogenital syndrome' describing these effects is usually attributed to Gallais (1912a,b); the first detailed description of such a case was that of DeCrecchio (1865). The problems of adrenocortical pathology at this time were compounded by several factors. The rare medullary and even rarer cortical tumours were not clearly distinguished from one another until the turn of the century, and the presence of symptoms such as hypertension with both types of tumour added to the confusion. Furthermore, the erroneous identification of renal clear cell adenocarcinomas (hypernephromas) as so-called adrenal-rest tumours by Grawitz (1883) did little to clarify the situation. Although Grawitz's theory was rejected by Stoerk in 1908 the distinction between these tumours and true adrenocortical lesions continued to cause problems for many years.

Evidence for the higher control of adrenal cortex began to accumulate in the early years of the 20th century although it was largely ignored in contemporary studies. Atrophy of the adrenals in anencephalic fetuses had been noted by Morgagni as early as 1719 but it remained for Ascoli and Legnani (1912) to provide the first experimental evidence of pituitary control with their observation of adrenocortical atrophy in hypophysectomised dogs. Simmonds (1919) noted a similar effect in man. It was Smith (1930) with his hypophysectomised rat assay who laid the foundation for the characterisation of the 'adrenotrophic hormone' as a separate principle by Collip et al. (1933), its subsequent isolation by Li et al. (1943) and by Sayers et al. (1943), its sequencing by Bell and co-workers (1954) and finally its total synthesis by Schwyzer and Seiber in 1963. The role of the adrenal gland in relation to stress was repeatedly emphasised by Selye (1946), who suggested that derangement of the pituitary-adrenal axis was involved in a wide variety of pathogenetic mechanisms. Along with these controversial theories Selye coined the terms 'mineralocorticoid' and 'glucocorticoid'.

In the search for the active principles of the adrenal cortex, 1930 was undoubtedly a turning point. In that year Swingle and Pfiffner published a detailed summary of their studies of active cortical extracts, relying on a time-consuming and difficult assay based on the survival time of adrenalectomised cats and dogs. Knowledge of the tissue-specific effects of putative cortical secretions was at that time largely non-existent, although Houssay had suspected that they were related to carbohydrate metabolism and an involvement in the regulation of kidney functions had been suggested by Marshall and Davis (1916).

In the late 1920s, however, considerable progress had been made in the development of a reliable survival-time assay of cortical activity, notably by Rogoff and Stewart (1928), and using these assays several groups soon claimed preparation of active cortical extracts. They included Rogoff and Stewart (1928) themselves with 'interrenalin' and Hartman and his colleagues (1928) with their adrenaline-free 'cortin'. All these studies were, however, superseded by Swingle and Pfiffner at Princeton, to whom the preparation of the first really potent cortical extract can be credited. Their material, which was prepared by organic solvent extraction, could be freed from residual adrenaline without loss of activity and supported adrenalectomised animals indefinitely, rather than merely postponing their demise. Dramatic remissions with this extract in cases of Addison's disease were obtained during 1930–32 by

Rowntree and Greene at the Mayo Clinic and by Harrop and Weinstein at Johns Hopkins Hospital.

The vast quantities of adrenal tissue used in these studies (usually of bovine origin) clearly precluded the routine clinical use of such extracts and no progress had been made at this time in identifying the chemical nature of the adrenocortical hormone(s). Szent-Györgi had isolated adrenal ascorbic acid in 1928 but it was not until 1934 when Kendall at the Mayo Clinic announced the preparation of a crystalline cortical extract with a molecular weight of 350 and a tentative empirical formula of $C_{20}H_{30}O_5$ that the road to the routine therapeutic use of cortical hormones was opened. During the period 1934–1938, his group, that of Wintersteiner and Pfiffner (1935) and Reichstein (1936) in Basel succeeded brilliantly in attaining these objectives. Using vast quantities of adrenal tissue (batches of 3000 lb were not uncommon) and methods of solvent extraction, countercurrent distribution and fractional crystallisation, the major products of the cortex were prepared. Compound A (11-dehydrocorticosterone) and and Compound E (cortisone) were characterised in 1936, Compound B (corticosterone) and Compound F (cortisol) in 1937, and Substance S (11-deoxycortisol) and Substance Q (deoxycorticosterone) in 1938. Chemical studies showed that these were all steroids with 21 carbon atoms, i.e., C_{21}-compounds. Their relationship to the then newly characterised sex steroids was readily apparent from their chemical degradation to steroids with 19 carbon atoms such as adrenosterone (Substance G). It was suspected from their structure that they might all be synthesised from cholesterol, although direct proof was lacking until the work of Hechter (1951).

These studies did not immediately resolve the problem of the identity of the active cortical hormone, although belief in a unitary hormone was gradually eroded by the multiplicity of products isolated from the gland. The precise role of individual compounds remained in doubt and Gaunt (1975) has recently published an entertaining personal account of this exciting era of research. Not only was it apparent that various steroids possessed widely differing levels of life-sustaining 'cortin' activity but it was also realised that the yields of various steroids obtained by the laborious processes then in use did not necessarily reflect tissue levels. In fact, it was not until 1953 that Bush and Sandberg showed that cortisol was the major free plasma steroid in man.

Returning to the chronological sequence, however, by 1940 a battery of tests of steroid bioactivity were now available. They included disturbance of electrolyte balance (Loeb), nitrogen balance (Harrop), hepatic gluconeogenesis (Britton and Silvette) and asthenia and work tests (e.g. Everse-de Fremery and Ingle tests). These assays revealed that a large part of the activity in cortical extracts, notably its salt-retaining activity, resided in an 'amorphous fraction' that had thus far resisted crystallisation and characterisation (Kendall 1941).

The objective of complete synthesis of the active steroids already isolated was nevertheless pursued, and in 1948 Sarett at Merck eventually announced the synthesis of cortisone in quantities sufficient for clinical use, in itself a major feat of organic synthesis. Cortisone was, in fact, largely ignored when first isolated as it was only weakly active as a 'life-sustaining' steroid in adrenalectomised animals; its potency was only revealed when it was tested for specific 'glucocorticoid' activity.

Cortisone was not the first chemically synthesised adrenal steroid to be used therapeutically. Both 11-dehydrocorticosterone and deoxycorticosterone (acetate) had been previously employed by Thorn and his associates (1942) in clinical trials in Addison's disease, but with only limited success. The widely publicised and dramatically successful use of cortisone by Hench and Kendall in rheumatoid arthritis in 1949, however, saw the culmination of a project initiated nearly 20 years earlier, albeit in a clinical context that had hardly been envisaged at the outset.

The most notable advance in understanding the pathophysiology of the adrenal cortex that took place during this era of chemical steroid research was the description, by Harvey Cushing in 1932, of symptoms of adrenal hyperfunction found in association with basophilic pituitary adenomas. Up to that time many clinical manifestations of cortical hyperfunction had escaped general recognition, with the exception of the adrenogenital syndrome to which we have already referred. Occasional cases of apparent endocrine imbalance of unknown aetiology had, however, surfaced from time to time.

Cushing's unique contribution was to describe both the precise physical changes and the pituitary alterations in a series of such previously obscure 'polyglandular syndromes'. Although he acknowledged that the adrenocortical hyperplasia noted in some cases might be responsible for some of the systemic manifestations of pituitary basophilism, his primary concern was to link all these effects to the pituitary tumours, which he considered their root cause. Bauer (1936) was probably the first to champion the role of the adrenal cortex in the aetiology of Cushing's syndrome, which he termed 'interrenalism', and he drew attention to the fact that an identical syndrome could be observed in many cases where no pituitary changes were demonstrable, thus distinguishing between what came to be known as Cushing's disease proper and Cushing's syndrome.

At this time no techniques for measuring directly physiological quantities of adrenal steroids, let alone adrenocorticotrophic hormone, existed. Proof of the excessive quantities of adrenal steroids secreted in Cushing's syndrome was obtained by Anderson and Haymaker (1937) when they prolonged the life of adrenalectomised rats with extracts of patients' sera. Further evidence of the inverse relationship between physiological changes in Cushing's syndrome and Addison's disease was forthcoming from studies such as those of McQuarrie, Johnson and Ziegler (1937) on electrolyte balance, and in 1938 Haymaker distinguished clearly for the first time between the concept of excessive adrenal androgen secretion as responsible for the adrenogenital syndrome and excess 'cortin' secretion in Cushing's syndrome. The latter was not finally identified until Mason and Sprague (1948) isolated cortisol in increased amounts from the urine of a patient with Cushing's syndrome. The 'adrenal theory' of Cushing's syndrome had, however, gained strength for many years previous to this finding, notably as propounded by Fuller Albright (1943), even to the point where the pituitary changes were deemed secondary in nature.

The clinical recognition of both the adrenogenital syndrome and Cushing's syndrome had preceded the isolation of the relevant hormones by several years. This was not, however, the case with the last member of the classic triad of hypercortical states, hyperaldosteronism. This was probably due in part at least to the fact that its symptoms, notably hypertension, overlapped those of many other disease states. By the late 1940's it was evident that an unidentified cortical steroid was a key factor in hydromineral regulation, notably the retention and excretion of sodium. There was, furthermore, good circumstantial evidence from animal studies that it originated in the zona glomerulosa, as suggested by Swann (1940). A salt requirement of adrenalecto-mised animals had been noted as long ago as 1927 by Marine and Baumann, but it was the studies of Loeb (1932) on electrolyte balance in Addison's disease that clinched the case and drew attention to the probable role of adrenal hormones in salt and water metabolism. Deoxycorticosterone (Substance Q) was potent in causing salt and water retention and for over a decade, therefore, it remained the most likely candidate for the adrenal 'mineralocorticoid'. Doubts as to its true physiological role persisted on account of the very limited amounts of this steroid in the gland. By the end of the 1940's several groups had begun to reinvestigate the 'amorphous fraction' of cortical extracts with the aim of finding a new mineralocorticoid. The prize fell to Simpson and Tait at the Middlesex Hospital, who observed that an unidentified component of a commercial adrenal extract had a marked effect on urinary electrolyte balance in adrenalectomised rats, and they have recently reviewed the interesting history of this discovery (Tait and Tait 1978). Their success came with the conjunction of two new methods, the paper chromatography systems of Bush and an elegant mineralocorticoid bioassay. 'Electrocortin' was isolated in 1952 and renamed aldosterone the following year after its structure had been determined in a collaborative effort between the Middlesex group and Reichstein, von Euw, Schindler, Wettstein and Neher in Basel (1954). Aldosterone was first isolated from man by Luetscher and Johnson (1954), and the symptoms of its pathophysiological excess were finally recognised in association with certain adrenocortical tumours the following year by Conn (1955) thus concluding what may be termed the historical era of adrenal research.

Part A
THE NORMAL ADRENAL CORTEX

Chapter 3
Origin and Development of the Adrenal Gland

Embryology

The adrenal cortex is of mesodermal origin with its parenchymal steroidogenic cells
arising from the coelomic mesothelium. The most extensive study of human adrenal
embryogenesis is that of Crowder, based on the Carnegie Embryological Collection
(Crowder 1957). The following resumé is taken largely from his descriptions which must
supersede, by virtue of their completeness, the earlier but still widely quoted studies of
Keene and Hewer (1927), Uotila (1940), and Velican (1948).

At about the 25th day of gestation (5–6 mm length), the coelomic epithelium lateral
to the gastric mesentery and medial to the mesonephros and urogenital ridge comes to
consist of cuboidal/columnar cells among which many mitoses occur during the next
5–7 days. This results in cords of large polyhedral epithelioid cells which extend into the
overlying mesenchyme to form the adrenal primordium. These processes take place
bilaterally between the levels of the 6th–12th thoracic segments in the so-called adrenal
groove (Fig. 3.1), medial to the contiguous zone of coelomic epithelium from which the
gonadal blastema arises.

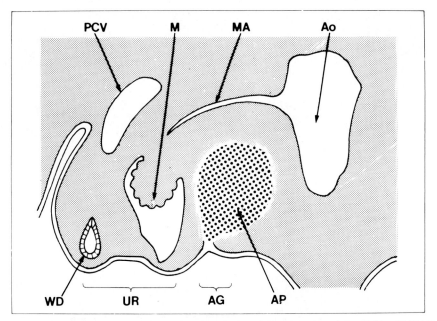

Fig. 3.1. Cross-section through the trunk region of a 4-week human embryo (after Velican 1948). The adrenal
primordium (AP) is situated above the adrenal groove (AG) next to the urogenital ridge (UR), and it is
bounded by the mesonephros (M), mesonephric artery (MA), and aorta (AO). Other adjacent structures
include the posterior cardinal vein (PCV) and the Wolffian duct (WD).

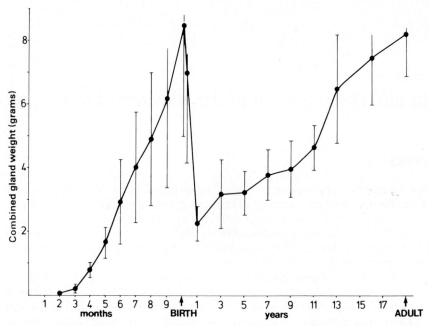

Fig. 3.2. Adrenal gland weights during development. The means (*points*) ± SD (*bars*) of prenatal gland weights are shown, from the data of Tanimura et al. (1971) and postnatal glands (sudden death cases) after Dhöm (1973).

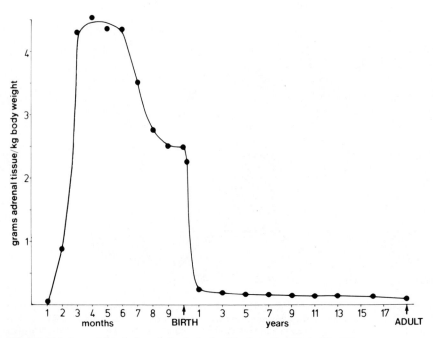

Fig. 3.3. Relative weight of adrenal glands during life, from the data in Fig. 3.2.

At about the 30th day of gestation (9 mm length) cells from the medial wall of the capsule of the mesonephric glomerulus begin to migrate towards the adrenal primordium. Some penetrate the enlarging gland and apparently give rise to intraglandular stromal cells; the remainder form its mesenchymal capsule. Around the 35th day the coelomic epithelial cells subadjacent to the adrenal primordium become smaller, more basophilic, while continuing to push upwards in cords and columns into the primordium. This is now contained within a quadrilateral area bounded by the medial face of the mesonephros, the mesonephric arteries and the aorta (Fig. 3.1). The ontological significance of these various types of coelomic adrenal primordial cells is obscure. Contrary to earlier studies, Crowder (1957) found no evidence of separate origin of the fetal and definitive cortex as the two mesothelial contributions appear to be intimately intermingled throughout the gland; similar conclusions were reached by Gruenwald (1946).

The developing gland enlarges rapidly between the 35th and 45th days of gestation, due in large part to the invasion of nerve tracts along which primitive sympathetic cells destined to form the medulla will later migrate. The cortex continues to receive contributions from the coelomic epithelium, however, until the embryo is 19–20 mm in length (45 days). By this time the gland is cigar-shaped, is totally enveloped by the mesenchymal capsule, and weighs approximately 1 mg.

By the eighth week of gestation each gland weighs 4–6 mg, the increase being due to internal proliferation through mitotic activity largely confined to the outer cortical zone. A clear morphological distinction is now apparent between the peripheral definitive cortex and the centrally-located fetal cortex, first described by Starkel and Wegrzynowski (1910), and Elliot and Armour (1911).

The adrenal circulation is also established at an early stage. Venous drainage from the adrenal gland is by segmental veins draining into the postcardinal and subcardinal veins, which become reduced progressively until by 60 days (30 mm) there are usually three main veins within each gland and a single vein leaving it. The adrenal arteries stem from the non-segmental lateral branches of the descending aorta and the capillary sinusoids within the gland are in functional continuity with the general circulation by the end of the second month of gestation (Hervonen and Suoranta 1972).

During the third month of gestation the greatest relative increase in adrenal weight takes place and by the 12th week of gestation, each gland weighs about 80 mg (Figs. 3.2 and 3.3). Active proliferation is, however, still confined largely to the outer, definitive cortex (Crowder 1957), although the fetal zone now comprises the majority of the overall cortical width.

These descriptions lead to the inescapable conclusion that the rapid enlargement of the fetal cortex during the first trimester stems largely from centripetal contributions from the definitive cortex, thus refuting the popular, but unsubstantiated, concept of a separate origin of the two prenatal cortical zones.

Fetal Development

The adrenals enlarge during the second trimester in direct proportion to the increase in total body weight. The relative weight of the glands at this time is over 4 g/kg or 35 times the adult value (Fig. 3.3). By the sixth month of gestation, each gland weighs about 1.5 g, the weight increase being due largely to the expansion of the inner fetal zone (Fig. 3.4). There is also a gradual transformation of the gland from an ovoid shape into a more extended, flattened form (Fig. 3.5).

During the third trimester, gland weights continue to increase, but at a slower rate than the rest of the body, resulting in a decline in relative weight to about 2.5 g/kg at the

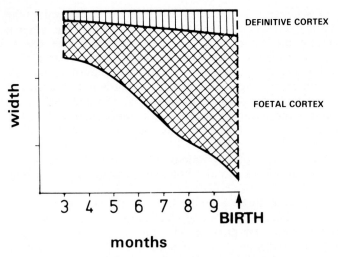

Fig. 3.4. Relative width of the prenatal zones of the adrenal gland. Modified from the data of Dhöm et al. (1958) and Dhöm (1965).

time of birth when each gland weighs just over 4 g (Figs. 3.2 and 3.3) (for histology see p. 41). No sex difference in adrenal size, shape, weight or zonal distribution has been detected in the human embryo at any stage of development.

The adrenal medulla is not prominent in the human fetus. Its constituent cells never occupy more than 10% of the total volume of the gland (Van Hale and Turkel 1979).

Postnatal Development

At birth, the adrenal glands show a relatively narrow yellow ring of definitive or adult zone cells over a deep brownish-red, hyperaemic, fetal zone. The most dramatic event in postnatal development of the gland is the involution of the fetal zone first described by Thomas (1911). The precise chronology of normal involution has not been accurately established, but qualitative observations indicate that cellular degeneration is substantial at two weeks and well established by the end of the first month when about 50% of the gland weight has been lost (Tähkä 1951; Dhöm 1965). By the end of the first year, only the stroma of the degenerated fetal cortex remains (see p. 50).

During the first six months of life there is also a substantial increase in the depth of the definitive cortex. The histological features of cortical development and the preadult gland will be discussed later (p. 41). In morphological terms, however, one of its consequences is the compaction of chromaffin cells to form a discrete medulla. The loss of substance also converts the plump distended gland of the neonate into a relatively shrunken, leaf-like organ, which weighs on average only about 1 g at the end of the first year of life (Fig. 3.2).

Dhöm (1973) has published a complete series of normal adrenal weights in sudden death from infancy through childhood to puberty (Fig. 3.2). It is apparent from these data that true normal weights in children are significantly lower than indicated by previous workers. Thus, up to age five years, mean unfixed weights do not exceed 2 g per gland, rising to just over 2 g in early puberty with a fairly substantial increase during the pubertal growth spurt. No sex differences in the postnatal gland and maturation of the cortex were detected by Dhöm. In cases of 'consuming illness' with

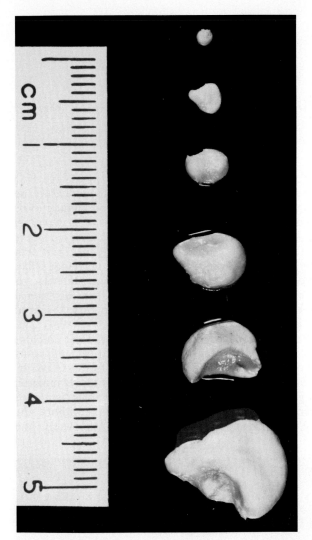

Fig. 3.5. The appearance of the fetal adrenal gland at different stages of gestation is shown. The stages illustrated range from $6\frac{1}{2}$ to 20 weeks (4 mg to 520 mg in weight).

antemortem stress and raised plasma ACTH levels, weights are increased by 0.5–1.0 g per gland, depending upon the age, i.e. a rise of 50%–75%. This weight increase of the young gland in response to the stress of the terminal illness thus equals or exceeds that of the adult (see p. 18).

Chapter 4
Structure of the Adult Adrenal Cortex

Gross Anatomy

The overall dimensions of the adult adrenal glands are similar; they measure on average, 5.0 cm by 2.5 cm along their major axes with the left gland tending to be slightly (2–3 mm) wider. The right gland is pyramidal in outline and is often described as resembling a cocked-hat; the left gland is crescentic in shape. Both have a concave posterior surface where they abut onto the kidneys, with a ridge-like crest that increases in prominence laterally (Fig. 4.1). The anterior surface of both glands is flat, except for the anterior groove from which the main adrenal vein emerges, and which is more prominent on the left adrenal. Computerised tomography (CT) of the adrenal glands tends to give linear or V-shaped profiles of the right gland with Y-shaped triradiate shapes formed by the left (Wilms et al. 1979).

On macroscopic examination each gland can be divided into a *head*, which contains the bulk of the medulla (Fig. 4.2) and which measures up to 6 mm in depth at its broadest part, a *body* with some medullary tissue and a *tail* which lies furthest from the midline of the body and which consists solely of cortical tissue (Dobbie and Symington 1966). On either side of the long axis of the gland there are 2–3 mm thick 'wings' or 'alae' where two opposed layers of cortex abut in sandwich fashion without any interposing medulla (Fig. 4.2). With increasing age, nodules of varying size, weight and

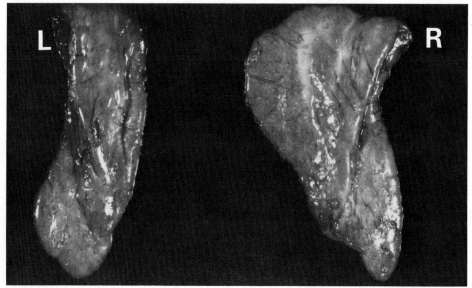

Fig. 4.1. The gross appearances of the left (**L**) and right (**R**) adult adrenal gland from their anterior aspects are shown. (× 1.1)

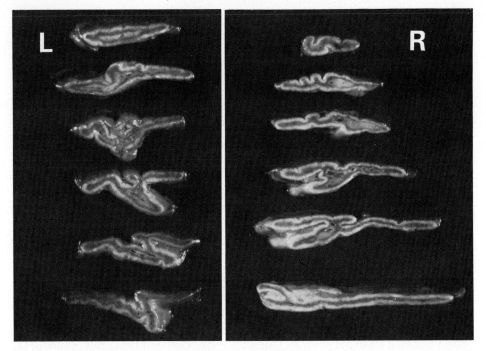

Fig. 4.2. A series of sections through the left (**L**) and right (**R**) adult adrenal glands is illustrated. Note the medulla is confined to the head of the gland (*upper sections*). (× 1.5)

appearance will also be detected on gross examination of many adrenals, as will be described in detail later (p. 53).

Weight

The precise weight of the normal adult adrenal gland has been significantly over-estimated for many years due to reliance on unselected autopsy series.

In cases of sudden death in adults without prior illness, the mean weight of individual glands is 4.0–4.2 g with a coefficient of variation of ±15% (95% limits of 2.8–5.5 g) (Fig. 4.3). Ninety percent of the total weight of the gland is accounted for by the cortex. The mean weight of adrenal glands of Negroes dying suddenly is 3.8 ± 0.8g (SD). These data do not, therefore, support the contention that negroid adrenals are intrinsically smaller than those of whites (Stirling and Keating 1958). There is no significant correlation between absolute body weight and adrenal weight (Gelfman 1964), and no significant differences in the mean weights of normal left and right glands have been recorded (Fig. 4.3). Neither pregnancy nor the menopause appear to result in significant adrenal weight changes in humans although pregnancy-related changes and indeed sex differences are common in other mammals (Chester Jones 1957).

Mean non-diseased adrenal weights in surgical cases (Fig. 4.3) in so far as breast cancer is concerned, do not differ from those of the sudden death series, provided glands with obvious metastatic deposits are excluded. One may conclude, therefore, that significant physiological adrenal enlargement probably occurs only during severe and/or prolonged stress (Symington 1969).

If death is preceded by a prolonged illness (i.e. stress) there is a significant increase in mean adrenal weight. Series in this category give individual mean gland weights

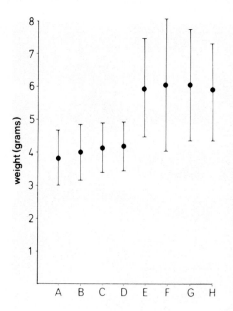

Fig. 4.3. Weights of the adult adrenal glands. Means (*points*) ± SD (*bars*) of single gland weights (n = 25–30) are given. From the series of: (A) Allbrook (1956), sudden death, males, East Africa; (B) Studzinski et al. (1963), surgical, females, U.K.; (C) Quinan and Berger (1933), sudden death, right gland, U.S.A.; (D) Quinan and Berger (1933), sudden death, left gland, U.S.A.; (E) Studzinski et al. (1963), unselected autopsy, males, right gland, U.K.; (F) Studzinski et al. (1963), unselected autopsy, males, left gland, U.K.; (G) Studzinski et al. (1963) unselected autopsy, females, right gland, U.K.; and (H) Studzinski et al. (1963) unselected autopsy, females, left gland, U.K.

ranging 5.8–6.2 with coefficients of variation of ±25% (95% limits 2.7–9.4 g) (Fig. 4.3). Unselected autopsy series composed solely or predominantly of Negroes show somewhat lower mean values (Allbrook 1956; Gelfman 1964), but in view of the fact that the weight of negroid glands in sudden death is not different from whites, it seems likely that this may result from a bias in respect of stress endured during terminal illness.

Assertions that the adrenal glands of males are heavier than females (absolute weight), or that their weight relative to body weight is greater in females are still to be found in various textbooks. These conclusions appear to have been based on one large autopsy series (Holmes et al. 1951), where the differences reported are not only small (<10%) but are unlikely to be significant given the totally unselected nature of this series. Several other series have shown no such differences (Fig. 4.3).

Blood Supply

The blood supply to the adrenal is unique as far as endocrine glands are concerned in that the main arteries and veins take, for the most part, quite separate courses.

The conventional description of the afferent vessels is that the superior, central and inferior aspects of each gland are supplied by multiple adrenal arteries arising, respectively, from the inferior phrenic artery (superior adrenal arteries, average number seven on each side), the aorta at the level of the superior mesenteric artery (medial adrenal arteries, average number one to two) and from the renal artery (inferior adrenal arteries, average number three). There are, however, wide variations in the number and size of such afferent vessels, some of which (medial and inferior) divide en route to the gland. Variations are commonly found in the source of the inferior phrenic artery, and additional adrenal arteries may stem from the gonadal, ureteric, hilar and extrahilar vessels (Gagnon 1957).

The overall result is that each adrenal gland sits in the centre of a web of incoming vessels (Fig. 4.4) which terminate in an anastomosing arcade over the entire surface of the gland and from which up to 50–60 small arterial twigs penetrate the capsule.

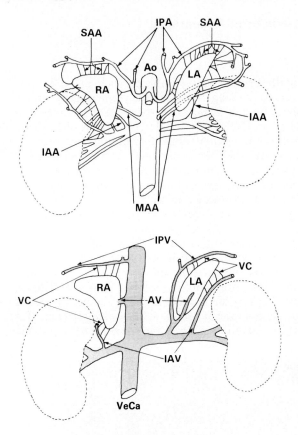

Fig. 4.4 Afferent (*top*) and efferent (*bottom*) vascularisation of the human adrenal glands. (After Gagnon 1956, 1957). LA, left adrenal; RA, right adrenal; IPA, inferior phrenic arteries; SAA superior adrenal arteries; Ao, aorta; IAA, inferior adrenal arteries; MAA, medial adrenal arteries; VeCa, vena cava; IPV, inferior phrenic veins; AV, adrenal veins; VC, venae comitantes; IAV, inferior adrenal veins.

In contrast, most of the effluent blood is collected within the gland into a single central vein which emerges on its anterior surface along the anterior groove. The right adrenal vein is short, passing directly from the gland to the inferior vena cava. The left adrenal vein runs medially to usually join the inferior phrenic vein before entering the left renal vein, although it may run directly into the latter in some cases (Gagnon 1956).

Anomalies and variations in the venous system such as duplication of the main renal vein are encountered, albeit less frequently than with the afferent blood supply (Johnstone 1957). It is important to recognise such anomalies in view of the diagnostic importance of adrenal venography (Field and Saxton 1974). It has been suggested that the shortness and consequent lack of compliance of the right adrenal vein may be responsible for the fact that perinatal adrenal haemorrhage is encountered more frequently in the right than the left gland (Black and Williams 1973).

The adrenal gland possesses an alternative drainage route which may assume considerable significance as a means of preserving adrenal function when either the main vein or the inferior vena cava is occluded by thrombosis. Emissary veins run centrifugally from the central vein and its branches through the cortex, notably in the tail region, to join the pericapsular veins which in turn collect into the venae comitantes (Dobbie and Symington 1966). These follow closely the routes of the superior and inferior groups of adrenal arteries, ultimately draining into a variety of contiguous veins including the inferior phrenic and inferior adrenal veins (Fig. 4.4). Collateral drainage through these vessels has been recognised for many years, although under normal circumstances this route is probably of minor significance.

Light-Microscopic and Ultrastructural Appearance

The Normal Gland

The adult adrenal cortex consists of three readily recognisable parenchymal cell types, arranged in concentric zones or layers comprising the outer zona glomerulosa (glomus ≡ a ball), the inner zona reticularis (rete ≡ a net) and, between them, the zona fasciculata (fascis ≡ a bundle). The appearance of the different zones is dictated by their respective cellular arrangements, differential lipid distribution and pigment accumulation, and the deployment of their vascular and stromal supporting framework (Fig. 4.5). The stromal framework is moderately conspicuous in man, but less so than in other large mammals (e.g. cow, sheep); the lipid content of the human gland, by contrast, is high compared with most other animals.

The classical appearances of the cortical zones are best seen in glands removed at operation, or from accident (sudden death) victims, rather than in typical post-mortem samples. Because of its morphological responses to stress (p. 35), the adrenal cortex is perhaps the most difficult endocrine gland to define in its 'normal' state. This is exemplified by figures given for the relative volumes occupied by the different zones. The normal glomerulosa seldom occupies more than 5% (not ~15% as is sometimes still quoted), the fasciculata about 70% and the reticularis 25%. The use of special stains does not, on the whole, provide any further useful or functionally meaningful distinctions between individual cortical cells although lipid and connective tissue stains

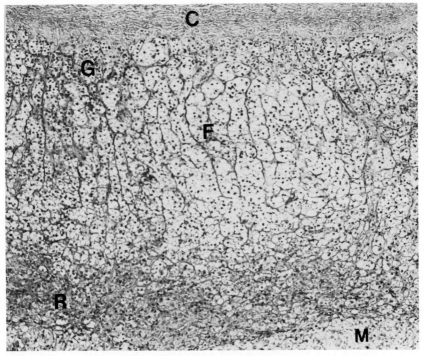

Fig. 4.5 The normal human adrenal cortex. This gland, removed from a woman aged 62 years with metastatic breast carcinoma, weighed 3.65 g. The outer zona glomerulosa (G) has a focal distribution beneath the capsule (C) while the zona reticularis (R) occupies the inner quarter of the cortex. The clear cells of the zona fasciculata (F) comprise the remainder. A small area of adrenal medulla (M) is present on the innermost aspect. (H + E × 90)

(Elias and Pauly 1956; Dobbie and Symington 1966) may sometimes be useful in delineating various features of the gland.

Capsule This is composed of several layers of elongated connective tissue cells disposed parallel to the surface of the gland and surrounded by collagen fibres; ultrastructurally the cells are unremarkable.

Zona glomerulosa The cells of this zone, which are the sole source of the mineralocorticoid aldosterone, are distributed in the human cortex in an ill-defined, focal manner. They form a zone which is situated around the periphery of the cortex immediately beneath the capsule (Fig. 4.5). Its component cells form rounded nests or clusters (Fig. 4.6) surrounded by a fine capillary network; they are small round cells with a high nuclear-cytoplasmic ratio and small, single dense rounded nuclei. The cytoplasm contains sparse amounts of visible lipid compared to the large liposomes found in the cells of the zona fasciculata.

Zona glomerulosa cells are characterised ultrastructurally by their abundant rounded or, more commonly, elongated mitochondria with internal regular tubulo-lamellar cristae (Fig. 4.7) (Table 4.1). The Golgi complex, but not the smooth endoplasmic reticulum, is prominent; lysosomes are few. The cell membranes, which may possess microvilli, frequently exhibit complex interdigitations between adjacent cell membranes with intercellular dilatations which can sometimes be seen at the light-microscopical level, and which are also sometimes present in the outer zona fasciculata. As in all zones of the cortex, specialised junctional complexes are not prominent, although more are seen with the glomerulosa than elsewhere. Basement membrane material may be seen surrounding each cell cluster in the zona glomerulosa. Under conditions of hypertension associated with elevated renin levels, the smooth endoplasmic reticulum increases in glomerulosa cells, there is a shift towards tubular mitochondrial cristae, and lysosome-like bodies increase in number (Hashida and Yunis 1972); reduced ACTH levels in vivo do not alter the ultrastructure of the cells (Mitschke and Saeger 1973).

Table 4.1. Electron microscopic appearances of human adrenocortical cells

	Zona glomerulosa	Zona fasciculata (clear cells)		Zona reticularis (compact cells)
		Outer	Inner	
Cytoplasmic volume	Small	Very large	Large	Intermediate
Smooth endo-plasmic reticulum (SER)	Scanty	Scanty	Increased	Densely packed
Mitochondria	Elongated, small, cristate	Ovoid, small, few internal tubules and vesicles	Spherical, variable size, sometimes large with many internal vesicles	Ovoid, medium-size tubulo-vesicular internum
Lipid	Scanty, free, osmiophilic	Many osmiophilic free droplets OR Many empty membrane-bound vacuoles		Very few vacuoles
Lysosomes	Few	Few	Increased	Many
Microvilli	Occasional	Occasional	Increased	Many

Adapted from Dobbie et al. 1967.

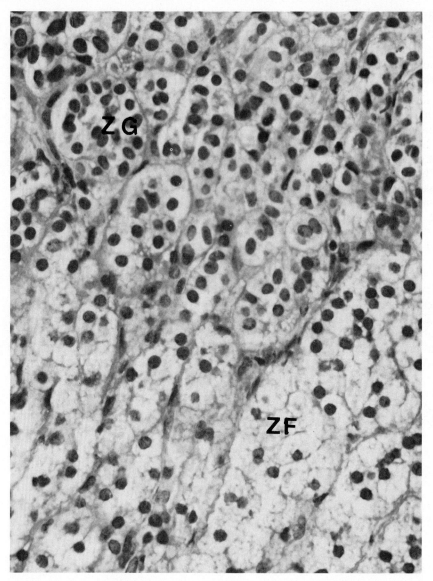

Fig. 4.6. The normal human adrenal cortex. The outer zona glomerulosa (ZG) consists of small cells with a high nuclear : cytoplasmic ratio and lipid-containing cytoplasm, arranged in rounded nests. This zone merges with the larger clear cells of the zona fasciculata (ZF) with their characteristic vacuolated cytoplasm, which are arranged in columns separated by fine fibrovascular trabeculae. (H + E × 500)

Zona fasciculata   Although the normal zona glomerulosa is often ill-defined and may appear to merge with the adjacent or underlying zona fasciculata there is normally no recognisable zona intermedia in the human gland although such exists in some other mammals (Idelman 1978). The zona fasciculata which, together with the zona reticularis, probably forms a single functioning unit for the production of glucocorticoid and such sex steroids as are produced by the gland, comprises the greater part (∼70%) of the normal cortex. This zone is readily recognised

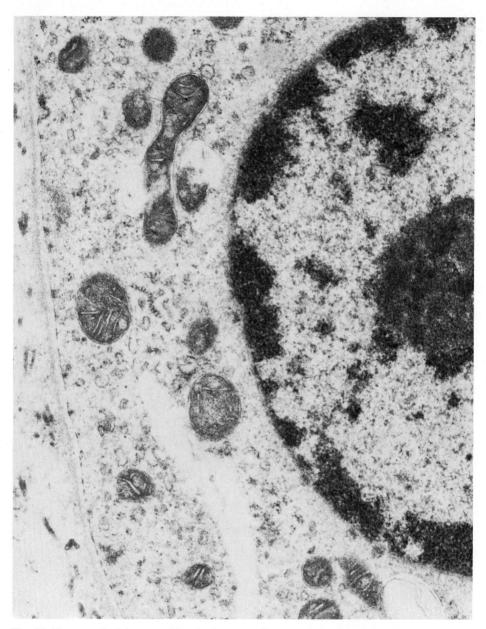

Fig. 4.7. The normal adult cortex. The ultrastructure of a zona glomerulosa cell is shown with typical ovoid/elongated mitochondria with dense matrix and lamellar cristae. The smooth endoplasmic reticulum is sparse but numerous ribosomes and polysomes can be seen throughout the cytoplasm (× 35 000). The cell is surrounded on its outer surface (*left*) by a continuous basement membrane. In this and all electron-micrographs illustrated herein the tissue was fixed in phosphate-buffered glutaraldehyde, post-fixed in osmium tetroxide, embedded in Epon/Araldite and sections stained with uranyl acetate and lead citrate.

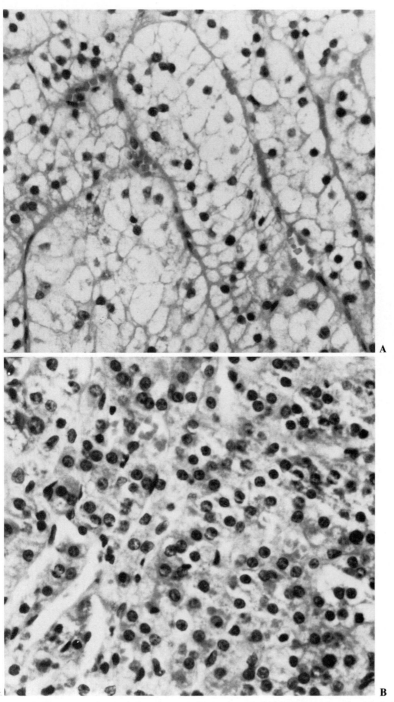

Fig. 4.8. The normal human adrenal cortex. The columns of clear lipid-rich cells with their single rounded hyperchromatic nuclei which comprise the zona fasciculata are shown above (**A**) while the smaller lipid-sparse compact cells of the zona reticularis with its prominent vascular sinusoids are illustrated below (**B**). The compact cells have a granular eosinophilic cytoplasm and indistinct cell membranes. (H + E × 500 [**A**]; × 510 [**B**])

macroscopically by its yellow colour, due to lipochrome pigments and high lipid, predominantly cholesterol ester (p. 70) content. Extraction of the lipid during preparation of typical paraffin-embedded sections results in the cells of the zona fasciculata having a vacuolated appearance. Hence the term 'clear cells' as used by Symington (1969) and the older 'spongiocytes' (Guieysse 1901) still used in the French and German literature.

The clear cells of the zona fasciculata are arranged in radially disposed columns extending from the zona glomerulosa or, where the latter is absent, from the connective tissue capsule to the zona reticularis (Fig. 4.5). They are large with prominent cell membranes and a low nuclear-cytoplasmic ratio; the nuclei are round and dense (Fig. 4.8). Between the fasciculata columns, there is a fine collagenous stroma, in which compressed capillary sinusoids may be seen; at intervals denser connective tissue trabeculae traverse the zone. At the light microscopical level, there is a relatively sharp line of demarcation between the zona fasciculata and the underlying zona reticularis, although this border may undulate with interdigitation of the two zones.

Two cell types have been described in ultrastructural studies of the zona fasciculata. In the outer part of this zone, the cells have features akin to those of zona glomerulosa cells (MacKay 1969). While such outer fasciculata cells have abundant liposomes, they still have uniformly-sized spheroidal mitochondria with tubulo-lamellar cristae and only a few internal vesicles. In the inner aspect of the zona fasciculata, on the other hand, the clear cells have mitochondria with predominantly lamellar internal arrays, while at the border with the zona reticularis the mitochondria not only vary considerably in size but have a tubulo-vesicular internal organisation (Fig. 4.9). Lysosomes are few in number in the outer fasciculata but increase at the interface zone with the zona reticularis. Atrophy of the adrenal cortex associated with reduced levels of ACTH in vivo results in almost total loss of the smooth endoplasmic reticulum in zona fasciculata and zona reticularis cells, together with a marked reduction in the complexity of the mitochondrial cristae (Mitschke and Saeger, 1973). Similar changes can be seen in vitro (Armato et al. 1975a, b).

Zona reticularis   The zona reticularis comprises the remainder of the cortex, normally occupying the inner one–quarter to one–third. It is brown in colour consisting of cells with relatively small amounts of cytoplasmic lipid which, after preparing paraffin sections and staining with haematoxylin and eosin, appear eosinophilic and finely granular. They are termed 'compact cells', and are arranged in anastomosing cords, between which prominent sinusoids may be seen (Fig. 4·8). In size compact cells of the zona reticularis are intermediate between those of the zona glomerulosa and the zona fasciculata. Many of the cells contain lipofuscin pigment, a form of peroxidised tissue lipid aptly described by Deane (1962) as the biological equivalent of linoleum, and which contributes to the brown colour of the zone.

At the ultrastructural level there is, as with the other zones, a gradual transition from the typical clear cells of the zona fasciculata to the compact cells of the zona reticularis. The typical compact cell possesses few liposomes, many lysosomes, numerous lipofucsin granules, and abundant mitochondria with predominantly tubular internal structures (Fig. 4.10). Some workers (Long and Jones 1967; Zwierzina 1979) have noted a predominance of vesicles in the mitochondria of zona reticularis cells; differences may be related to prior stress and ACTH levels and/or the precise mode of fixation employed. The smooth endoplasmic reticulum is densely packed and stacks of rough endoplasmic reticulum can frequently be seen. The cells show numerous microvilli at their cell membranes and micropinocytotic vesicles can also be seen (MacKay 1969). 'Light' and 'dark' cells seen under the EM are probably without physiological significance and may be related to fixative penetration.

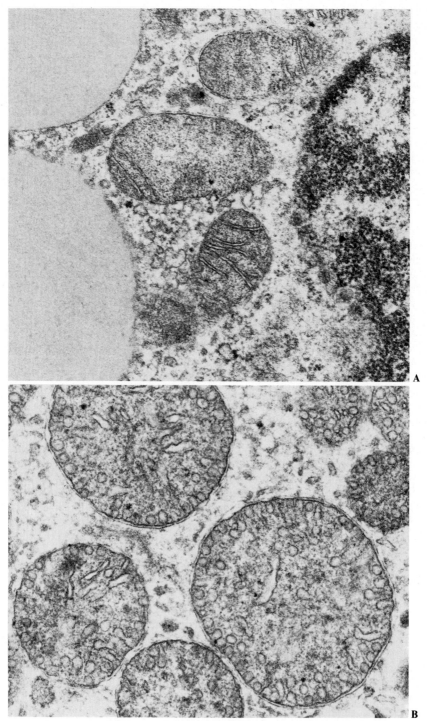

Fig. 4.9. The normal adult cortex. The ultrastructural appearances of mitochondria in the outer (**A**) and inner (**B**) zona fasciculata are shown. Note the lamellar cristae in the outer region and enlarged spherical mitochondria with tubules and vesicles in the inner region of the zone. ($\times 45\,000$)

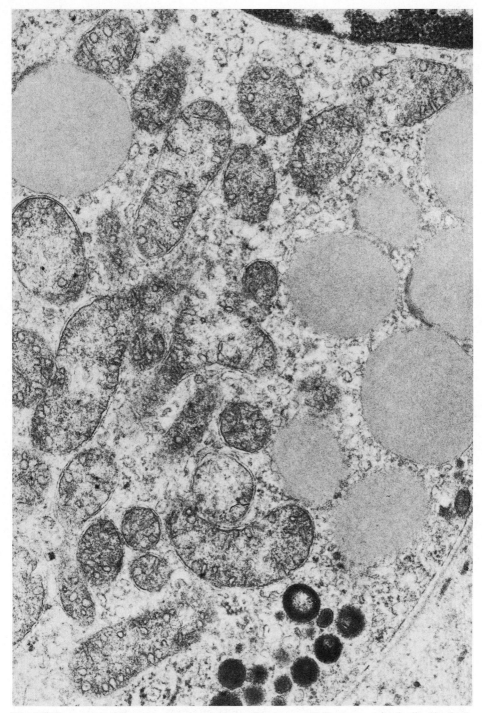

Fig. 4.10 The normal adult cortex. A zona reticularis cell is shown with liposomes, microbodies (lipofuscin granules) and elongated mitochondria with tubulo-vesicular cristae. (× 35 000)

In general, therefore, the precise ultrastructure of the adult human adrenal cortex is somewhat less well defined than in many animals (Idelman 1978). The gradual ultrastructural transition between the various zones is, however, noteworthy as it suggests a functional contiguity and relationship between them. Further details of human adrenal ultrastructure can be seen in MacKay (1969), Neville and MacKay (1972) and Tannenbaum (1973).

These then comprise the major cell types recognisable within the human adrenal cortex. Minor components may include lipid-laden macrophages (lipophages) superficially resembling clear cells and common in certain types of pharmacologically-induced lipoid hyperplasia (Marek and Mötlik 1975). At the boundary of the zona reticularis and the adrenal medulla occasional catecholamine-type granules in otherwise typical cortical cells have been noted (Hashida and Yunis 1972; Kovacs and Horvath 1973). The latter so-called 'corticomedullary' cells probably represent cortical cells which have pinocytosed refluxed amine granules released by medullary cells. Focal collections of adrenocortical cells, usually of the clear cell type, are also commonly found within the medulla (Fig 4.11).

Magalháes (1972) has described cells in the cortex which contain paracrystalline arrays reminiscent of the Reinke crystalloids of Leydig cells. However, neither the perivascular (subendothelial) location of these cells nor their lack of typical cortical cell ultrastructure lends credence to the suggestion that they are steroidogenic or specifically involved in adrenal androgen synthesis (Idelman 1978); they may, in fact, be a form of sympatheticotrophic cell (see p. 286).

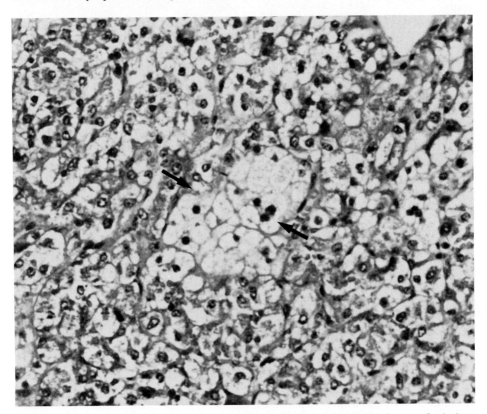

Fig. 4.11. The normal human adrenal gland. A small focal collection of clear lipid-laden zona fasciculata-type cells (*arrows*) is seen within the adrenal medulla. (H + E × 250).

The Cortical Cuff In addition to the classical zones described above, further cortical tissue is found in the gland itself around the central vein and its main branches. Here it forms the so-called 'cortical cuff' (Fig. 4.12) which separates the medulla from the central vein. The three zones are also readily recognisable in this cuff with focal groups of zona glomerulosa cells adjacent to the central vein and reticularis cells next to the medulla. Where the vein leaves the gland, these cuff elements are reflected back in continuity with the remainder of the cortex. This cuff is supplied with blood derived from the arteriae comitantes which run in the wall of the large veins and blood flows centrifugally through the cuff to enter the medulla (see p. 32).

The Effects of Adrenocorticotrophic Hormone (ACTH)

A knowledge of the effect of ACTH on the structure and functions of the normal adult human adrenal cortex is a prerequisite and central to an understanding of the pathological changes observed in both hyper- and hypocorticalism.

Our present understanding of the relevant effects of ACTH in man is almost exclusively derived from studies employing two-stage bilateral adrenalectomy as a

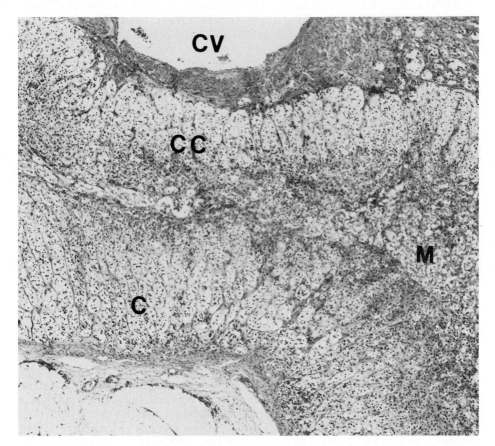

Fig. 4.12. The normal human adrenal gland. The cortical cuff (CC) is seen to surround the central vein (CV) and to separate it from the remainder of the cortex (C) and the medulla (M). Note that compact cells are found in the cortical cuff next to the medulla and not on its innermost aspect next to the central vein. (H + E × 50)

therapeutic modality for breast cancer, which were carried out by the Glasgow group in the late 1950s and 1960s. In this protocol, 10–20 days elapsed between the removal of the first and second glands, during which time ACTH preparations could be administered. During surgery, the adrenal vein was also cannulated and the acute effects of hormone administration examined.

ACTH may be regarded as having three principal effects in man relevant to adrenocortical pathology, namely on (1) adrenal weight, (2) adrenocortical morphology, and (3) adrenocortical steroidogenesis and secretion.

Histochemical investigations (Symington et al. 1956) have shown that the compact cells of the zona reticularis compared to the clear cells of the zona fasciculata contain large amounts of cytoplasmic RNA (corresponding to rough endoplasmic reticulum and ribosomes), acid and alkaline phosphatases (derived presumably from their abundant lysosomes) and enzymes of the Krebs' (citric acid) cycle. Within four minutes of the in vivo administration of ACTH, adrenal blood flow rises and there is a 2–3-fold increase in steroid production, notably cortisol (Grant et al. 1957a). No morphological, histochemical or weight changes are noted within this time span apart from ascorbic acid depletion.

Commencing at about 48 h and becoming well established by the fourth day of ACTH treatment, adrenal weight begins to rise from the normal mean value of about 4 g, and increases of the order of 115 % have been observed (Studzinski et al. 1962). At this stage the greater part of the increased weight is probably accounted for by hypertrophy of pre-existing cells, although hyperaemia may also play a part.

Histologically the clear cells at the junction of the zona fasciculata and zona reticularis, referred to by Symington (1969) as the *interface zone*, lose much of their visible lipid and are converted into compact cells morphologically identical to the pre-existing compact cells of the zona reticularis. This conversion from clear to compact cells gradually extends outwards and thus results in an apparent broadening of the zona reticularis. With administration of high amounts of ACTH for as little as four days (Symington 1962), the whole cortex can come to be composed of compact cells extending out to reach the zona glomerulosa, or the capsule where this zone is absent (Fig. 4.13). These morphological changes are accompanied by these former clear cells of the zona fasciculata acquiring increased levels of cytoplasmic RNA, Krebs' cycle enzymes (Studzinski et al. 1962) and also many of the ultrastructural features of zona reticularis cells (Carr 1960; Symington, 1962). There are also demonstrable increases in the activity of various steroid-metabolising enzymes (Grant et al. 1957b). Collectively, these functional changes and the increased mass of cortical tissue account for the substantially higher total steroid output ($\sim$ 10-fold increase) which results as a trophic response to ACTH.

Intraglandular Vascularisation

An important feature of adrenal vascularisation in so far as function is concerned, is the lack of a significant direct arterial supply to the deeper cortical layers (Dobbie and Symington 1966). They depend principally on blood that has already passed through the outer zones and which, therefore, contains their accumulated secreted steroids, a factor which may be of crucial importance for functional zonation (see p. 105). The importance of this arrangement is evident from the fact that even in the largest mammals, such as the elephant (Krumrey and Buss 1969) and whale (Race and Wu 1961), this relationship is preserved. The overall depth of the cortex does not exceed 5 mm (compared with 1–2 mm in man); its bulk is provided by lateral expansion and folding, as in man.

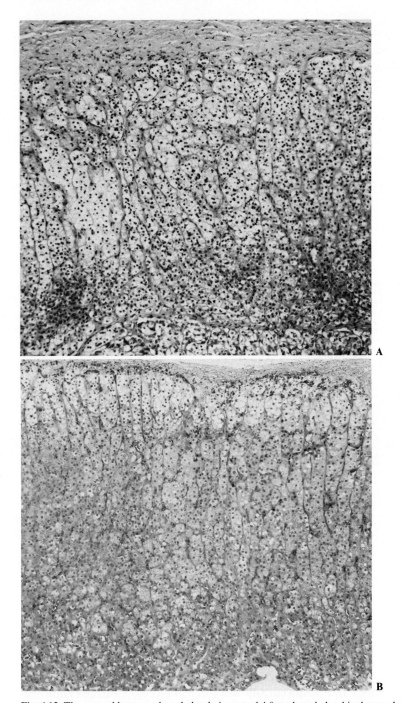

Fig. 4.13. The normal human adrenal gland. A normal 4.0 g adrenal gland is shown above (**A**) and is to be compared with the lower gland (**B**) removed from a female patient given ACTH (80 U/day) for 4 days and which weighed 6.79 g. The latter (**B**) consists of compact lipid-sparse cells which extend outwards almost to reach the capsule. A small residual area of clear cells remains below the capsule. (H + E × 120 [**A**]; × 90 [**B**])

The major part of the cortical tissue in man is perfused by blood that enters the parenchyma from the capsular arterial plexus (see p. 19). It passes through the cortex in thin-walled capillaries arranged in loops around the outer zona glomerulosa passing in more or less straight channels with limited lateral interconnections through the zona fasciculata, and ending in an anastomising dense plexus in the deepest part of the cortex (zona reticularis) (Fig. 4.14).

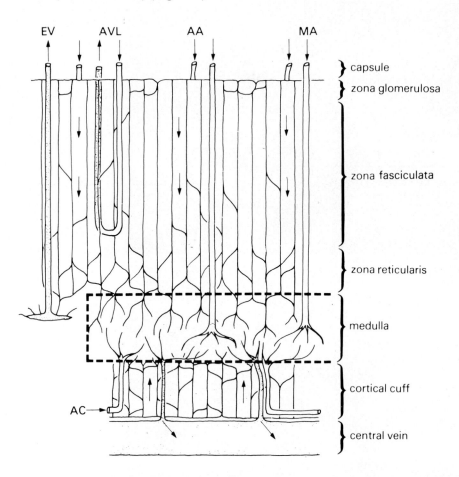

Fig. 4.14. Intraglandular vascularisation of the human adult adrenal cortex (after Dobbie and Symington 1966 and Lazorthes et al 1959). Details of the vascular pattern on the *left* illustrate the regions of the gland without interposed medulla and on the *right* the patterns found in the head of the gland where there is medulla. The *arrows* represent the direction of normal blood flow. EV: emissary vein; AVL: arterio-venous loop; AA: adrenal artery; MA: medullary artery; AC: arteriae comitantes.

The blood supply to the cortical cells is, therefore, derived from a series of capillary sinusoids which are lined by endothelial cells with attenuated cytoplasm and numerous fenestrae or 'pores' closed by a single membrane (Neville and MacKay 1972). These capillaries are usually referred to as 'sinusoids' although the endothelium lacks phagocytic capabilities. Complete gaps in the endothelium are occasionally seen but are probably preservation artifacts. In the narrow perivascular spaces there are usually two basement membranes, one closely applied to the endothelium and the other to the cortical cells, between which a few fibroblasts, occasional macrophages and small amounts of collagen may be discerned (MacKay 1969).

Most blood entering the cortex in the head of the gland ultimately runs into the medulla. It is generally believed that this creates a corticomedullary portal system. In the wings of the gland, and especially the tail, where medullary elements are reduced or absent, effluent cortical blood is collected into venules and veins running longitudinally between the apposed cortical layers (e.g. in the alar raphe). Such veins ultimately merge into the larger central vein, but they also connect with the centrifugal emissary veins which return blood to the capsule (Fig. 4.14).

The only significant deviation from this pattern occurs in the sleeves or cuffs of cortical tissue that invaginate from the outer cortex to surround the central vein and its major branches where they penetrate the gland (Fig. 4.12). Here the cortex is supplied by small arteries around the wall of the major veins. These give rise to an inverted capillary plexus identical to that seen in the major part of the cortex, except that the blood passes centrifugally, rather than centripetally, to drain into an overlying, rather than underlying, medulla. At all times, however, the zona glomerulosa lies nearest to the source of arterial blood (Fig. 4.12).

In addition to the corticomedullary portal plexus, the medulla is also supplied by the arteriae medullae, which pass directly to the medulla from the capsular arterial plexus (Fig. 4.14), and from corresponding vessels traversing the cortical cuff.

Ultimately all cortical effluent blood passing across the medulla collects into venules which enter the central vein and its major branches. These major effluent vessels are equipped with a series of eccentrically arranged bundles of longitudinally disposed smooth muscle. Their function has provoked some speculation over the years (Coupland 1975), but Dobbie and Symington (1966) have concluded from their reconstructions of the gland that their contraction occludes the lumen of the thin-walled venules that collect blood from the medullary sinusoids and drain into the main veins by passing between the muscle bundles. Longitudinal muscle bundles as such are, however, absent in the newborn and present only in small amounts in children, increasing with age (Symington 1969; Payan and Gilbert 1972). They would appear to assume pathophysiological importance in relation to haemorrhage (see p. 278).

The total flow of blood through the adrenal gland is high and can be increased by ACTH (Grant et al. 1957a). In most large mammals rates of up to 5 ml/min/g have been measured (Wright 1963); the maximum rate of blood flow through each human gland may reach 10 ml/min, a flow rate approached only by the thyroid gland.

Lymphatic Supply

The best available evidence (Merklin 1966) indicates that adrenal lymphatics are confined for the most part to the capsule of the gland, lying beneath an extensive subserous network in the periadrenal loose connective tissue in which pairs of lymphatic vessels tend to be associated with a small artery and a vein (Feyrter and Holczabek 1978b). As with some of the periadrenal veins, the periadrenal lymphatic vessels possess longitudinal muscle bundles in their walls that appear to regulate the inflow of lymph from the lymph capillaries. Cortical (and medullary) parenchymal tissue is, however, completely devoid of lymphatics, which reappear only in the adventitia of the central veins and its major tributaries. Lymphatic drainage from the adrenal is medial into the thoracic duct or cysterna chyli directly or by way of regional lymph nodes. Adrenal lymphatic abnormalities may be one cause of adrenal cysts (p. 294).

Innervation

It has long been believed that the parenchymal steroidogenic cortical cells are not directly innervated and are consequently not subject to direct neural influences. Some recent evidence tends, however, to suggest that there is a possibility of neurotropic effects on the cortex.

The adrenal gland receives an abundant nerve supply. A capsular nerve plexus is formed from a mixture of medullated and non-medullated fibres originating in the greater splachnic nerve and associated abdominal plexus of the sympathetic autonomic nervous system, probably combined with parasympathetic contributions from the phrenic and vagal nerves (Mitchell 1953; Coupland 1975). From this plexus, nerve bundles traverse the cortex mostly in association with the arteriae medullae and the connective tissue trabeculae that penetrate the gland.

The vast majority of these nerves terminate either in the medulla, or in the smooth muscle of the major adrenal vessels. They include pre-ganglionic sympathetic fibres which innervate the phaeochromocytes, and postganglionic fibres originating outside the cortex or from the occasional ganglion cells found around the capsule or in relation to the medulla (Mikhail and Amin 1969). The adventitia of the central vein has a rich nervous plexus and also contains ganglion cells (Symington 1969). However, except for a small number of postganglionic fibres which probably innervate the muscular elements of the larger blood vessels traversing the cortex, none of these autonomic nerves appear to terminate in the cortex itself. The distribution of cholinergic fibres in the human adrenal cortex has been described by Coupland (1961).

Some recent electron microscopic investigations have suggested that cortical cells may be subject to neural influence. Some non-myelinated axons pass very close to cortical cell membranes (200 Å) and on occasions displace the basal lamina (Garcia-Alvarez, 1970). The fibres contain dense-core granules and it has been suggested that they represent so-called 'vegetative synapses' of a type purportedly present in the cortex of rats and pigs (Unsicker 1971). However, no specialised pre- or post-synaptic structures have been reported.

Feyrter and Holczabek (1978a) have recently described rarely observed associations between what appear to be cortical parenchymal cells and nerve bundles (so-called 'cortico-neuronal complexes') and ganglion cells ('corticoganglionic complexes') in the capsule and adjacent adipose tissue of the human adrenal gland. These are reminiscent of the tendency of hilar steroidogenic cells in the ovary and testis to be found in the vicinity of nerve tracts (sympatheticotropic cells).

Chapter 5
The Effect of Stress on the Structure of the Adrenal Cortex

The appearances of the normal adrenal gland are different at autopsy from those of operatively removed glands and are explicable on the basis of the effects of ACTH upon the adrenal cortex (p. 29). The changes are caused by the increased circulating levels of ACTH which rise because of antemortem stress induced by such conditions such as trauma, burns, infection, myocardial infarction, etc (Symington 1969). Thus the changes take the form of an increase in adrenal weight and an alteration in morphology, which will commence with lipid loss at the *interface zone* between the zona reticularis and the zona fasciculata. The precise changes seen at postmortem examination, however, will depend upon the length and the severity of the stress.

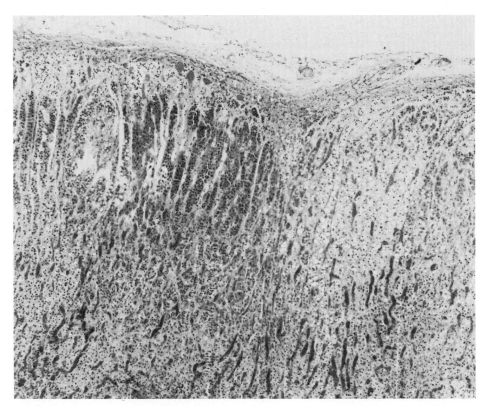

Fig. 5.1. The human adult cortex. Response to stress. Focal lipid depletion. The broadened cortex consists of segments with inner compact cells and outer clear cells together with areas where the compact cells extend out to reach the capsule, or zona glomerulosa (H + E × 60)

These reactions to stress with lipid loss have been classified by Symington and his colleagues (1955) as focal lipid depletion, focal lipid depletion with degeneration, complete lipid depletion and lipid reversion. It is important to appreciate that each is not a separate entity but reflects part of a spectrum of change in response to stress.

In *focal lipid depletion*, the clear cells of certain segments of the zona fasciculata are converted to compact cells. This process is said to commence focally at the interface between the two zones. As a result, areas of the cortex will consist solely of compact cells extending out towards or reaching the capsule or the zona glomerulosa where it is present, thereby forming a homogeneous compact cell layer. Between such foci areas of zona fasciculata with their clear cells will remain (Fig. 5.1).

When stress is severe and/or prolonged, the entire cortex may lose its visible lipid content and be converted to compact cells. This is called *complete lipid depletion* (Fig. 5.2) and in our recent experience is the commonest autopsy pattern. Various degenerative changes may be superimposed upon these appearances. One consists of cytolytic degeneration of the adrenocortical cells in the zona fasciculata, especially immediately below the capsule, Such cells come to have a pale cytoplasm with the H&E stains due to a low RNA content. In other instances, cords of either clear or compact cells may be separated from the stroma by spaces, giving rise to the so-called

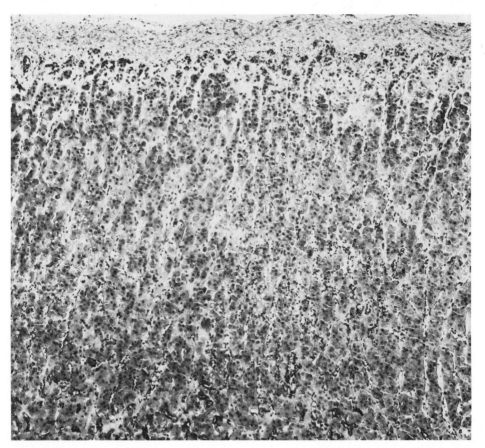

Fig. 5.2. The human adrenal cortex. Response to stress. Complete lipid depletion. The cortex consists exclusively of compact cell columns which extend from the innermost areas to reach the outer zona glomerulosa. Note the prominent vascular sinusoids. (H + E × 90)

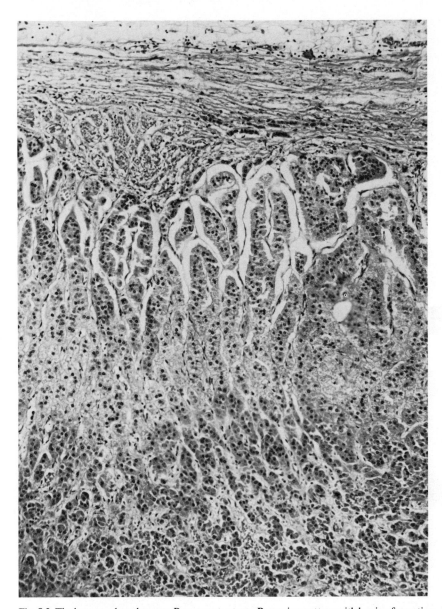

Fig. 5.3. The human adrenal cortex. Response to stress. Reversion pattern with lumina formation. A zone of compact cells lies immediately below the capsule. The inner compact zona reticularis is seen below and between them an area of clear lipid-laden cells. Between the outermost compact cell columns there are prominent spaces referred to as pseudotubules or lumina (H + E × 150)

'pseudotubules' or 'lumina' (Fig. 5.3) as described by Wilbur and Rich (1953). In our studies of both normal adult human and rodent adrenocortical cells in monolayer tissue culture, we have noted that the addition of high levels of ACTH results in a marked retraction of the adrenal cells away from one another so that spaces begin to appear between them (Fig. 5.4) (O'Hare and Neville 1973a; Neville and O'Hare 1978). It may well be, therefore, that this so-called pseudotubular change is not due

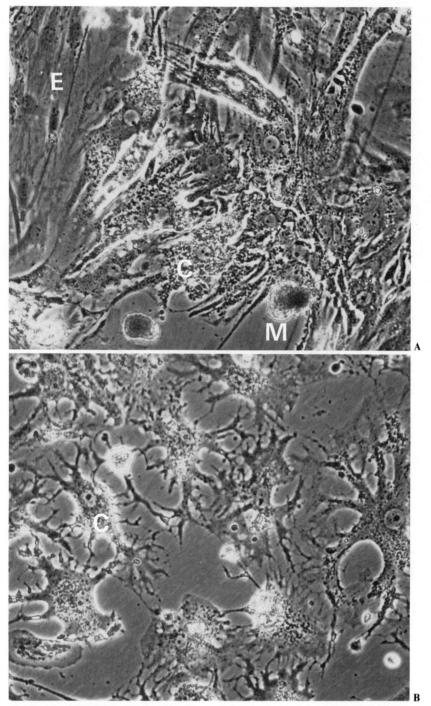

Fig. 5.4. Normal adult human adrenocortical cells in monolayer culture. Phase contrast photomicrograph or cortical cells (C) maintained in absence (**A**) and presence (**B**) of ACTH $_{1-24}$ (1 μg/ml). Note the 'retraction' of the adrenal cells in response to ACTH. Other cell types are also present, including endothelial cells (E) and macrophages (M). (× 200 [**A**]; × 200 [**B**])

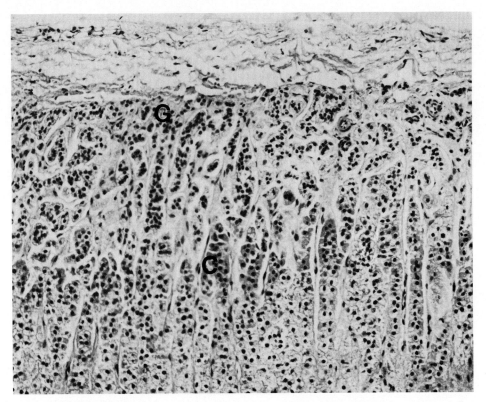

Fig. 5.5. The human adrenal cortex. Response to stress. Reversion pattern. Note the so-called 'reversion pattern' is present in this autopsy gland, and the outer compact cells (C) are separated from the capsule by a prominent zona glomerulosa (G). (H + E × 90)

solely to degeneration but may also represent the in vivo morphological equivalent of a cell retraction response induced by ACTH in monolayer culture.

Infarction and haemorrhage may also be superimposed on the pattern of complete lipid depletion which appearance was once referred to as that of an 'exhausted adrenal'. Extensive biochemical studies have shown, however, that the levels of steroid hormones in the plasma and urine are raised in such subjects and that the in vivo administration of ACTH may increase the steroid output to an even greater level (Sandberg et al. 1956). Even under the chronic stress of hunger cachexia, hyperplasia and increased functional activity are the rule.

In some adrenals, foci of cellular hypertrophy normally involving the compact cells will be seen. Those appearances represent, in our opinion, a further response to ACTH and stress and are not premalignant in nature. They are particularly frequent in the adrenals in the 'ectopic' ACTH syndrome (p. 131).

In children, by contrast, stress results in an apparently random change of the clear cells into compact cells so bestowing a speckled appearance of intermittent clear and compact cells throughout the cortex (Symington 1969). When stress is severe complete lipid depletion may ensue.

Frequently at autopsy, groups of strongly eosinophilic cells are situated beneath the capsule or the zona glomerulosa. This zone of compact cells has often been mistaken by others for a prominent zona glomerulosa (Fig. 5.5). The remainder of the cortex consists of a clear cell zona fasciculata and an inner compact cell zona reticularis. The name applied to this appearance is *lipid reversion* (Sarason 1943). It has often been suggested that this process represents a stage in the recovery from stress with a centrifugal replenishing of the lipid content of the zona fasciculata, which commences at the interface zone and extends progressively outwards towards the capsule, leaving, for a time, a rim of lipid-poor cells at the periphery. However, we have personally found these features not infrequently at autopsy in patients who are presumably still under the influence of stress, and in operation-removed glands from subjects with hyperaldosteronism (Fig. 15.16).

With increasing age, nodules will be detected more frequently in the adrenal cortex. Their appearance, significance and response to stress will be discussed later (see p. 53).

Chapter 6
Morphological Changes in the Adrenal Cortex with Age

The Prenatal Cortex

The definitive and fetal zones become apparent in the prenatal cortex by the sixth week of gestation (Fig. 6.1). The outer definitive zone which comprises 30%–15% of the gland volume depending on age is composed of small (10–20 μm) basophilic cells arranged in arched cords (Fig. 6.2). They have densely-staining nuclei, with high

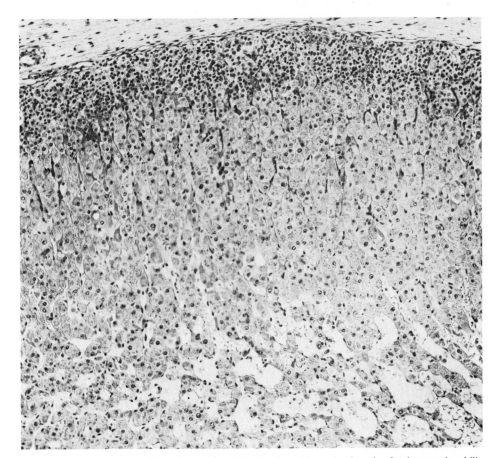

Fig. 6.1. The prenatal cortex: 16 weeks gestation. This gland consists predominantly of an inner eosinophilic fetal zone capped by a rim of smaller cells which comprise the definitive cortex. (H + E × 100)

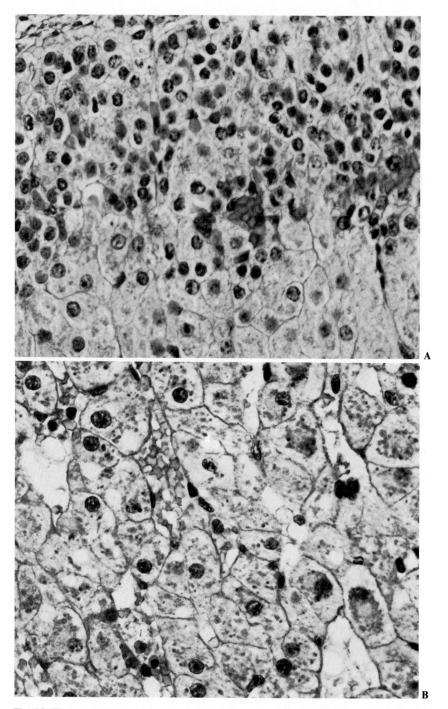

Fig. 6.2. The prenatal cortex: 16 weeks gestation. The cells of the definitive cortex (**A**) have a high nuclear: cytoplasmic ratio and some cytoplasmic lipid. They are arranged in arched cords and which merge gradually with the more irregularly arranged fetal zone cells. On the inner aspect of the fetal zone (**B**), the cells are larger, have eosinophilic granular cytoplasm and are arranged in cords separated by prominent vascular spaces. (H + E × 600 [**A**]; × 600 [**B**])

nuclear: cytoplasmic ratio and, although lipid-poor at the outset, accumulate some cytoplasmic lipid with increasing age (Dhöm et al. 1958).

Cavities similar to those described as 'microcysts' in postnatal glands (see p. 294) are common in this outer zone of the prenatal cortex (Gruenwald 1946); their developmental and/or pathological significance is obscure.

The inner eosinophilic fetal zone which constitutes the core of the gland is composed of larger (20–50 μm) cells, arranged in tightly-packed cords towards the outer aspect of the zone but more widely spaced in its innermost regions where there is increased prominence of vascular sinusoidal spaces (Fig. 6.2). Islands of immature neuroblasts destined to form the medulla can be seen between the innermost fetal zone cells (Fig. 6.3).

Ultrastructural observations (Johannisson 1968; McNutt and Jones 1970; Fujita and Ihara 1973) show significant differences between definitive and fetal zone cells throughout gestation, but also demonstrate a transitional zone with intermediate characteristics. During the first trimester, the definitive zone cells exhibit features associated with active protein synthesis consistent with their role as germinative cells. They contain numerous free ribosomes and many glycogen particles; the SER is poorly developed consisting of a few isolated tubules and saccules. The mitochondria have predominantly lamellar cristae (Fig. 6.4). During the second trimester, the mitochon-

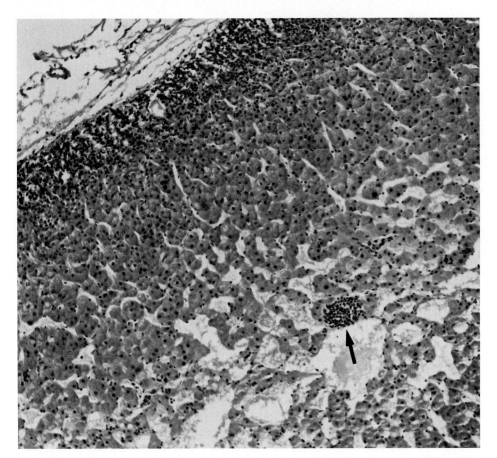

Fig. 6.3. Prenatal cortex: 18 weeks gestation. A small nest of neuroblasts (*arrow*) is seen on the innermost aspect next to a prominent vascular space. (H + E × 120)

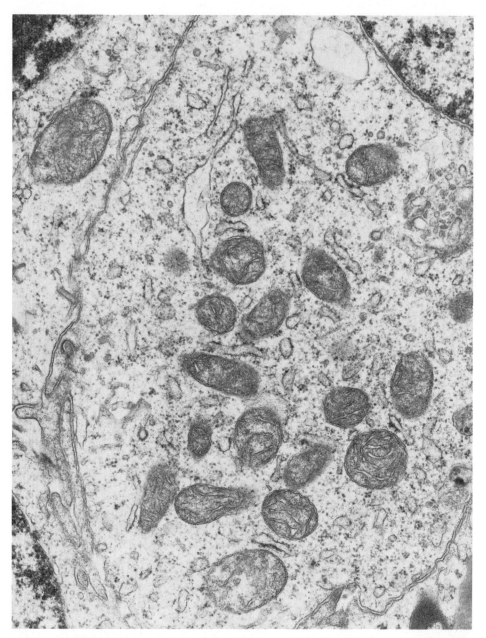

Fig. 6.4. Ultrastructure of the prenatal cortex, definitive zone: 10 weeks gestation. The definitive zone cell contains many ribosomes, abundant small mitochondria with lamellar cristae. The smooth endoplasmic reticulum is inconspicuous. Note also the interdigitating plasma membranes of adjacent cells. (× 27 650)

dria assume a tubular internal structure, glycogen diminishes, and osmiophilic lipid droplets begin to appear in the cytoplasm. By the end of the second trimester the SER of definitive zone cells increases in amount, although it never achieves the prominence found in the fetal zone cells. 'Light' and 'dark' cells have been described in the definitive zone of the prenatal cortex (Johannisson 1968) but may be fixation artifacts.

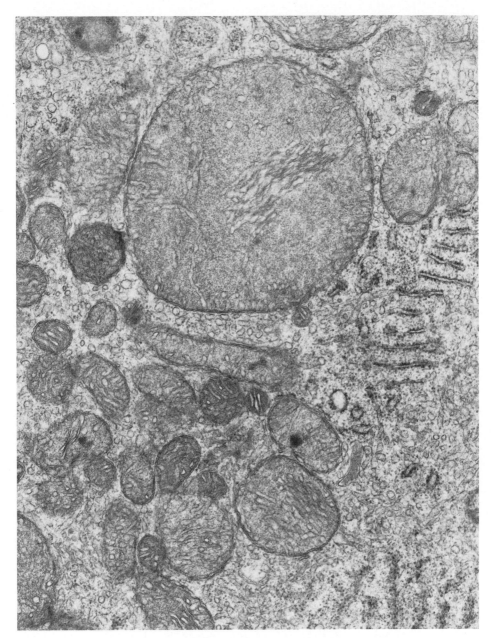

Fig. 6.5. Ultrastructure of the prenatal cortex, fetal zone. 10 weeks gestation. The fetal zone cell contains numerous large mitochondria with tubulo-vesicular internal structures, parallel stacks of rough endoplasmic reticulum and a prominent smooth endoplasmic reticulum. ($\times$ 27 000)

At all stages of development the fetal zone cells have a prominent SER forming a tightly packed network of convoluted tubules. The Golgi apparatus is also prominent. In early embryos the mitochondria of fetal zone cells vary in size and contain irregularly organised tubular cristae (Fig. 6.5); during the second trimester the mitochondria enlarge and show a predominantly tubulo-vesicular internal structure.

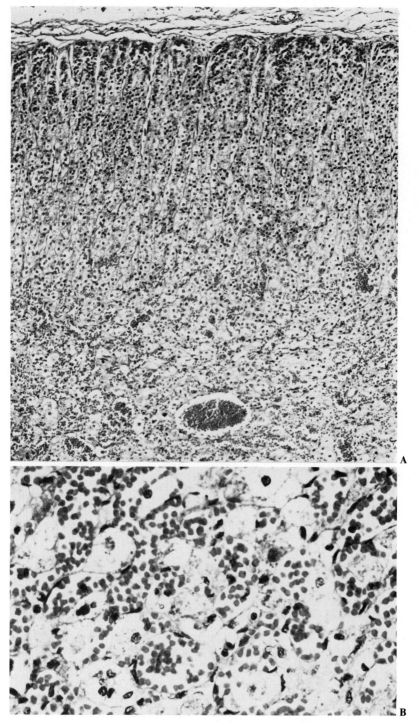

Fig. 6.6. Neonatal cortex. 1 week old. The cortex (**A**) consists of a narrow outer lipid-rich zone with cells arranged in arches and which merge with the inner fetal zone cells. At higher power (**B**) it can be seen that these exhibit degenerative changes together with marked vascular congestion. (H + E × 100 [**A**]; × 500 [**B**])

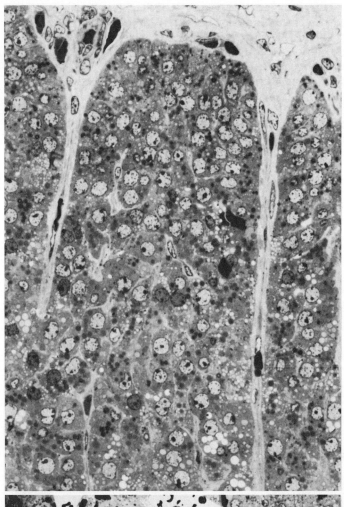

A

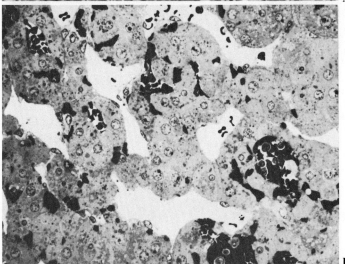

B

Fig. 6.7. Neonatal cortex. The definitive zone (**A**) consists of arched cellular columns while the fetal zone (**B**) is markedly vascular. (Reproduced by kind permission of Mäusle 1972). (Semithin sections from Epon-embedded material; Methylene blue ×640 **A** and **B**)

Later in pregnancy, the RER in fetal zone cells consists of characteristic large stacks or parallel arrays of cisternae and membrane-bound dense granules are common. Cells at the boundary with the definitive zone show closely apposed membranes but in the inner part of the gland they possess numerous interdigitating microvilli; specialised junctional complexes are, however, rare.

Electron microscopy reveals a transitional zone between the definitive and fetal zones. In this area, the cells have mitochondria of the fetal zone type but the SER and RER are less abundant (McNutt and Jones 1970). These observations emphasise the continuity of cortical zonation in the fetus, and illustrate the precocious structural differentiation of the fetal zone as compared with the definitive cortex at all stages of gestation.

The Neonatal and Prepubertal Cortex

The changes in macroscopic appearance and weight of the adrenal glands after birth and through to puberty have already been discussed (Figs. 3.2 and 3.3; p. 12). At birth the cortex consists of a narrow outer yellow zone and a deep brownish-red hyperaemic inner zone. With the postnatal loss of the fetal zone, the gland loses up to 50% of its birth weight within a month and then gradually shrinks to just over 1 g in weight at 1–2 years of age. It grows only slowly thereafter to reach 2 g by the tenth year but doubles in weight during puberty and adolescence to reach the mean adult weight of just over 4 g by 15–18 years of age (Fig. 3.2). No sex differences have been noted in this process.

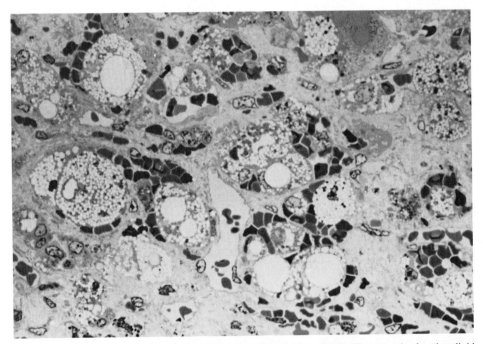

Fig. 6.8. Neonatal cortex. There is advanced involution of the fetal zone cells. They contain abundant lipid vacuoles. Red blood cell extravasation and interstitial oedema are marked. (Reproduced by kind permission of Mäusle 1972) (Semithin sections from Epon-embedded material; Methylene blue × 640)

Cytologically the key events in prepubertal cortical development are first, the involution of the fetal zone, second the establishment of zonation in the outer cortex and, finally, the later emergence of a recognisable zona reticularis.

The outermost cells are relatively lipid-rich (although not to the same extent as the adult zona fasciculata), they have a high nuclear: cytoplasmic ratio and are organized in broad arches or arcades from which extend inwards radially disposed columns of similar cells, without overt zonation (Figs. 6.6 and 6.7).

Prior to involution the innermost cells of the newborn cortex are still strongly eosinophilic and relatively lipid-sparse, very similar in fact to early third trimester fetal zone cells. Within the first few days after birth a degenerative change in this zone that signals the start of involution can be detected ultrastructurally (Mäusle 1971). There is disruption of cell membranes and accumulation of myelin-whorls in the cytoplasm and, at the light microscopic level, interstitial oedema and red cell extravasation is observed (Fig. 6.6). As cellular degeneration proceeds the fetal zone cells develop giant mitochondria, and abundant liposomes (not seen in the pre-involutionary inner cortex); membrane-bound dense granules become especially prominent. At the light microscopic level, large droplets of stainable lipid can be observed accumulating in the centre of the gland and numerous macrophages enter the tissue and engulf the damaged cortical cells until they too become laden with lipid droplets (Mäusle 1972) (Fig. 6.8). This process of heterophagocytosis can usually be observed to start within 3–10 days after birth. Although instances of delayed involution have been noted (Benner 1940) (see also page 133), the process is established in almost all instances by the end of the first month and by six months little if any of the original fetal zone of the cortex remains (Fig. 6.9). The collapse of the inner parenchyma and its replacement by connective tissue elements leads to the formation of a so-called 'medullary capsule' which separates the newly compacted phaeochromocytes from the cortex (Fig. 6.10), and also the two apposed layers of cortex in those parts of the gland where the medulla is absent (Fig. 6.9).

The development of the outer 'arcuate' zone during the first year of postnatal life follows a different pattern. During the first six months, the original broad arches of definitive cortex cells remain compressed and subdivided by radially disposed connective tissue elements (Gruenwald 1946). Lipid continues to accumulate in all the cells in the form of small droplets (Dhöm 1965), notably in the parallel cords of cells that extend downwards to make up, in part, for the loss of inner zone cells (Fig. 6.11). Typically, during the second half of the first year, connective tissue elements come to separate the cells immediately beneath the capsule into first ovoid and then rounded 'glomeruloid' structures. Cytologically, although these cells do not yet have the typical characteristics of adult zona glomerulosa cells, they do constitute a diffuse continuous concentric zone that can now be described as a zona glomerulosa. They are, however, somewhat more lipid-sparse compared to the underlying fasciculata type cells. According to Kreiner and Dhöm (1979), the zona glomerulosa remains diffuse during childhood and adolescence. At some time during early adult life, therefore, it must assume the focal distribution characteristic of the adult gland, presumably being displaced by the outward 'extension' of lipid-rich zona fasciculata cell columns.

The final stage in the development of the adult gland involves the evolution of the zona reticularis. The time of appearance of compact cells constituting a recognisable zona reticularis is apparently very variable and the archetype is difficult to assess, even in the sudden death type of gland. The most extensive study of this type of gland is that of Dhöm (1973) who believes that in adrenals up to about three years of age a zona reticularis is seldom if ever seen. By five years he reports focal accumulations of compact cells on the innermost aspect of the cortex in the majority of glands examined as the medullary capsule gradually undergoes dissolution, and with a further year or two

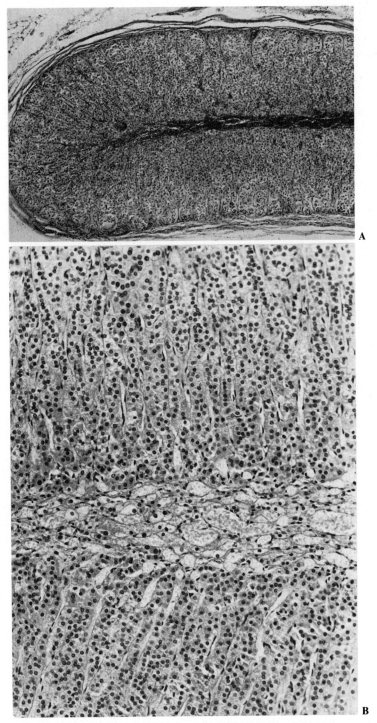

Fig. 6.9. Infant cortex. 6 months of age. The cortex (**A** and **B**) consists of columns of relatively uniform cells. The fetal zone has involuted leaving collagen fibres and a network of capillaries (**B**) in the centre. No medulla is present in this illustration. (Reproduced by kind permission of Dhöm 1965) (H + E × 50 [**A**]; × 125 [**B**])

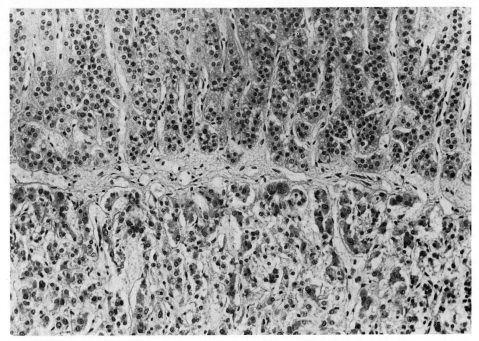

Fig. 6.10. Infant cortex. 12 months of age. A thin medullary 'capsule' separates the cortex (*above*) from the medulla (*below*). (Reproduced by kind permission of Dhöm 1965) (H + E × 160)

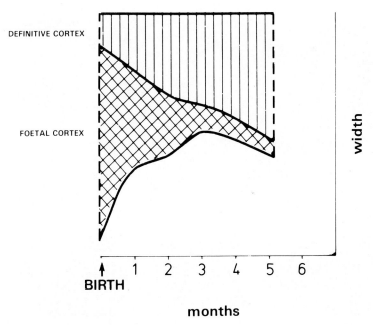

Fig. 6.11. Postnatal development of the cortex. The relative widths of the fetal and definitive zones are shown during the first six months of life. (After Dhöm 1965)

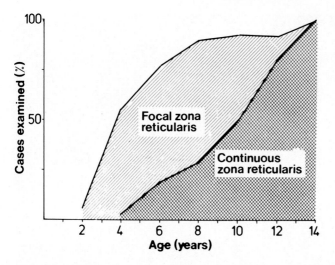

Fig. 6.12. Development of zonation according to Dhöm (1973).

some glands already show a continuous zona reticularis. During the next five years during the pubertal and immediate postpubertal period an increasing proportion of glands examined by Dhöm showed a continuous zone (Fig. 6.12) and the numbers with only focal accumulations of compact cells diminished, until by the 14th year virtually all glands possessed a continuous, concentric zona reticularis. The definitive adult pattern of zonation is apparently established at this age and the developmental phase of cortical growth completed. Our personal experience of the cortex in childhood has been confined to pathological cases or hospital deaths where it is clear that substantial zonal changes including a prominent compact cell zona reticularis can occur as the result of stress (Fig. 6.13) and increased levels of circulating ACTH.

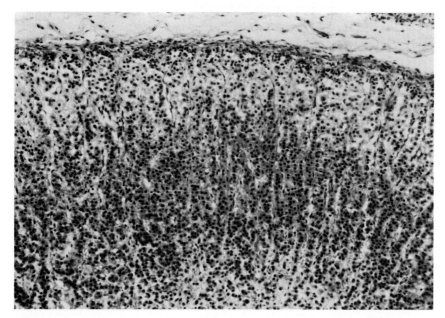

Fig. 6.13. Infant cortex. 18 months of age. The inner aspect of the cortex contains a prominent inner zone of compact lipid-sparse cells in this hospital death case. (H + E × 125)

Postpubertal Cortex

Generalised changes in the postpubertal cortex during the normal process of ageing have not been extensively studied. Lipofucsin pigment increases with age (Kreiner and Dhöm 1979). Fibrosis of the stroma does not appear to be specifically associated with ageing, although fibromyomatous nodules have been noted in association with the longitudinal muscle bundles of the larger veins, especially in patients with cardiovascular disease (Payan and Gilbert 1967). Kreiner and Dhöm (1979) report the zonation as becoming increasingly irregular with advancing years, although the zona reticularis is always preserved as a well-developed zone, irrespective of age. Irregularity of cortical zonation is, in part, associated with the increased frequency with which cortical nodules are observed in older persons (vide infra).

Adrenocortical Nodules

Adrenocortical nodules are interesting lesions. We still lack convincing explanations of their physiological and pathological functional properties in vivo, despite numerous recent advances in our knowledge of their structure (Dobbie 1969). Not only do they occur in association with a variety of adrenal-induced and adrenal-associated disorders but they have caused many pathologists diagnostic and interpretative difficulty (Neville 1978).

Nodules are localised overgrowths of adrenocortical cells that in our opinion, are not true neoplasms. They are best regarded as representing a variation of adrenal structure occurring predominantly as part of the ageing process. Nodules continue to be recognised most frequently at autopsy in patients without apparent functional adrenal abnormalities, when they may confusingly still be referred to as 'non-functioning' adenomas (e.g. Tang and Grey 1975). However, it is important to remember that they can also occur in association with the various pathological changes associated with hypercorticalism (see pp. 125, 226).

While the existence of the larger forms has been known for many years (Letulle 1889), only recently has it been recognised that a similar basic pathological process results in the formation of small microscopic nodules, the typical large, so-called 'non-functioning adenoma', and all sizes between these two extremes (Dobbie 1969). All forms of nodules tend to be bilateral and have been stated to be more frequent in Negroes (Russell and Masi 1973). The various types and stages of nodule development have been described by Dobbie (1969), and recently reviewed in detail (Neville 1978). The earliest abnormality appears to be a microscopic rounded lesion, usually yellow in colour situated wholly within the cortex, towards its periphery or in the centre of the gland in relation to the main vein (Fig. 6.14). Continued enlargement results in compression of the surrounding tissue. They may grow to form mushroom-like masses protruding through the capsule or expand within the gland until a large lesion of 2–3 cm diameter is formed (Fig. 6.15).

A variety of terms has been applied, in the past, to describe the occurrence and evolution of such lesions. They include 'non-functioning' adenomas, adenomatous hyperplasia, nodular hyperplasia and, when small, micronodular hyperplasia. In some series, the difference between an adenoma and a nodule has been taken to be one of size, nodules being defined <0.8 cm diameter and adenomas >0.8 cm diameter (Granger and Genest 1970). Tchertkoff et al. (1979) concur with us that all such terms are best disregarded now that it is appreciated that a similar disease process results in the genesis of all such lesions and that time may be the important factor in determining their size. They are all, in our opinion, best referred to simply as nodules. In

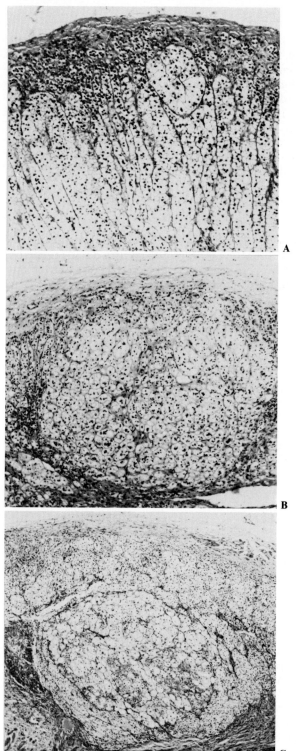

Fig. 6.14. The nodular adrenal gland. A series of clear-cell nodules of varying size, the larger of which are distorting the normal architecture of the gland, is shown. Note their different intraglandular locations. (H + E × 70 [**A**]; × 60 [**B**]; × 55 [**C**])

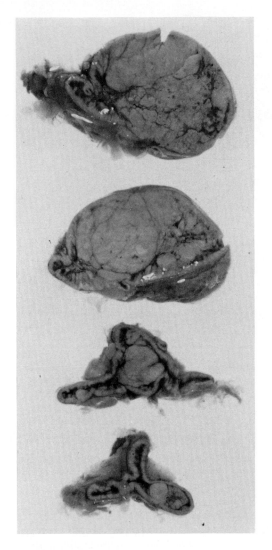

Fig. 6.15. The nodular adrenal gland. A series of nodules in one gland is illustrated. They range from 8 cm in diameter down, and in their position in the cortex from entirely intraglandular to projecting from one pole. (×0·6)

normotensive subjects they may be recognisable macroscopically in up to 3% of adrenals examined, without a marked sex bias (Granger and Genest 1970). However, their frequency and size undoubtedly increase with age (Russell et al. 1972) and with hypertensive disease. Micronodular changes, on the other hand, may be seen in at least two-thirds of adrenals examined from normotensives (Salomon and Tchertkoff 1968).

Generally nodules consist of clear-lipid-laden cells similar in size and appearance to those of the normal zona fasciculata. The cells are arranged in cords and clusters separated by prominent fibrovascular trabeculae (Fig. 6.16A). On occasion, so-called 'non-functioning black nodules' composed of compact cells may be detected (see below). It is important to distinguish both types of nodule from their morphologically similar neoplastic counterparts which may cause hypercorticalism (Figs. 12.5, 12.17).

Larger nodules at autopsy may reveal a variety of further morphological changes including extensive areas of fibrosis and hyalinization, and even myxomatous change. Occasionally numerous dilated sinusoidal spaces are present imparting an angiomatous appearance, and into which haemorrhage may occur to cause one type of

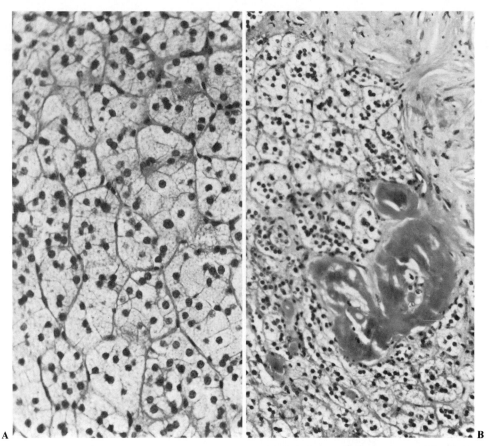

Fig. 6.16. The nodular adrenal gland. On the *left* (**A**), the nodule may be seen to consist of nests of clear lipid-laden zona fasciculata-type cells with minimal pleomorphism. In relation to many such lesions, a marked arteriopathy is frequently seen (**B**). (H + E × 240 [**A**]; × 160 [**B**])

cystic change (see p. 294). Nodules are also a favoured site for the deposition of metastatic carcinoma and infective lesions such as tuberculosis. Finally, larger nodules, particularly after prolonged stress, may reveal areas of myelolipomatous change (p. 291) and even osseous metaplasia.

There is still dispute as to the functional and pathological importance of nodules. Salomon and Tchertkoff (1968) who found nodules at all age groups, believed that they were of an innocuous nature and a consequence rather than a cause of disease. However, Russell and Masi (1973) who, like many others (e.g. Granger and Genest 1970), found them to be more frequent in association with hypertension, believed that they played an aetiological role in this context (see p. 240). Dobbie (1969), on the other hand, believed that they resulted from vascular damage rather than causing hypertension with such changes. He noted a high incidence of hyalinisation and intimal proliferation with luminal obliteration in the capsular arteries of nodule-containing adrenal glands (Fig. 6.16B), and has proposed that the resulting ischaemia causes focal cortical atrophy. Surrounding the central vein are clear cells forming a perivenous cuff (Fig. 4.12), supplied by arteries accompanying the central vein. These arteries are apparently less compromised by the arteriopathy so that those central cortical cells may be able to undergo hyperplasia to form nodules and come to fill the ischaemic defect of the outer cortex. This might account for the high frequency with which nodules are related to the central vein, but does not explain why the total weight of adrenal plus nodules often greatly exceeds that of the normal gland.

Nodules are, in fact, capable of producing steroids in vitro (Symington 1969; Honn et al. 1977), and of responding to prolonged ACTH treatment in culture (Fig. 6.17), although they do not appear to be responsive in short-term in vitro experiments (Honn et al. 1977). Studies in monolayer culture have shown that their component cells possess the inherent ability to form the same spectrum of steroids, including cortisol, in approximately similar amounts on a per cell basis as normal human zona fasciculata cells (Fig. 6.18). However, despite the size that they can sometimes reach, they do not appear to exert a significant effect in vivo, as no specific derangement of corticosteroid metabolism has ever been demonstrated unless there are concomitant hyperplastic changes in the uninvolved cortex. Moreover, if they were fully functional and producing cortisol in vivo, the attached cortex would show atrophy. The clear cells of a nodule frequently fail to respond to ACTH administration in vivo, or stress, but sometimes undergo the compact cell conversion that occurs in the surrounding cortex (Fig. 6.19). This apparent anomaly, and the lack of detectable excess steroids, may be due to their abnormal vascular supply inhibiting the response to ACTH and/or the synthesis of steroid hormones. It has also been noted that many such nodules show much lower levels of glucose-6-phosphate dehydrogenase activity than the surrounding cortex (Cohen 1966) a feature emphasising their functional distinction from normal cortical cells, and related to their possible low in vivo steroid output. Ultrastructural studies concur with this concept as their component cells are not exceptionally well-endowed with characteristic steroidogenic organelles (Tannenbaum 1973).

The Autopsy 'Black' Nodule

The occurrence of pigmented ('black') nodules in the human adrenal gland (Baker, 1938) has, until recently, been regarded as rare (MacAdam 1971; Garret and Ames 1973). Although large nodules (>2 cm) are uncommon, a recent study of a consecutive series of 100 autopsies has shown that smaller nodules of this type can be found in over one-third of glands when carefully sought (Robinson et al. 1972). Their incidence is, therefore, similar to that of the well recognised yellow nodule discussed above, and like yellow nodules, black nodules are common in older patients of both sexes, and are not, in the great majority of cases associated with any detectable abnormalities of adrenocortical function.

In size and distribution black nodules are also similar to the yellow nodules. They vary typically from 0.1–1.5 cm in diameter and from light brown to black in colour. The majority reported by Robinson et al. (1972) were single but multiple black nodules were seen. They occurred bilaterally in 30% of cases. When small they are most frequently located at the corticomedullary boundary.

Microscopically such nodules consist of compact zona reticularis-type cells arranged in short cords, trabeculae and acinar clusters, and are remarkable only in the concentration of irregular (1–2 μm) electron-dense, membrane-bound lipofucsin pigment bodies therein; other ultrastructural features closely resemble normal zona reticularis cells.

It is important to distinguish these non-hormone syndrome-inducing nodules from other pigmented lesions which can involve the adrenal gland. These include myelolipoma, haematoma, haemangioma, melanoma and phaeochromocytoma. In addition to general morphology, appropriate histochemical procedures can be of assistance.

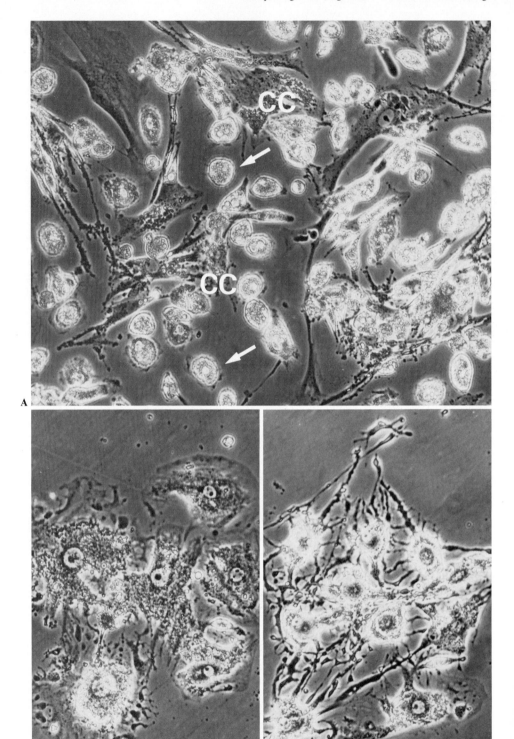

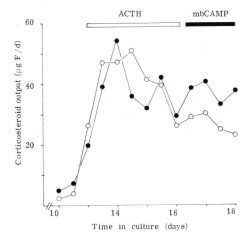

Fig. 6.18. Steroidogenesis by monolayer cultures of an adrenocortical nodule (*open circles*) and the attached gland (*closed circles*) containing equal numbers of cells and treated with ACTH$_{1-24}$ (1 µg/ml) followed by monobutyryl cyclic AMP (mbCAMP, 0.5 mmol/l). Note that the glucocorticoid output of the nodule fully matches that the remainder of the gland when the cells are exposed to a trophic stimulus in a uniform culture environment.

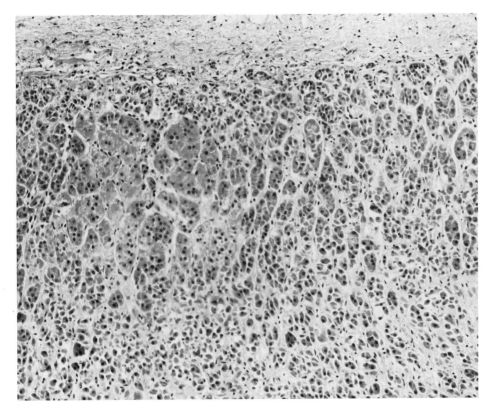

Fig. 6.19. The nodular adrenal gland. An autopsy gland showing complete lipid depletion. In this instance, the small nodule also consists of compact cells. (H + E × 90)

◁ **Fig. 6.17.** The nodular adrenal gland in monolayer cell culture. In addition to the cortical cells (CC), numerous macrophages (*arrows*) are found in cultures prepared from the macronodules similar to those illustrated in Fig. 6.15. The adrenal cells, nonetheless, show a retraction response on exposure to ACTH for 3–4 days in culture (**B** without, **C** with ACTH). (PC × 100 [**A**]; × 200 [**B**]; × 200 [**C**])

It should also be remembered that darkly pigmented benign tumours (true adenomas) can also occur in the adrenal cortex and examples associated with Cushing's syndrome (Bahu et al. 1974; Uras et al. 1978) and primary aldosteronism (Caplan and Virata 1974) have recently been recorded. These lesions are usually at least 2–3 cm diameter when removed and apart from the associated symptomology of hypercorticalism, the appearance of the attached and contralateral adrenal glands will enable an accurate diagnosis to be made; with for example atrophy when such tumours are responsible for Cushing's syndrome. Such black adenomas do not, in our opinion, constitute a specific clinicopathological entity (Visser et al. 1974), as it seems likely that the excessive pigment accumulation, possibly due to disordered lysosomal function, is a fortuitous circumstance occurring in a small minority of such benign lesions, apparently irrespective of their functional attributes.

Chapter 7
Iatrogenic Changes

ACTH

The structural and functional effects of in vivo ACTH administration upon the adrenal cortex have been described previously (p. 29); therapeutic administration of ACTH is now seldom encountered although it may be employed in the differential diagnosis of pituitary-adrenal disease.

Steroid Therapy

The systemic and topical administration of the glucocorticoid hormones, cortisol and cortisone and analogues such as prednisone, prednisolone, betamethasone and dexamethasone is still widely practised for a variety of non-endocrine disorders. In pharmacological doses, they can result in the development of iatrogenic Cushing's syndrome. Because of their inhibitory effects on the hypothalamo-pituitary axis, ACTH secretion declines, plasma ACTH falls to low or undetectable levels and the

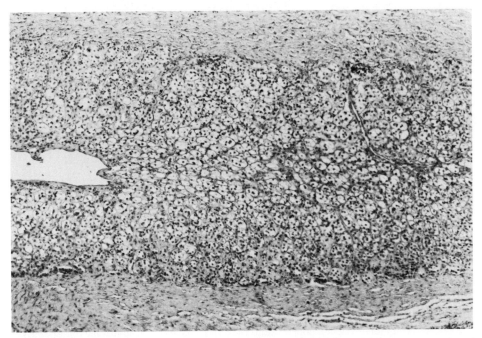

Fig. 7.1. Atrophic adrenal cortex. The cortex is narrowed due to steroid-induced atrophy. It consists solely of clear lipid-laden cells of the zona fasciculata type. A thickened capsule is also apparent. (H + E × 240)

adrenal cortex undergoes atrophy. Iatrogenic atrophy of this type may also occur in the newborn where the mother has received steroid therapy (Oppenheimer 1964).

In the fully developed state, the adrenal gland is smaller than normal, lighter and has a thinned leaf-like appearance. On section, the cortex is diffusely yellow in colour and consists for the most part of clear lipid-laden cells of the zona fasciculata-type (Fig. 7.1). The capsule is oedematous, and the zona glomerulosa where present may also appear to be more prominent than normal due to cortical shrinkage.

These atrophic changes associated with iatrogenic Cushing's syndrome are quite distinct from the appearance of the adrenal in Cushing's syndrome due to primary

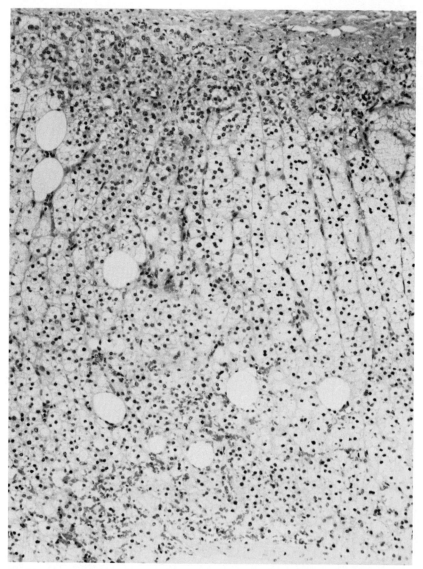

Fig. 7.2. Aminoglutethimide-treated gland. This female subject received aminoglutethimide and prednisone replacement therapy for two months prior to death. The cortex is broader than normal and consists solely of lipid-laden clear cells of the zona fasciculata type with occasional adipose spaces. The zona glomerulosa is also more prominent than normal. (H + E × 90)

hypothalamo-pituitary causes (p. 00). With cortisol or other glucocorticoid hormone-producing adrenal tumours, plasma ACTH levels will also be reduced and ipsilateral and contralateral adrenal atrophy will be present. However, these disparate aetiologies for adrenal atrophy are readily distinguished by the clinical history.

Inhibitors of Adrenal Steroidogenesis

Aminoglutethimide

There is a current vogue to administer a variety of inhibitors of adrenal steroidogenesis to effect medical 'adrenalectomy' as part of the overall management of breast cancer (Coombes et al. 1980). These agents are sometimes also used to control excessive hormone secretion by unresectable or recurrent adrenal neoplasms and occasionally in non-tumorous Cushing's syndrome.

One such drug is aminoglutethimide. This inhibits both the conversion of cholesterol to pregnenolone, and of androgens to oestrogens (p. 76). Thus, the production of all adrenal steroids will be reduced and cholesterol accumulates within the gland. This is the picture presented by glands with non-tumorous Cushing's syndrome treated with aminoglutethimide, the only material of this type to have received detailed morphological examination to date (Mötlik et al. 1973; Marek and Mötlik 1975). Apart from this lipoid transformation and the concomitant accumulation of

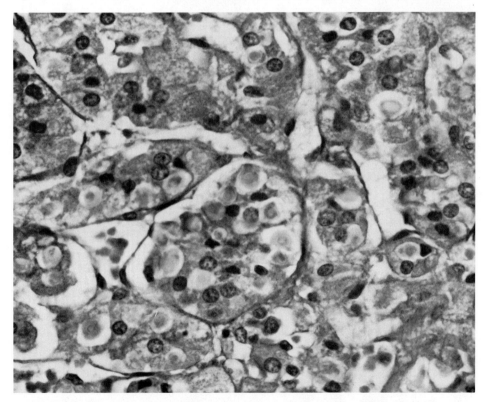

Fig. 7.3. Spironolactone bodies. A series of eosinophilic whorled structures are seen in the hyperplastic zona glomerulosa in the cortex attached to an adenoma causing Conn's syndrome in a patient given spironolactone preoperatively. (H + E × 700)

macrophages/histocytes which engulf lipids to form 'lipophages' which superficially resemble cortical cells, there are a few other structural changes discernable at the EM level in man following aminoglutethimide administration, apart from rarefaction of some mitochondrial cristae in the zona fasciculata (Mötlik et al. 1973; Marek and Mötlik 1975).

In the absence of additional therapy, hyperplasia would eventually occur as the result of raised plasma ACTH levels and a picture rather akin to that of congenital lipoid hyperplasia due to enzymic deficiencies would be expected in normal glands (see p. 167). However, as replacement steroid therapy is required in these patients, who had normal adrenal function originally, e.g. in breast cancer, one might anticipate that hyperplasia would not ensue and suppression of endogenous ACTH would result in varying degrees of cortical atrophy. In cases we have seen, however, the cortex has been broader than normal, but the cells have shown lipid accumulation (Fig. 7.2).

Spironolactone

The antihypertensive drug spironolactone (Aldactone) (see p. 76 for mechanism of action) is commonly used to lower the blood pressure of patients with hyper-

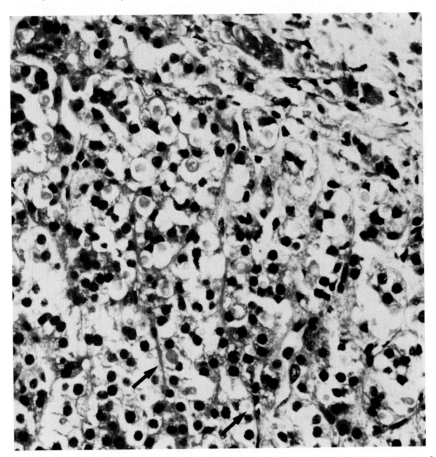

Fig. 7.4. Spironolactone bodies. These bodies extend to involve the clear cells of the outer zona fasciculata (*arrows*) in a gland attached to an adrenal adenoma causing Conn's syndrome. (H + E × 430)

aldosteronism and low plasma renin (Conn's syndrome) diagnostically and therapeutically prior to operation. In such circumstances, and when used as a diuretic, small rounded, birefringent, haloed eosinophilic inclusions appear in the adrenal cortex (Fig. 7.3) as first noted by Janigan (1963). These are the so-called 'spironolactone bodies' which are commonly about the size of a red blood cell but can range from

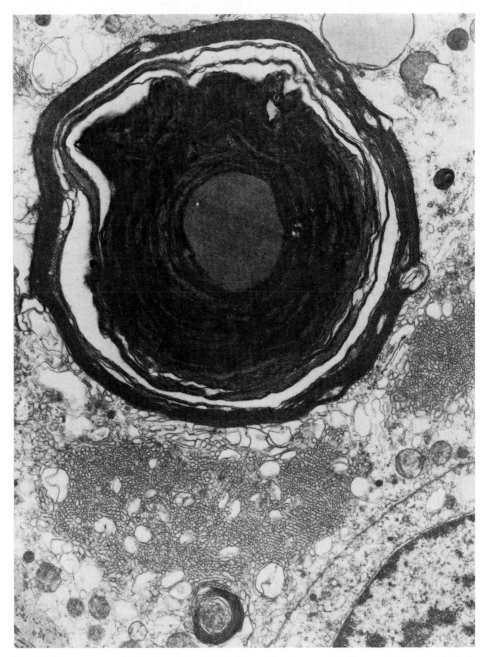

Fig. 7.5. Ultrastructure of the spironolactone body. These structures consist of concentric laminated whorls of membrane usually with a lipid centre. (× 14 550)

2–20 μm diameter. They are usually found in the cytoplasm of cells of the zona glomerulosa. On occasion they are also seen in adjacent cells of the outer zona fasciculata which are possibly those cells with ultrastructural features akin to zona glomerulosa cells (Fig. 7.4) (see p. 22).

Histochemically spironolactone bodies react as a phospholipid-protein complex, staining intensely with Sudan black and Luxol fast blue (Jenis and Herzog 1969). Ultrastructurally they consist of intensely osmiophilic laminated concentric whorls of double-layered, smooth-surfaced membranes, often enclosing a lipidic core (Jenis and Herzog 1969; Davis and Medline 1970). They probably arise from the smooth endoplasmic reticulum as a direct response to the drug (Fig. 7.5).

It is generally believed that spironolactone bodies afford a specific marker of aldosterone-producing cells (Conn and Hinerman 1977) and hence it is not surprising to find them in some analogous cells with adenomas producing aldosterone and associated with Conn's syndrome (p. 212) (Cain et al. 1974; Shrago et al. 1975). Personal experience has failed to detect them in the nodules also found in Conn's syndrome. This can have important diagnostic implications (p. 212).

Spironolactone bodies appear within about a week after spironolactone therapy is started (Jenis and Hertzog 1969), increase steadily in number up to about 50 days of treatment but apparently decline in number thereafter despite its continued administration (Conn and Hinerman 1977). No structures resembling spironolactone bodies have ever been reported in the adrenals of normal subjects or patients receiving other forms of therapy, or in other organs in spironolactone-treated cases. They disappear within 2–3 weeks of ceasing therapy.

O, p′-DDD (Mitotane, Lysodren)

The fat-soluble drug o,p′-DDD is a special case, having a marked and specific cytolytic effect on adrenocortical cells in some, but not all mammals. It can be used to treat unresectable adrenocortical carcinomas (Bergenstal et al. 1959). In this role, 35%–60% of treated cases respond to some degree with a significant, albeit small, increase in mean survival times (Hutter and Kayhoe 1966b; Lubitz et al. 1973). It has also been administered in non-tumorous Cushing's disease (Southren et al. 1961; Luton et al. 1979) although gastrointestinal and neural side effects limit its use.

The morphological effects of o,p′-DDD in man are poorly documented. Administration of cumulative doses of over 2 kg results in significant atrophy of the normal gland, which shows extensive destruction and fibrosis of virtually all the cells of the cortex (Bergenstal et al. 1960) and thus differs from adrenal atrophy caused by steroids (see p. 61). In many cases, however, it is clear that o,p′-DDD treatment in lesser doses does not cause atrophy on this scale (e.g. Hertz 1962; Touitou et al. 1978), and the adrenolytic effects of the drug in man cannot be as profound as in the dog where massive cytolysis and atrophy occur within a few weeks (Vilar and Tullner 1959). The adrenolytic effect of o,p′-DDD is of course demonstrable in adrenocortical tumours, and may predispose them to haemorrhage and infarction.

The mechanism of adrenolysis is obscure. In the dog the lesions commence in the zona reticularis, extend to the zona fasciculata but spare the zona glomerulosa, at least in short term experiments. Ultrastructural observations (Kaminsky et al. 1962) show rapid damage to mitochondria and in the absence of comparable observations in man, it must be assumed that such damage also eventually kills human adrenocortical cells. Similar changes have been noted with paraquat (Nagi 1970).

Other Inhibitors

Several other drugs with effects on pituitary-adrenal function are now used for therapeutic and diagnostic purposes; all are, therefore, potential causes of iatrogenic changes in cortical morphology. They include metyrapone and trilostane, which are direct inhibitors of adrenal steroidogenisis (see Table 8.3). The antiandrogens, danazol and cyproterone acetate, have recently been shown to be potential direct inhibitors of adrenal steroidogenesis (Barbieri et al. 1980) and, in the case of cyproterone acetate, also to inhibit ACTH secretion (Girard et al. 1978). However, adrenal morphological changes in response to these drugs have not been recorded. Metyrapone, for example, causes no detectable changes in cortical ultrastructure (MacKay 1969) in spite of its profound effect on steroidogenisis (see p. 76).

Chapter 8
Functional Activity of the Adrenal Cortex

All known hormones synthesised and secreted by the adult human adrenal cortex are steroids (Fig. 8.1) which in man are derived by a series of enzymatic steps from cholesterol. The most important and/or quantitatively dominant hormones produced are illustrated in Fig. 8.1.

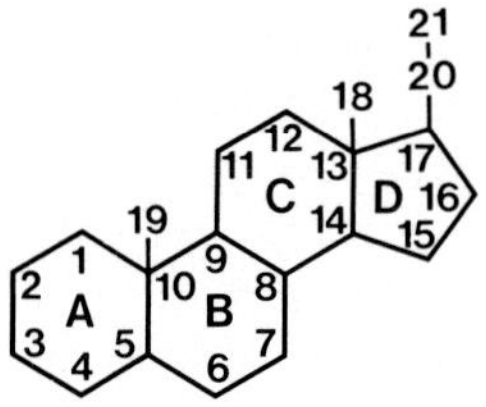

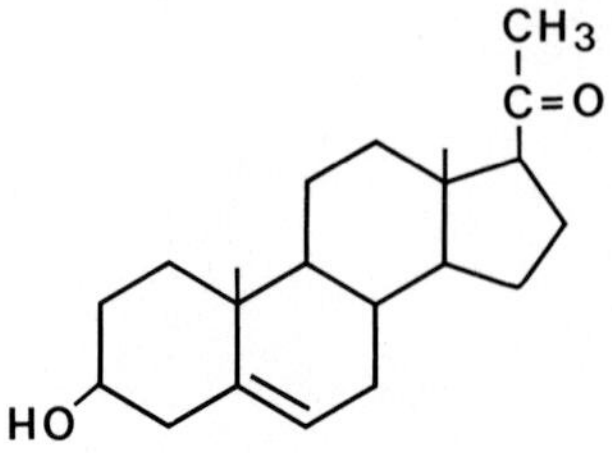

Pregnenolone

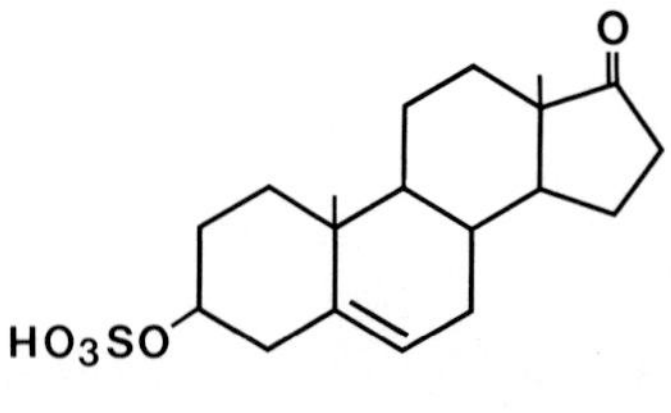

DHA Sulphate

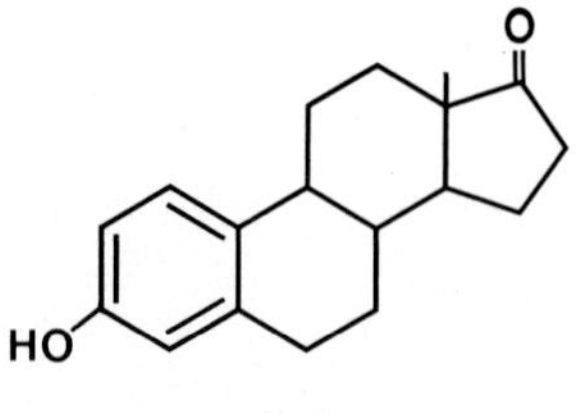

Oestrone

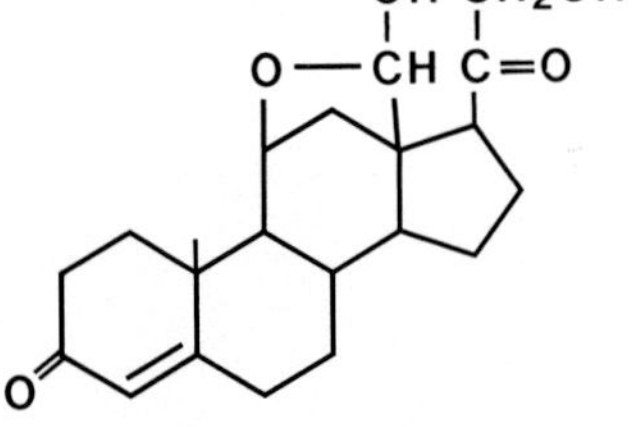

Aldosterone

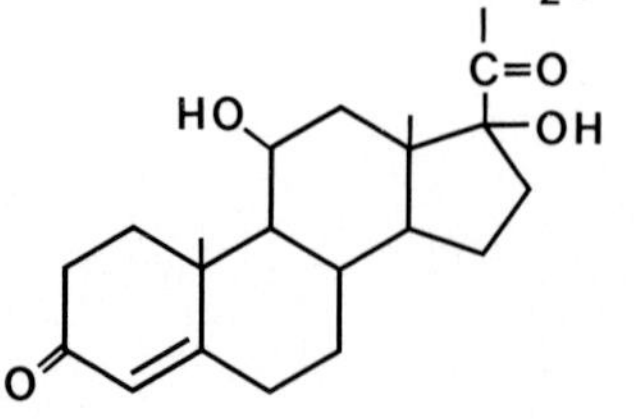

Cortisol

Fig. 8.1. Structures of the quantitatively predominant steroid hormones of different classes secreted by the human adrenal cortex.

Adrenal Chemistry

Steroids

Adrenal steroids may possess 21 carbon atoms (C_{21} steroids), examples being the potent glucocorticoids, cortisol and corticosterone, or the mineralocorticoid aldosterone (Fig. 8.1). Other adrenal steroids with androgenic properties such as DHA and testosterone are C_{19} steroids while the oestrogens are C_{18} steroids.

Steroid concentrations in the normal human adrenal cortex are low. Cortisol occurs in amounts varying from 5–20 μg/g wet weight using recently developed HPLC techniques for steroid analysis (O'Hare and Nice 1981). A typical scan of UV-absorbing steroids in the gland is illustrated in Fig. 8.2. These figures indicate that little storage of steroid hormones occurs in the tissue with its total content typically representing only about five minutes production at normal secretion rates.

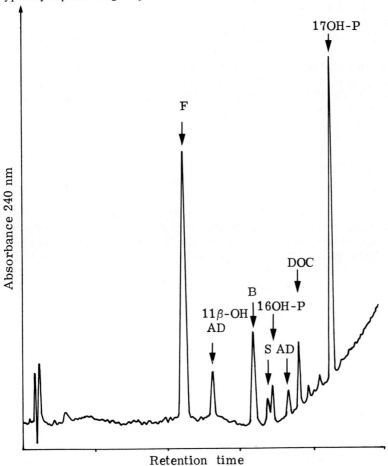

Fig. 8.2. High performance liquid chromatography (HPLC) of UV-absorbing steroid hormones extracted from the normal adult human adrenal cortex, according to the methods described in O'Hare and Nice (1981). In this, as in all HPLC's illustrated herein separations of the steroids were achieved using a reversed-phase (RP) method with gradient elution (water/methanol or water/dioxane) on an octadecylsilane-bonded (C_{18}) column packing, as described by O'Hare et al. (1976); the identities of the eluted compounds were established by comparison with consecutive chromatograms of steroid hormone standards (see Table 8.1 for abbreviations, 16OH-P: 16α-hydroxyprogesterone, 17OH-P: 17-hydroxyprogesterone).

Lipids

In cases of instantaneous death, the total adrenal lipid represents 50%–60% of the dry weight of the gland, but only 15%–25% in cases of fatal fulminating infections (Adams and Baxter 1949) due to stress-induced changes in cortical morphology (see p. 36). Neither sex nor age influence the lipid content of the adult gland. During the stress-induced lipid depletion the bulk of the loss is accounted for by sterol esters, free sterol remains relatively unchanged, as do triglycerides (Riley 1963). The detailed composition of adrenal lipid is as follows: oleate accounts for approximately 45% of sterol esters and palmitate, linoleate and stearate about 8%–10% each, with arachidonate contributing about 4% of the total. This pattern of adrenal sterol esters differs significantly from that of blood, notably in the smaller contribution of linoleate. Oleate and palmitate each represent about 25% of the adrenal triglycerides, with 15% as stearate and 10% arachidonate. The adrenal triglycerides are thus very similar in type to those found in depot fat in other parts of the body. Oleate, palmitate and stearate contribute equally (20%–25% each) to the fatty acid component of adrenal phospholipids. These components of adrenal lipid are susceptible to dietary influences as studies on Japanese have shown reduced concentrations of palmitate and a higher proportion of unsaturated fatty acids than in Western patients (Takayasu et al. 1970).

The sterol component of the adrenal lipids is almost exclusively cholesterol (40 mg/g total) with concentrations of hydroxycholesterols 3–4 orders of magnitude lower (Raggatt et al. 1972). Under treatment with the cholesterol side-chain cleavage inhibitor aminoglutethimide (see p. 76) levels of adrenal esterified cholesterol rise by a factor of up to three. Free cholesterol levels, however, remain normal in the gland under these conditions, and there is no detectable accumulation of hydroxycholesterols (Raggatt et al. 1972). Compact cells contain a higher proportion of free cholesterol, compared with cholesterol ester, than clear cells, according to Grant (1960).

The only other significant alteration in the chemistry of adrenal lipids in man that has been detected is a tendency of arachidonate concentrations to rise in glands with reduced steroid secretion rates, and a slight relative decline in this unsaturated fatty acid in hyperplastic glands (Raggatt et al. 1972). This association suggests the preferential formation of the steroid hormones in the human adrenal cortex from cholesterol esterified with arachidonate (see p. 71).

Vitamins

Concentrations of ascorbic acid range up to 1.3 mg/g in fresh adrenal tissue (Agate et al. 1953), higher than any other tissue except the corpus luteum, with correspondingly high concentrations of reduced glutathione (Pirani 1952). This vitamin is rapidly released from the gland into the blood in response to acute stress or exogenous ACTH administration (Agate et al. 1953). The total ascorbate content of the adrenal represents, however, only about 1% of the total body store in man. It is, therefore, most improbable that its release materially influences distant tissues. It may act on the medulla, however, to stabilise catecholamines and possibly facilitate their synthesis (Weiner 1975). The functional role of these high ascorbate (and dehydroascorbate) levels in the adrenal cortex itself still remains incompletely understood. Hornsby (1980) has recently suggested that the redox balance of the adrenal cell plays an important role in protecting cytochromes involved in steroid biosynthesis from free radical damage, and ascorbate may play a part in such mechanisms, as well as generating reducing equivalents for steroid hydroxylations. There is, however, no evidence of impaired steroidogenesis in old age when ascorbic acid levels are low (Dubin et al. 1978) or in human scurvy (Treager et al. 1950).

The human adrenal cortex also contains relatively high concentrations of the lipid-soluble vitamin A and its carotene precursors (Popper 1941). Animal studies (Schor and Glick 1970; Gruber et al. 1976) indicate, however, that this vitamin does not play an obligatory role in adrenal steroidogenesis.

Hormonogenesis by the Adult Adrenal Cortex

Pathways of Steroidogenesis

Adrenal steroids in man originate from cholesterol via the C_{21} steroid pregnenolone (Fig. 8.1). Alternative pathways via other sterols such as desmosterol are enzymatically feasible but insignificant under normal conditions (Goodman et al. 1962). Cholesterol for steroid biosynthesis is generated from stored lipid by ACTH-stimulated hydrolysis of cholesterol esters, with arachidonate especially prominent, which then may serve as the precursor of prostaglandins (Grant 1978). The kinetics of cholesterol metabolism in man indicate that steroid hormones are formed within the cortex primarily from cholesterol taken up from the plasma (Borkowski et al. 1972; Bolte et al. 1974), probably in the form of low density lipoprotein (Carr et al. 1980d). This cholesterol undergoes rapid exchange with adrenal cholesterol esters; de novo sterol formation from acetate is of minor significance for normal steroidogenesis (Fig. 8.3). ACTH-stimulated lipid depletion (see p. 36) cannot, however, be due entirely to steroidogenesis as the quantities of cholesterol esters involved (~ 3 g) are far too great (equivalent to 100 days continuous cortisol production); thus direct release of cholesterol probably also occurs (Grant 1978).

Pregnenolone, therefore, stands as the key steroid intermediate in the synthesis of all classes of adrenal hormone, irrespective of whether they are C_{21}, C_{19} or C_{18} compounds (Fig. 8.1). Pregnenolone is metabolised principally by one of two routes (Fig. 8.4). One involves 17α-hydroxypregnenolone which is a major intermediate in the synthesis of both cortisol (Cameron et al. 1968; Grant 1978; Whitehouse and Vinson 1968) and DHA (Cameron et al. 1969) i.e. the so-called Δ^5-pathway. Cortisol is the major 17-hydroxysteroid. Alternatively, pregnenolone is metabolised via pro-

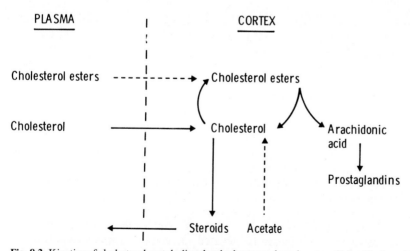

Fig. 8.3. Kinetics of cholesterol metabolism by the human adrenal cortex. (After Borkowski et al. 1972)

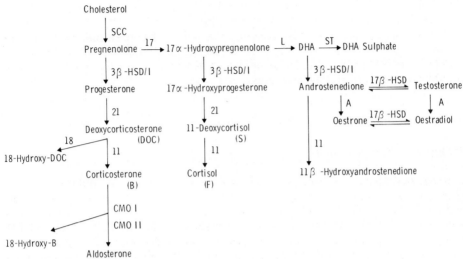

Fig. 8.4. Major pathways of steroidogenesis in the adult human adrenal cortex. See Table 8.2 for details of enzymes involved, and Griffiths and Cameron (1970) for the kinetic evidence on which it is based.

gesterone and deoxycorticosterone (the Δ^4-pathway) to form corticosterone, which is the main 17-deoxysteroid. The preferred pathway of aldosterone synthesis (Fig. 8.4) in man is almost certainly via corticosterone, although minor routes via 18-hydroxy-corticosterone (Pasqualini 1964) and 18-hydroxydeoxycorticosterone (Grekin et al. 1973) cannot be entirely excluded. Our own studies of cultured adult adrenal cells (O'Hare et al. 1980a) have provided no evidence for the direct formation of C_{19} steroids such as 11β-hydroxyandrostenedione from glucocorticoids such as cortisol, contrary to the homogenate studies of Hudson and Killinger (1972). The preferred pathways indicated by these data are illustrated in Fig. 8.4.

Although a total of about 50 different steroids have been isolated from the human adrenal gland, less than 20 are sufficiently active as mineralocorticoids, glucocorticoids, androgens or oestrogens to be regarded as physiologically significant. A list of these steroids together with their relative secretion rates is given in Table 8.1. Their plasma levels are given in Appendix A and normal values for urinary steroids in Appendix B.

Other minor compounds formed by the adult gland include 16-hydroxysteroids, such as 16α-hydroxyprogesterone (Ramseyer et al. 1974), 16α,18-dihydroxy-deoxycorticosterone (Dale and Melby 1973) and 16β-hydroxydehydroepiandro-sterone and its sulphate (16βOH-DHA) (Sekihara et al. 1976; Yamaji et al. 1980), 20α- and 20β-hydroxycorticoids (Touchstone et al. 1965; Touchstone and Kasparow 1970), 5α-reduced steroids (Charreau et al. 1968) and 11-dehydrocorticosteroids including cortisone (Compound E), 11-dehydrocorticosterone (Compound A) and adrenosterone (Compound G). A limited amount of steroid hydroxylation at positions 1α, 2α, 2β, 6α and 6β has also been demonstrated with human material (Jenkins 1965; Plasse and Lisboa 1973) and 7-keto steroids have been described (Neville and Webb 1965). Few, if any, of these minor adrenal steroids seem to exert significant biological effects and most represent catabolic products. As with the more proximal precursors of the major adrenal steroids illustrated in Fig. 8.4, including pregnenolone, pro-gesterone, 17α-hydroxypregnenolone and 17α-hydroxyprogesterone (Bermudez and Lipsett 1972), all are normally secreted only in very small amounts. Several have, however, been shown to be significantly elevated under pathological conditions of hyperplasia and neoplasia (Fantl et al. 1973; McKenna et al. 1977).

Table 8.1. Human adrenal steroid production rates relative to cortisol[a]

Steroid	Abbreviation[b]	Rate
Cortisol	F	100
Dehydroepiandrosterone sulphate	DHAS	125
Corticosterone	B	5
Dehydroepiandrosterone	DHA	8
11-Deoxycortisol	S	3
Androstenedione	AD	3
11β-Hydroxyandrostenedione	11βOH-AD	N.A.[b]
18-Hydroxycorticosterone	18OH-B	1.7
Deoxycorticosterone	DOC	1.2
Aldosterone	ALDO	0.75
18-Hydroxy-11-deoxycorticosterone	18OH-DOC	0.6
Testosterone	T	0.06
Oestrone	E$_1$	0.02
Oestradiol-17β	E$_2$	<0.002

[a]Values for uniquely adrenal C_{21} corticosteroids were obtained from mean daily production rates (Sandor et al. 1976) and for other C_{19} and C_{18} steroids from adrenal arteriovenous concentrations relative to cortisol (Baird et al. 1969; Saez et al. 1972) and production rates in vitro (Keymolen et al. 1976). Note that peripheral plasma ratios are significantly different in some cases (e.g. B/F, DHAS/F) owing to differences in metabolic clearance rates (Table 8.5). Normal cortisol production rates are 18–30 mg/day; for further details see Sandberg and Slaunwhite (1975).
[b]Not available in the literature, but plasma levels are similar to those of androstenedione (Appendix A).

Steroid sulphates (primarily DHAS) are, on the other hand, a major product of the adult human adrenal cortex (Table 8.1); glucuronides do not seem to be formed in the gland. Sulphotransferase activity in the adult gland responsible for sulphate formation is present at approximately half the level of the liver (Böstrom et al. 1964); a separate steroid sulphatase can also be detected in the adrenal (Dominguez et al. 1970), which is responsible for the hydrolysis of sulphurylated compounds. Cholesteryl sulphate has been detected within the adrenal gland (Drayer et al. 1964) and can be synthesised therein (Adams and Edwards 1968). Direct pathways of steroid sulphate metabolism are not, however, thought to be of major significance and most sulphurylated steroids are probably formed directly from their free steroid precursors, although contrary opinions have been expressed (Dominguez et al. 1975). Roberts and Lieberman (1970) give an extensive review of steroid sulphate biochemistry.

Steroid sulphotransferase has recently been isolated in substantially pure form from the cytosolic fraction of human adrenal glands (Adams and McDonald 1979) and appears to be the rate-limiting step in steroid sulphate formation. The substrate affinity of the enzyme (Böstrom et al. 1964; Adams and McDonald 1979), is such that of the steroids listed in Table 8.2 only DHA (and pregnenolone), and to a much lesser degree testosterone, oestradiol and deoxycorticosterone are sulphurylated to any extent. Adrenal secretion rates of, for example, corticosterone-21-sulphate (Kielman et al. 1966) and cortisol-21-sulphate (Kornel and Ezzeraimi 1980) are only a few percent of those for corresponding free steroids.

The role of steroid sulphurylation in the adult human adrenal cortex, therefore, appears to be the generation of what are generally regarded as physiologically inactive compounds from potentially hormonally active steroids such as DHA, thus limiting the inappropriate androgenisation that would otherwise occur. This, in our opinion, is the most logical way in which the massive production of DHAS by the adult human cortex can be rationalised, and this may be of even greater importance in the fetus (see p. 93).

The lipid solubility of the steroid hormones, together with the lack of significant storage within the gland indicate that they probably cross the cell membrane primarily by diffusion; exocytosis and specific transport mechanisms seem unlikely to be

Table 8.2. Location, kinetics and cofactor requirements of adrenal steroid metabolising enzymes

	Cofactors	Reversibility	Localisation	Abbreviation[a]
Cholesterol side-chain cleavage system	NADPH + H+ + O2	−	Mitochondrial	SCC
17α-Hydroxylase	NADPH + H+ + O2	−	Microsomal (SER)	17
C17–20 Lyase (desmolase)	NADPH + H+ + O2	−	Microsomal	L
3β-Hydroxysteroid dehydrogenase	NAD+	+	Mainly microsomal but possibly some mitochondrial	3β-HSD
5-En-4-en-isomerase	None	+	Mainly microsomal but possibly some mitochondrial	I
11β-Hydroxylase	NADPH + H+ + O2	−	Mitochondrial	11
18-Hydroxylase	NADPH + H+ + O2	−	Mitochondrial	18
Corticosterone methyl oxidase I (18-hydroxylase)[b]	NADPH + H+ + O2	−	Mitochondrial	CMOI
Corticosterone methyl oxidase II (18-dehydrogenase)[b]	NADPH + H+ + O2	−	Mitochondrial	CMOII
Aromatase	NADPH + H+ + O2	−	Probably microsomal	A
17β-Hydroxysteroid dehydrogenase	NADP+ or NAD+	+	Cytosolic	17β-HSD
Steroid sulphotransferase	Adenosine 3-phosphate 5′-phosphosulphate	−	Cytosolic	ST

[a]Fig. 8.4.
[b]Ulick (1976b)

involved in this process. Steroid release into the blood is, nevertheless, probably facilitated by their binding to plasma proteins such as cortisol binding globulin (CBG) and albumin which decrease the effective free extracellular concentrations of the hormones (Westphal 1971). This hypothesis has been experimentally confirmed for testicular hormones (Ewing et al. 1976) and probably applies to the adrenal as well. The biologically active fraction of the hormone in the blood is the free fraction, which in the case of cortisol typically represents about 10% of total plasma hormone levels (Brien 1980). A recent case of an apparent abnormality in the binding affinity of CBG has been described in a patient with pituitary-dependent Cushing's syndrome (Barragry et al. 1980). Changes in the amounts and properties of such binding proteins can, therefore, potentially influence the clinical picture in cases of adrenocortical dysfunction.

Molecular Mechanisms of Steroidogenesis

Ultimately, all defects in steroidogenesis encountered in pathological tissue must stem from changes in the molecular mechanisms that govern steroid biosynthesis, and its control. These, therefore, merit some consideration, although we must rely in a large part on evidence accrued from animal experiments in constructing a model of human adrenal steroidogenesis at the molecular level.

The biosynthesis of all the major adrenal steroids involves a co-ordinated series of reactions carried out by membrane-bound enzymes located in the smooth endoplasmic reticulum or the mitochondria (Table 8.2). These enzymes, whose sites of action in the

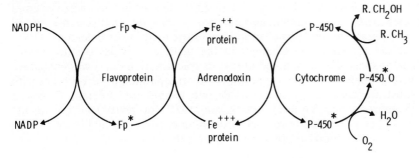

Fig. 8.5. Pathways of electron transport for mitochondrial steroid hydroxylation. (After Omura et al. 1965)

hormonal pathways of steroid biosynthesis have already been illustrated in Fig. 8.4, are listed in Table 8.2, together with their preferred cofactors; they comprise dehydrogenases, isomerases, lyases (desmolases) and hydroxylases (see Simpson and Mason (1976) for review).

Hydroxylating systems of the cortex are composed of several moeities. Thus a protoporphyrin haemoprotein (cytochrome P-450) located on the inner membrane of the mitochondria, and a FAD-containing flavoprotein (adrenodoxin reductase) associate with an iron-sulphur protein (adrenodoxin) which is soluable and is in the mitochondrial matrix, to form an electron-transport system for steroid hydroxylation (Fig. 8.5). The mitochondrial cholesterol side-chain cleavage system, 11β-hydroxylase and probably 18-hydroxylase conform to this pattern.

Microsomal hydroxylases, including 17α-hydroxylase, 21-hydroxylase, and C_{17-20} desmolase also involve cytochrome P-450s in association with phospholipids and another flavoprotein, immunochemically distinct from that in the mitochondria. Together they probably form a large micellar complex (Grant 1978). Both mitochondrial and microsomal hydroxylases appear to utilise molecular oxygen for their reaction, i.e. they are mixed function oxidases (Fig. 8.5), the specificity of which probably resides in the cytochrome P-450, which appears to bind the steroid substrate (Orme-Johnson et al. 1979). The reducing equivalents for these reactions originate in the pentose phosphate pathway and cytosolic malic enzyme for microsomal hydroxylases, and from Kreb's cycle intermediates via an energy-linked trans-hydrogenation and mitochondrial malic enzyme activity in the mitochondria (Simpson and Mason 1976). The co-ordination of these reactions as the steroid intermediates shuttle backwards and forwards between the different subcellular compartments affords an interesting problem. It should be noted that the reaction mechanisms detailed above have been determined largely with non-human adrenal preparations and differences in detail may occur in the human cortex.

Despite these considerable advances in our knowledge of steroid biosynthesis there remains a major question of substantial potential relevance to human adrenocortical pathophysiology viz. the possible existence of multiple steroid-metabolising enzymes carrying out the same reaction but with different substrate affinities. Thus pathological human adrenocortical tissues have been examined in which 3β-hydroxysteroid dehydrogenase activity for only one potential substrate had apparently been lost (Weliky and Engel 1963; Neville et al. 1969a) and similar effects have recently been observed in vivo in patients treated with 3β-hydroxysteroid dehydrogenase inhibitors (Komanicky et al. 1978). Enzyme kinetic data, however, have tended to support the alternative hypothesis of a single steroid dehydrogenase in both bovine (Neville et al. 1969b) and human glands (Yates and Deshpande 1975). Recent studies by Eastman and Neville (1977) have failed to separate substrate-specific 3β-hydroxysteroid dehydrogenases from adult human adrenal glands, despite extensive use of gel filtration, density gradient centrifugation and isoelectric focusing on detergent (Triton X-100)-solubilised preparations. Changes in the relative activities of the enzyme towards different substrates were noted during its fractionation but it was concluded that these were probably due to allotypes rather than separate dehydrogenases with restricted substrate specificity. Likewise, despite claims for different 5-en-4-en oxosteroid isomerases (see Samuels and Nelson 1975, for review) no convincing evidence has yet been obtained in respect of the human cortex; solubilisation of the enzyme prior to fractionation has posed major problems in the past (Neville and Engel 1968).

There is circumstantial evidence in man for the existence of more than one 21-hydroxylase (Degenhart et al. 1965) and 11β-hydroxylase (Zachmann et al. 1971) in certain types of congenital adrenal hyperplasia (see p. 158), but the in vitro kinetic evidence is weak (Klein et al. 1974). Purification of this type of enzyme (21-hydroxylase) has only been achieved very recently with bovine adrenals (Kominami et al. 1980). Hydroxylating systems are notoriously difficult to study in the human adrenal as they are extremely labile (Sinterhauf et al. 1974a,b).

The question of possible multiple steroid-metabolising dehydrogenases, isomerases and hydroxylases in the human adrenal cortex must, therefore, remain unanswered for the present. It is important to bear in mind, however, that different moeities may be responsible for the same reaction in different zones of the cortex (see p. 105).

Inhibitors of Steroidogenesis

The major sites of action of various clinically used inhibitors of human adrenal steroidogenesis, as revealed by studies in vivo and in vitro are listed in Table 8.3. The consequences of their use can be readily deduced from the pathways illustrated in Fig. 8.4, bearing in mind that precursors will accumulate above the level of the block and alternative pathways circumventing the inhibition, if available, will become operative.

Table 8.3. Mechanism of action of inhibitors of adrenal steroidogenesis in man

Inhibitor	Major site of action	Other effects	Reference
O,p'-DDD	11β-Hydroxylase		Brown et al. 1973
		18-Hydroxylase	Touitou et al. 1978
Aminoglutethimide	Cholesterol side-chain cleavage		Dexter et al. 1967
		Aromatase[a]	Samojlik et al. 1977
Trilostane	3β-Hydroxysteroid dehydrogenase		Komanicky et al. 1978
Spironolactone	11β-Hydroxylase	18-Hydroxylase	Cheng et al. 1976
		18-Dehydrogenase	Aupetit et al. 1978
		17α-Hydroxylase	Menard et al. 1979
		21-Hydroxylase	Menard et al. 1976
Metyrapone	11β-Hydroxylase		Dominguez and Samuels 1963
		Cholesterol side-chain cleavage	Carballeira et al. 1974
		18-Hydroxylase	Schöneshöfer et al. 1979

[a]D-Isomer 40 times more potent than L-enantiomer (Graves and Salhanick 1979).

   The molecular mechanisms of action of most of these inhibitors are not fully understood. Their structure as aromatic or heterocyclic compounds or straightforward cyclopentenophenanthrene-based steroid analogues (e.g. trilostane) presumably enables them to bind to the enzymes involved. Hydroxylase inhibitors interact with the steroid-binding cytochrome P-450 apparently via the haeme ligand; in the case of spironolactone (Menard et al. 1979) this may lead to the actual destruction of the cytochrome. Damage of this sort presumably relates in some way to the formation of the SER-derived spironolactone bodies (see p. 64), although it is interesting in this case that mitochondrial hydroxylases are its major biochemical sites of action (Table 8.3). It should be noted that the majority of these inhibitors have multiple sites of action, the most proximal affected adrenal enzymes dominating the clinical effect. Occasionally, unexpected adrenal effects will be encountered when steroid analogues are used for totally different reasons. Thus the antigonadotrophin danazol has recently been shown to inhibit human adrenal steroidogenesis (11β- and 18-hydroxylation) in vitro (Barbieri et al. 1980). Human cell cultures are an extremely valuable tool in these pharmacological studies, and may reveal quite unexpected effects of widely used drugs (Morgan and O'Hare 1979).

   Lastly, it should be remembered that a number of these drugs (e.g. metyrapone and spironolactone) have significant extra-adrenal effects which may indirectly modify circulating steroid levels, sometimes by binding to specific steroid receptors; and in the case of o,p′-DDD by modifying the extra-adrenal metabolism of cortisol (Bledsoe et al. 1964).

Control of Adult Steroidogenesis

Glucocorticoids

ACTH   The physiological control of adrenal glucocorticoid secretion depends on pituitary ACTH, whose secretion is in turn subject to feed-back regulation via the hypothalamo-pituitary axis by endogenous glucocorticoids and analogues such as dexamethasone. Steroidogenesis is not, however, totally dependent on ACTH as all glucocorticoid secretion does not cease in its absence. In panhypopituitarism and long-term steroid therapy when ACTH levels are often <0.2 pg/ml (Holdaway et al. 1973) small but measurable levels of glucocorticoids can be detected (~ 2 μg/100 ml, 55 nmoles/l) (James et al. 1968). Although the very low residual ACTH levels in vivo might be held responsible for this output, more direct evidence for an ACTH-independent 'baseline' of glucocorticoid secretion comes from studies of cultured adult human adrenal cells, which continue to secrete steroids at between 3%–10% of ACTH-stimulated levels (Fig. 8.6) even in its prolonged (1–2 months) absence (O'Hare et al. 1980a). Stimulation with $ACTH_{1-24}$ results typically in an 8–12-fold increment in steroid secretion in culture (Neville and O'Hare 1978), figures which are in good agreement with normal plasma cortisol levels which range from 4 up to 50 μg/100 ml (100–1,400 nmoles/l) with exogenous ACTH administration. In short-term experiments with isolated adult human adrenal cells a half-maximal steroidogenic response is elicited by ~ 20 pg/ml $ACTH_{1-24}$ (Kolanowski and Crabbe 1976) compared with typical circulating ACTH levels of 8–50 pg/ml (Berson and Yalow 1968; Holdaway et al. 1973).

   Activity-entrained nycthemeral rhythmicity of glucocorticoid secretion in normal subjects results in peak levels (~ 25 μg/100 ml, 690 nmoles/l) at between 4.00 and 8.00 a.m., with a nadir (~ 7 μg/100 ml, 190 nmoles/l) at about midnight. No sex- or age-dependent differences in rhythms have been detected in vivo (Krieger 1980).

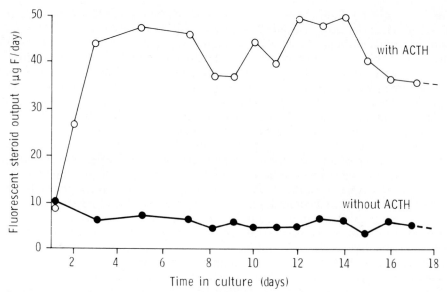

Fig. 8.6. Corticosteroid output of normal adult human adrenocortical cells in monolayer culture in the presence (*open rings*) and absence (*closed rings*) of $ACTH_{1-24}$ (1μg/ml). Reprinted with kind permission of Academic Press.

Cortisol levels do not, however, vary smoothly during the diurnal cycle. Short ($\frac{1}{2}$–1 h) ultradian secretory episodes ('spikes') occur, of which 5–10 may be identified in a single 24-h cycle (Krieger et al. 1971). These patterns correlate well with similar variations in plasma ACTH, bearing in mind its very short plasma half-life ($\sim$ 5 min) compared with that of cortisol (70 min). Isolated adrenal cell preparations show no evidence of intrinsic rhythmicity (O'Hare and Hornsby 1975). The secretion rate of various glucocorticoids is shown in Table 8.1.

ACTH administration not only increases the total glucocorticoid output of the gland but it also causes some changes in the proportions of different steroids secreted. This effect is clearly seen in cultured human cells (Fig. 8.7). Short-term ($<$24 h) hormone treatment increases corticosterone secretion to a greater extent than cortisol, while further stimulation eventually causes the ratio to shift strongly in favour of cortisol. Corresponding changes in the 17-hydroxy:17-deoxysteroid ratio have been noted in both short (Mason et al. 1975; Nishida et al. 1977) and long-term studies (Grant et al. 1957a,b) of ACTH administration in vivo and in hyperplastic glands (Sinterhauf et al. 1974a,b). Corticosterone levels compared with cortisol are considerably higher in adrenal venous effluent than in the peripheral plasma, owing to the rapid clearance and hepatic metabolism of the corticosterone. Since it possesses significant mineralocorticoid as well as glucocorticoid potency (Table 8.4), this rapid metabolism in the normal subject diminishes its potentially ambiguous physiological significance.

There is no evidence in adult man that the different pathways of glucocorticoid secretion are stimulated to a different degree by different molecular forms of ACTH and its precursors or its cogeners, such as β-endorphin, CLIP or αMSH, produced from the pituitary 31 kD pro-opiocortin precursor (Fig. 8.8), although Boiti and Yalow (1978) have suggested that this may happen in some other species.

Small changes in steroid secretion rates, including corticosterone, and to a lesser extent cortisol, have been observed in the elderly male (Romanoff and Baxter 1975). ACTH responses are however fully preserved and it seems likely that any difference is

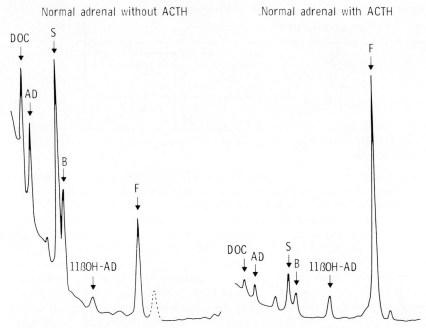

Normal adrenal without ACTH   Normal adrenal with ACTH

Fig. 8.7. HPLC scans of UV-absorbing (250 nm) steroids secreted by cultured adult human adrenocortical cells before and after 7 days continuous exposure to $ACTH_{1-24}$. Note the shift in the steroid secretion pattern in favour of 17-hydroxysteroids (e.g. F) after prolonged exposure to the hormone. For further details of the methods used see O'Hare et al. (1976).

Table 8.4. Relative biological potency of major adrenocortical steroids in vivo (from various sources)

	Glucocorticoid activity
Cortisol	100
Cortisone	65
Corticosterone	30
Aldosterone	20
11-Deoxycortisol	6
Deoxycorticosterone	0.5
	Mineralocorticoid activity
Aldosterone	100
Deoxycorticosterone	3
Corticosterone	0.5
18-Hydroxydeoxycorticosterone	0.2
Cortisol	0.1
11-Deoxycortisol	<0.1
	Androgenic activity
Testosterone	100
Androstenedione	20
Dehydroepiandrosterone	5
11β-Hydroxyandrostenedione	1

due to an alteration in feedback mechanisms and rates of peripheral metabolism rather than any intrinsic age-related diminution in the functional capacity of the cortex, as is probably also the case with the small sex differences in plasma glucocorticoid levels (Zumoff et al. 1974; Schöneshöfer and Wagner 1977).

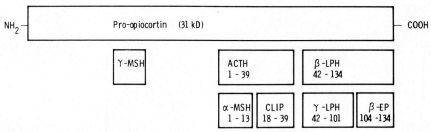

Fig. 8.8. The relationship of ACTH$_{1-39}$ and various peptide cogeners to their 31 kD precursor (pro-opiocortin). (After Nakanishi et al. 1979)

Intracellular mechanism of ACTH action   The ACTH-induced changes in the relative and absolute levels of secreted steroids are a consequence of its multiple effects which involve both acute and trophic responses of the steroidogenic mechanisms within the cell. The primary interaction with the cortex of the hormone (whose biological activity resides in its N-terminal sequence) is via a specific glycoprotein receptor located on the cell membrane and dependent for its integrity on its phospholipid environment. The hormone-receptor complex activates an adenylate cyclase moeity also found in the membrane. A detailed review of heterotopic effectors regulating adrenal adenylate cyclase has recently been compiled by Glynn et al. (1979). The resulting increased production of intracellular cyclic AMP (Fig. 8.9) then interacts with a protein kinase composed of a regulatory cyclic AMP-receptor subunit and a catalytic kinase unit; binding of cyclic AMP to the receptor results in allosteric alteration with dissociation and subsequent activity of the catalytic subunit (see for review, Gill 1976). The phosphorylation of a variety of cellular proteins (Koroscil and Gallant 1980) by the active kinase appears to initiate co-ordinated cellular metabolic processes that collectively enhance and sustain the steroid output of the gland.

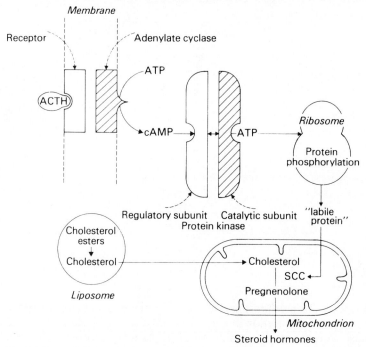

Fig. 8.9. Intracellular mechanism of the acute effect of ACTH on adrenocortical steroidogenesis.

Although the primary role of cyclic AMP in ACTH action has frequently been challenged (e.g. Perchellet and Sharma 1979) there is little data to support alternate potential intracellular regulators or second messengers such as cyclic GMP (O'Hare 1976). The ACTH-cyclic AMP model remains the most satisfactory, with powerful support from genetic studies of adenylate cyclase and protein-kinase-deficient mutants of adrenal cells (Rae et al. 1979), and studies of hormone-induced protein phosphorylation (Koroscil and Gallant 1980).

The normal rate-limiting steroidogenic step is the conversion of cholesterol to pregnenolone (Fig. 8.4). This process is swiftly modified by ACTH and appears to be mediated by a short-lived protein. It has been suggested that either transport of cholesterol into, or pregnenolone out of the mitochondria (Koritz-Hall hypothesis), are the processes immediately modified. Neither hypothesis has been convincingly proved, however, and a direct effect of some allosteric modulator on the side-chain cleavage enzyme system itself may be the mechanism whereby ACTH acutely increases the steroid output (Simpson et al. 1978; Farese and Sabir 1980). There is also some evidence that microtubules and microfilaments may be involved (Crivello and Jefcoate 1980). The acute effects of ACTH stimulation of the cortex, which do not involve changes in the levels of the steroid-metabolising enzymes themselves, are summarised in Fig. 8.9.

Long-term ACTH administration, however, increases the activity of several of the adrenal steroid-metabolising enzymes further down the pathway (e.g. 11β-hydroxylase and probably 17α-hydroxylase as well) and correspondingly enhanced levels of cytochrome P-450 can be detected in the hyperplastic human cortex (deAlvare et al. 1977). These changes occur slowly as the relevant enzymes have half-lives of 3–4 days (Purvis et al. 1973) and they probably account for the changes in relative levels of different glucocorticoids (i.e. 17-hydroxy and 17-deoxysteroids) that occur with prolonged hormone treatment.

Other factors   Despite clear evidence from animal studies that cortisol-secreting cells can respond, under some circumstances, to the octapeptide angiotensin II via increases in intracellular cyclic AMP (Peytremann et al. 1973), its seems improbable that a similar effect is obtained in man, or is of physiological significance. The majority of experiments in man have observed no stimulation of cortisol secretion in vitro (Williams and Braley 1977) or in vivo (Ames et al. 1965; Brown et al. 1972b; Kono et al. 1975; Mason et al. 1977) other than those accountable for by concurrent changes in ACTH levels. The only study in conflict with these conclusions is that of McKenna et al. (1978), these workers used 'Hypertensin', (^{5}-valine) angiotensin II amide, and measured short-term cortisol responses in vitro to concentrations of $<10^{-5}$ M. We ourselves have noted a slight response of cultured adult human adrenal cells to this pharmacological preparation in long-term experiments, but never to HPLC-pure (5-isoleucine) angiotensin II at the same concentration (Fig. 8. 10). It therefore seems likely that the naturally occurring form of the angiotensin peptide in man has, in its pure form, no significant capacity to stimulate human cortisol secretion.

While increased cortisol excretion and secretion has been noted in acromegaly (Charro et al. 1973) and the glands may be heavier than normal (Symington 1969), there is good evidence that the enhanced levels of hormones are an indirect rather than a direct response of the cortex to growth hormone (Lindholm et al. 1980). No other direct physiological stimuli of adrenal glucocorticoid secretion have been identified.

Mineralocorticoids

Aldosterone is the physiologically dominant mineralocorticoid secreted by the normal

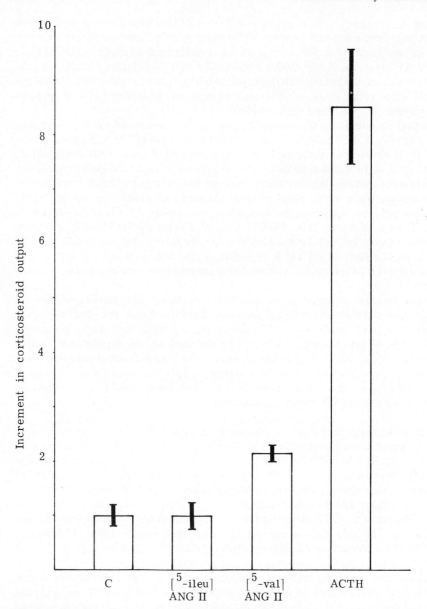

Fig. 8.10. Steroidogenic responses of the normal adult human adrenal cortex in monolayer culture to ACTH$_{1-24}$ (1μg/ml) and to [^{5}-isoleucine] angiotensin II (10μg/ml) and [^{5}-valine] angiotensin II amide (10μg /ml ('Hypertensin'). The means and standard deviations (*bar*) of the daily corticosteroid output during 5 days of consecutive exposure to the polypeptides are shown in comparison with a replicate culture prior to hormonal addition (C), and the results expressed in terms of the increment in steroid output observed.

adult human adrenal cortex; its principal function is to conserve sodium. It is 30–40 times more potent than deoxycorticosterone (DOC), over 150 and 200 times more active as a mineralocorticoid than corticosterone and 18-hydroxydeoxycorticosterone (18OH-DOC) respectively on Na$^+$/K$^+$ balance (see Table 8.4). Normal circulating levels of aldosterone vary from 5–50 ng/100 ml (0.14–1.4 nmoles/l) and are strongly influenced by posture, being higher in erect compared with recumbent subjects. Daily secretion rates in adults are $\sim 100 \ \mu g/day$, although they may rise to over $1000 \ \mu g/day$ in late pregnancy (see Table 8.1 and Appendix B).

Control of aldosterone secretion is a complex multifactoral process with pituitary hormones playing a relatively minor, permissive, role. The kidney was identified as a source of aldosterone-stimulating activity by Gross (1960), Davis et al. (1960) and Tobian (1960) on the basis of both physiological and histological studies, and the relationship of renin to aldosterone secretion was revealed when Genest et al. (1960) and Laragh et al. (1960) demonstrated that the vasoconstrictor peptide, angiotensin II, stimulated aldosterone.

The intimate relationship between aldosterone, blood pressure and the pathophysiology of hypertension has ensured intensive investigation of the control of mineralocorticoid secretion in man during the past two decades. While a number of questions regarding the aetiology of specific hypertensive states remain unanswered, it is now clear that the most important factors concerned with the normal control of aldosterone secretion in man are the plasma electrolytes and certain peptide hormones.

Electrolytes Sodium: Luetscher and Axelrad (1954) were the first to note that changes in sodium balance in man altered levels of aldosterone secretion, an effect mediated primarily by alterations in extracellular fluid volume and the renin-angiotensin system (Brown et al. 1964). Although animal experiments (Blair-West et al. 1962; Davis et al. 1963) demonstrated that lowering plasma Na^+ by 10–20 mEq stimulated aldosterone, these changes are far too great to constitute a physiological mechanism. Thus plasma Na^+ levels are often normal in man during sodium depletion and there is no evidence that hyponatraemia is a primary mechanism leading to hyperaldosteronism.

Potassium: Potassium has a direct acute and trophic effect (Dluhy et al. 1972) in man on aldosterone secretion, independent of changes in blood volume (Laragh and Stoerk 1957; Gann et al. 1964) and without involving the renin-angiotensin system (Brunner et al. 1970). The direct effect of this ion on aldosterone-secreting cells is well illustrated in tissue culture. When applied in supraphysiological levels to cultured aldosterone-producing cells, potassium can direct almost all of their steroidogenic potential into the production of aldosterone and 18-hydroxycorticosterone (18OH-B) (Hornsby and O'Hare 1977). Normally, however, physiological changes in plasma K^+ are not as important as the renin-angiotensin system although its effects are dominant in primary aldosteronism.

Polypeptide hormones Angiotensin II: The renin-angiotensin system is the major physiological regulator of aldosterone secretion in man (Davis 1975). Thus, to a very large extent renin/angiotensin levels and the aldosterone secretion rate change in parallel with changes in posture, blood volume or sodium intake, and the infusion of renin or angiotensin stimulates its secretion. The relevant physiological mechanisms are illustrated in Fig. 8.11.

The octapeptide angiotensin II is formed from the decapeptide angiotensin I by the action of a 'converting enzyme' present in most tissues but especially the lung; angiotensin I is in turn derived from a circulating 110 kD α_2-globulin (angiotensinogen) by the action of the enzyme renin secreted mainly (but not exclusively) by the renal juxtaglomerular apparatus (Peach 1977). Circulating angiotensin II levels are ~ 50 pg/ml in normal recumbent subjects (Emanuel et al. 1973) and its half-life in the plasma is of the order of 30 s, being rapidly inactivated by plasma 'angiotensinases'. Infusion studies in man have demonstrated that both the pharmacological ([5]-valine) angiotensin II amide (Hypertensin) and the naturally occurring ([5]-isoleucine) angiotensin II have an equal effect on adrenal steroidogenesis (Oelkers et al. 1975). The

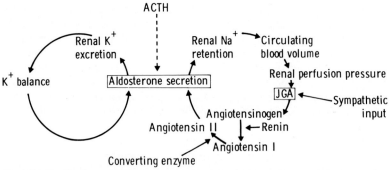

Fig. 8.11. Feedback mechanisms of aldosterone regulation in man. (Modified after Williams and Dluhy 1972)

(des-[1]asp) angiotensin II (so-called angiotensin III) produced in plasma and possibly in the cortex itself is somewhat less active when infused, probably because of its more rapid catabolism (Carey et al. 1978; Zager et al. 1980).

The direct effects of angiotensin II infusion in man are confined to a parallel increase in aldosterone and 18OH-B secretion (Mason et al. 1976, 1977). Although sodium repletion diminishes aldosterone secretion, extremely high levels of sodium intake (<1500 mEq/day) do not reduce it below 10–30 μg/day (Pratt and Luft 1979); this probably represents the 'baseline' levels of secretion under conditions of minimal physiological demand. Studies with inhibitors of converting enzyme activity have recently confirmed that the effects of sodium depletion in man are mediated primarily by angiotensin II (Sancho et al. 1976; Williams et al. 1978).

ACTH: The precise role of ACTH in the control of aldosterone secretion in man has provoked debate for some time, investigations being complicated by marked variations between individuals and the concurrent effects of activity and posture on mineralocorticoid output. It would appear that although ACTH is not a major regulator of aldosterone secretion in man, there is nevertheless good evidence that it plays an important role in maintaining the metabolic integrity of the mineralocorticoid-secreting cells, enabling them to respond to appropriate physiological stimuli such as changes in electrolyte balance.

Thus, although it was once believed that only pharmacological doses of ACTH could influence aldosterone, recent studies have clearly demonstrated significant responses to low-dose 'physiological' stimulation (Nicholls et al. 1975a). Further evidence for a physiological role of ACTH in mineralocorticoid regulation is the partial concordance of aldosterone levels with circadian variations of plasma glucocorticoids observed in recumbent subjects (Williams et al 1972; Katz et al. 1972; Kowarski et al 1975), both reaching a nadir in the late evening. It should be noted, however, that episodic variations in aldosterone do not always appear to correlate well with either changes in ACTH or renin-angiotensin levels (Weinberger et al. 1975) and some workers have suggested that another, as yet unidentified, stimulus is involved (James et al. 1976).

Although under certain circumstances the proportional response of aldosterone to ACTH can equal that of the glucocorticoids (Kem et al. 1975) this is not usually the case, and a notable feature of the aldosterone response is its transient nature (Liddle et al. 1956; Tucci et al. 1967). The initial stimulation is followed after 2–3 days by a marked suppression. Possible mechanisms whereby this effect is obtained will be discussed later (p. 108).

The most direct evidence for a physiological role of ACTH in aldosterone secretion in man comes from observations of hypophysectomised subjects and panhypopituitary conditions. Thus, while acute hypophysectomy does not significantly influence mineralocorticoid regulation (Ross et al. 1960) in the longer term there is a diminution of aldosterone excretion of up to 50% (Lieberman and Luetscher 1960). While high dose steroid therapy or dexamethasone suppression of ACTH does not always modify aldosterone secretion in response to sodium depletion (Williams et al. 1971), blunting (Spark et al. 1968) as well as total abolition of these responses has been noted in similar studies (McCaa et al. 1974). While some of the discrepancies between these reports are difficult to explain except on the basis of individual variation it would seem that in the longer term the absence of ACTH does result in a diminution of baseline levels of aldosterone secretion and responses to physiological stimuli, although the physical integrity of the aldosterone-secreting cells themselves may not be compromised (Jessiman et al. 1959).

ACTH is the main stimulus to secretion of other steroids with mineralocorticoid activity produced by the human adrenal gland. Thus plasma levels of corticosterone, deoxycorticosterone and 18OH-DOC are more responsive to ACTH (18–20-fold increases) than to angiotensin (two-fold increase) (Williams et al. 1976; Tuck et al. 1977) and 18OH-DOC and corticosterone levels show a striking parallelism in vitro and in vivo (Ulick 1976a; Sonino et al. 1980). These steroids are not, however, exclusively under ACTH control as in the presence of a sustained infusion of ACTH, administration of angiotensin II will enhance corticosterone, DOC and 18OH-DOC levels in vivo (Mason et al. 1979) and in vitro studies with isolated human adrenal cells have shown direct effects of angiotensin II on 18OH-DOC production by the aldosterone-secreting cells (Braley and Williams 1979). Interpretation of the concurrent effects of ACTH and angiotensin in vivo may, however, be complicated by the direct effects of angiotensin on ACTH secretion (Semple et al. 1979) and the alteration in metabolic clearance rates of corticosteroids caused by the extra-adrenal effects of angiotensin II (Messerli et al. 1977).

Other factors   The interaction of the acute and trophic effects of K^+, angiotensin II and ACTH would seem in principle to be sufficiently complex to permit all observed changes in aldosterone levels in man to be explained. Nevertheless, various workers in this field have, over the years, felt impelled to postulate the existence of additional unknown aldosterone-stimulating factor(s) (McCaa et al. 1974; Nicholls et al. 1975b). Since, however, Farrell's (1960) pineal carboline 'adrenoglomerulotropin' was abandoned, little progress has been made in identifying these postulated factors; both growth hormone (McCaa et al. 1978) and prolactin (Holland et al. 1977; Re et al. 1979) have now been convincingly discounted as direct stimulators of aldosterone secretion. Recently claims have been advanced on behalf of β-lipotropin (Matsuoka et al. 1980), α-MSH (Vinson et al. 1980) and β-melanotropin (Matsuoka et al. 1981) despite earlier work discounting these hormones (Davis et al. 1960), as well as another pro-opiocortin-derived peptide, γ-MSH (Al-Dujaili et al. 1981) (Fig. 8.8). The intimate biosynthetic relationship of these peptides and their occurrence within the same pituitary cells as ACTH makes it unlikely, however, that they are physiologically independent adrenoglomerulotrophins; no pituitary lesions specifically causing hyper-aldosteronism have, for example, been described. The origin and physiological significance of the proteinaceous 'aldosterone-stimulating factor' described by Sen et al. (1981) remain to be determined.

Molecular mechanisms of aldosterone regulation   Control of aldosterone synthesis is effected at two major points on the biosynthetic sequence, one early and one late (Fig. 8.12). There is also a clear distinction between the acute and trophic effects of angiotensin II and potassium. There is considerable evidence that the acute (3–5 min)

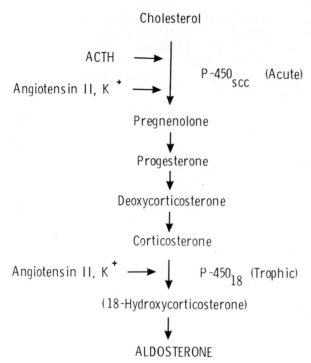

Fig. 8.12. Probable sites of action of regulators of aldosterone biosynthesis.

changes in aldosterone output are caused by an increased rate of cholesterol side-chain cleavage, i.e. the conversion of cholesterol to pregnenolone (Kaplan and Bartter 1962; Müller 1971; McKenna et al. 1978; Aguilera and Catt 1979), and this effect is mediated by increased association of the substrate with the mitochondrial cytochrome P-450$_{scc}$ moeity (Kramer et al. 1979; 1980).

Under such conditions of acute stimulation, the rate-limiting step in aldosterone synthesis probably shifts from the cholesterol-pregnenolone step to the later conversion of corticosterone to aldosterone, and acute stimulation by angiotensin II (or potassium) does not alter the latter reaction (Aguilera and Marusic 1971; Haning et al. 1970). Chronic (3–4 days) exposure does, however, enhance the conversion of corticosterone to aldosterone (Marusic and Mulrow 1967; Müller 1971; Aguilera and Marusic 1971; Aguilera and Catt 1979). These trophic effects are not limited to the peptide hormone but can, for example, be observed in cultures of aldosterone-secreting cells exposed to elevated potassium (Hornsby and O'Hare 1977) and in human cells from patients subject to prior potassium loading (Williams and Braley 1977). Trophic effects of this type are mediated by increased association of corticosterone with mitochondrial cytochrome P-450$_{18}$ (Kramer et al. 1979; 1980). While these glomerulotrophic stimuli do not increase cytochrome P-450 levels in intact animals, in hypophysectomised animals angiotensin II can mimic some of the effects of ACTH and increases in both 11β- and 21-hydroxylase activity have been reported (Aguilera et al. 1980).

The molecular mechanism of the last step in aldosterone biosynthesis is also interesting and has relevance to various congenital defects in mineralocorticoid production (p. 166). Ulick (1976b) has proposed that it proceeds by a double hydroxylation (corticosterone methyl oxidase, step I and II) and is followed by a spontaneous dehydration to give the aldehyde function (Fig. 8.13). Dissociation of the

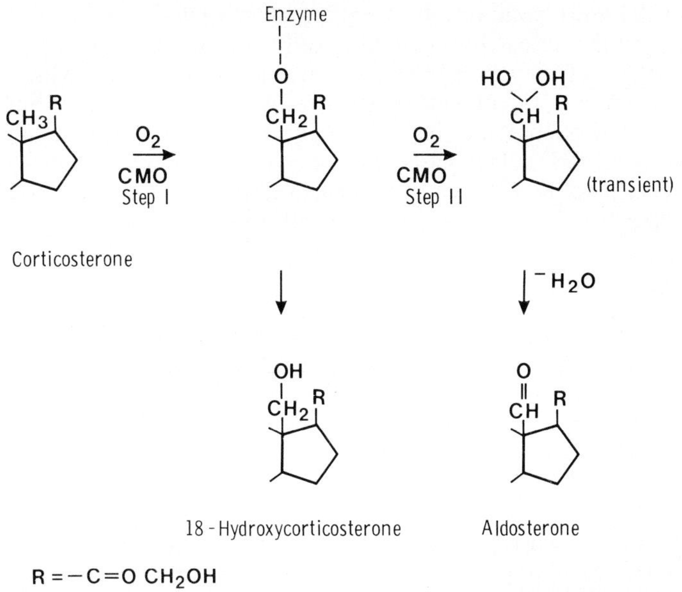

Fig. 8.13. Mechanism of corticosterone methyl oxidase (CMO) actions. (After Ulick 1976 b)

mono-oxygenated substrate at step I will yield 18-hydroxycorticosterone, but as a corollary the free steroid will not be an efficient substrate for aldosterone biosynthesis. This is consistent with experimental observations, which do not accord as well with the alternative proposition of separate enzymatically catalyzed 18-hydroxylation and 18-dehydrogenation.

Our knowledge of the intracellular mechanisms whereby angiotensin II and potassium influence these early and late steps in aldosterone formation is meagre. High affinity, high specificity angiotensin II receptors have been found in rat, bovine and human adrenal plasma membrane preparations (Glossman et al. 1974; Brown et al. 1980), and the peptide may itself increase the numbers of these receptors. Thus, angiotensin II infusion enhances the sensitivity of the human cortex to this peptide (Oelkers et al. 1974) and studies in the rat have shown direct increases in angiotensin receptor numbers as a result of sodium depletion (Aguilera and Catt 1978), and angiotensin infusion (Aguilera et al. 1980), this effect being synergised by concurrent increases in plasma K^+ (Hollenberg et al. 1974; Fredlund et al. 1977).

By analogy with other plasma membrane-receptor systems it might be anticipated that angiotensin II binding would generate an intracellular 'second message'. However, attempts to link this peptide with cyclic AMP have not been convincing, in so far as aldosterone-secreting cells are concerned (Saruta et al. 1972; Albano et al. 1974).

Prostaglandins (notably prostaglandin A_1) have been proposed as potential regulators of aldosterone secretion (Fichman et al. 1972). In vitro studies (Saruta and Kaplan 1972) do not, however, support the proposition that these compounds are direct mediators of angiotensin II activity on the adrenal cortex, and studies of the direct effects of PGA_1 and PGA_2 on aldosterone secretion by short-term in vitro preparations of human adrenal glands have given equivocal results (Honn and Chavin 1977).

Another possibility that merits consideration is the proposition that the effects of angiotensin II are mediated by changes in intracellular K^+ (Baumber et al. 1971). Such a mechanism would explain the concordance between both acute and trophic effects of the peptide and the ion at all known points on the steroidogenic pathway. It would also obviate the problem of how the aldosterone-secreting cells distinguish between the effects of ACTH and angiotensin II if cyclic AMP were to mediate the responses to both peptides. How precisely angiotensin II could influence intracellular K^+ is not clear, but effects on both membrane and microsomal Na^+-K^+-ATPase have been reported in animal systems (Gutman et al. 1972). The major drawback to this theory is that the small changes in extracellular K^+ known to influence aldosterone secretion (0.2–1 mEq) would not appear able to alter significantly intracellular K^+ levels.

Sex Steroids

The normal adrenal output of testosterone is small (Table 8.1), and it is not a significant source of oestradiol-17β. Nevertheless, the adrenal synthesis of androgens and oestrogens and their precursors is of significance in relation to pathological virilisation and feminisation associated with various adrenocortical disorders. The probable preferred pathways of synthesis of these compounds in the gland, and their relationship to the glucocorticoids are illustrated in Fig. 8.4.

Adrenal androgens   Naturally occurring adrenal steroids with significant androgenic activity in man are all C_{19} compounds of which dehydroepiandrosterone (secreted mainly as its 3-sulphate. Fig. 8.1), androstenedione, 11β-hydroxyandrostenedione, androst-5-ene-3β, 17β-diol and testosterone are the main examples. Their relative secretion rates are given in Table 8.1.

Androstenedione and testosterone together account for 85%–90% of the total androgenic activity (the 'androgenic index'), with DHA and androstenediol representing about 10%, and only 5% due to 11β-hydroxyandrostenedione (Table 8.4). Although the latter is secreted in greater amounts than some C_{19} adrenal steroids, its rapid metabolic clearance rate, which it shares with androstenedione (Table 8.5) results in low circulating levels (Lejeune-Lenain et al. 1980). Much of the activity of the adrenal 'androgens' is due to the facility, or otherwise, with which they can be converted peripherally to 'active' hormones such as testosterone or 5α-dihydrotestosterone.

Table 8.5. Metabolic clearance rate (MCR) of adrenal androgens[a] and other steroids

Steroid	MCR (litres/day)
DHA	2100
Androstenedione	1800
Androstenediol	750
Testosterone	730
DHA sulphate	22
Cortisol	200
Aldosterone	2000

[a]Poortman et al. 1980.

11β-Hydroxyandrostenedione is the only C_{19} steroid that can be considered an exclusive product of the adrenal cortex; the remainder are all secreted in greater or lesser amounts by the gonads. Thus, while about 80% of the circulating unconjugated DHA originates in the cortex (Horton and Tait 1967) all other unconjugated C_{19} steroids are secreted in substantially greater quantities by the testis. In females the adrenal contribution to circulating androgens is more significant and its relative importance

Table 8.6. Plasma androgen levels in women (nmol/l)[a]

	Premenopausal[b]	Postmenopausal[c]
Testosterone[d]	1.3	1.0
5α-Dihydrotestosterone (DHT)	0.9	—
Androstenedione[d]	5.8	2.0
DHA	20	8.5
DHA sulphate	3100	1660
Androstenediol	2.6	1.4

[a]Vermeulen and Rubens 1979.
[b]Mean of all phases of menstrual cycle.
[c]10–20 years after menopause.
[d]Show significant variations within menstrual cycle, being highest at midcycle.

depends on both menstrual and menopausal status (Table 8.6); up to 80% of circulating androstenediol has been estimated to be adrenal in origin in women (Vermeulen and Rubens 1979).

DHA sulphate is a special case as it is not only the major C_{19} compound secreted by the human cortex but it is also the steroid secreted in the greatest amounts, irrespective of class, accounting for about half the total steroid output of the gland (Table 8.1). The very high circulating levels of DHA sulphate (90–180 $\mu g/ml$, 2–4 mmoles/1) are principally a consequence of its very low metabolic clearance rate (Table 8.5). DHA sulphate itself is generally considered to be devoid of significant physiological activity, although some may be converted peripherally to DHA by tissues with significant sulphatase activity (e.g. breast).

Control of adrenal androgen output   ACTH plays a major role in the control of adrenal androgen secretion. This is evident from the concordance between the levels of the glucocorticoids and C_{19} compounds such as androstenedione (Huq et al. 1976; James et al. 1978b) and 11β-hydroxyandrostenedione (Lejeune-Lenain et al. 1980) in the adrenal venous effluent, including nycthemeral variations and episodic secretion. Nevertheless, ever since Reifenstein et al. (1945) suggested that the adrenal might be influenced by gonadotrophins, the evidence for and against the existence of a specific adrenal androgen-stimulating hormone has provoked much discussion.

Setting aside for the moment the possibility of occasional ectopic gonadal cells within the cortex (p. 285), almost all recent studies have shown no influence of pituitary or placental gonadotrophins on the steroid output of the adult gland, including C_{19} steroids (Marshall et al. 1973; Lee et al. 1975; Polansky 1975; Kolanowski et al. 1977). Thus while earlier reports have claimed a specific stimulation of adrenal DHA by LH (Pauerstein and Solomon 1968), its synchronised episodic secretion with cortisol (Rosenfeld et al. 1975) implicates ACTH as its major controlling factor.

The status of other putative androgen-stimulating factors remains equivocal at this time; we and others (Anderson 1980) do not find evidence for their existence convincing. Nevertheless, this topic has continued to attract much interest, not least in respect of the role of the cortex during puberty and abnormalities thereof, and the proceedings of an entire symposium have recently been devoted to the adrenal androgens (Genazzani et al. 1980).

The evidence with respect to prolactin as an adrenal androgen-stimulating hormone can be summarised as follows. Hyperprolactinaemia has been associated with elevated plasma levels of DHA and/or DHA sulphate in several studies (Bassi et al. 1977; Carter et al. 1977; Vermeulen et al. 1977; Kandeel et al. 1978; Vermeulen and Ando 1978). Recent studies have confirmed this effect (Genazzani et al. 1980) although in some cases the correlation is poor and the extent of the rise is often small and observed only after prolonged hyperprolactinaemia. By contrast, in vitro studies (O'Hare et al. 1980a; Serio et al. 1980) have failed to demonstrate any effect of either bovine or human prolactin on cultured normal adult human adrenocortical cells, and short-term infusion studies in vivo (Varma et al. 1977) have likewise proved negative. Older studies claiming such effects (Boyns et al. 1972) can probably be discounted on the grounds of residual ACTH contamination of the hormone preparations used (O'Hare et al. 1980a). The evidence of favour of prolactin stimulation of adrenal androgens in vivo depends on the assumption that all DHA sulphate is always adrenal in origin. This may not, in fact, be the case (Vihko and Ruokonen 1975; Peretti and Forest 1978) and 11β-hydroxyandrostenedione may be a better marker in this context.

There is also clinical and physiological evidence that prolactin is not involved in adrenal androgen control. This has been summarised recently by Grumbach et al. (1978) and consists essentially of the observation that while adrenal androgen levels rise early in puberty (p. 91) no corresponding increase in prolactine levels has been detected. An alternative unidentified 'adrenal androgen stimulating hormone' (AASH) has been postulated, and Parker and Odell (1979) have recently claimed the identification of such a factor in bovine pituitary extracts. Equally powerful arguments against the existence of such a factor have been proposed by Anderson (1980). As the relevant evidence stems largely from observations of adrenal steroidogenesis at puberty, its consideration will be postponed until this phase of adrenal function (p. 91) and the mechanisms of functional zonation (p. 108) are discussed in greater detail. It has recently been observed, however, that 'adrenal androgens', whose concentrations in plasma undoubtedly decline with age (Table 8.6), do not respond to ACTH in the elderly to the same extent as corticosteroids and mineralocorticoids (Parker et al 1981). The mechanism of this effect remains obscure as morphological studies (Kreiner and Dhöm 1979) have not revealed marked changes in overt zonation with age.

It should be noted, nevertheless, that no pituitary lesions specifically associated with adrenal virilism without concurrent changes in glucocorticoid secretion have ever been described, although a case of nodular hyperplasia has been noted, probably fortuitously, in hyperprolactinaemia with a pituitary adenoma (Boyar and Hellman 1974).

Adrenal oestrogens   The isolation of oestrone from bovine adrenal glands by Beall (1939) provided the first evidence that the cortex was capable of forming C_{18} steroids. During the 1950's enhanced oestrogen secretion was demonstrated in several adrenocortical carcinomas (Wallach et al. 1957) and West et al. (1958) showed that both oestrone and oestradiol-17β were excreted in ovariectomised women. As levels were raised by ACTH it was suggested that they may have originated in the normal cortex; most were, however, probably derived from peripheral conversion of adrenal androgens. Conclusive proof of the adrenal synthesis of oestrogens therefore awaited the advent of radioimmunoassay methods and the measurement of the hormones in arterial and adrenal venous blood. These methods demonstrated that oestrone was produced at about 1/5000th the level of cortisol (Baird et al. 1969). Adrenal gradients of oestradiol-17β have not been detected (Greenblatt et al. 1976) and its secretion rate must, therefore, be at least ten times lower than that of oestrone (Table 8.1).

Conjugated oestrogens, such as oestrone sulphate, may be formed in the gland but they do not contribute significantly to circulating levels (Ruder et al. 1972). There is no evidence of sex differences in adrenal C_{18} steroid synthesis.

Although oestrogen formation by both short- and long-term in vitro preparations from feminising adrenocortical carcinomas (Millington et al. 1976; Fang et al. 1978) has been reported to be enhanced by prolactin, the purity of the hormone was not confirmed in either case. Thus at the present time there is no conclusive evidence of the separate control of adrenal oestrogen secretion in the normal human cortex by this or any other hormone, except ACTH.

Adrenal progestogens   Progesterone is secreted by the human adrenal gland at levels ~1% of those of cortisol, having been first detected in the adrenal venous effluent in man by Short (1960) and in males this adrenal output accounts for most of the circulating progesterone. No sex differences in secretion rates have been noted and there is no evidence for its separate control by hormones other than ACTH (Bermudez and Lipsett 1972; Vermeulen and Verdonck 1976).

Hormonogenesis by the Prepubertal and Pubertal Cortex

Except for the immediate post-natal period the secretion rates of glucocorticoids and mineralocorticoids do not change with age or stage of sexual maturation when they are expressed as a function of body mass (Kenney et al. 1966; New et al. 1966). At puberty, however, there is a marked increase, relative to corticosteroids, in the circulating levels of the C_{19} steroids, particularly DHA and DHA sulphate. Both these steroids normally regarded as being predominantly adrenal in origin, are present in the serum in high amounts at birth but decline rapidly to reach their lowest levels by the end of the first year, when the fetal zone of the gland has involuted (p. 51). They remain low ($<2\,\mu g/$ 100 ml for DHA-S) up to about the sixth year (Peretti and Forest 1976; 1978). The adrenal androgens begin to rise about 1–2 years before pituitary gonadotrophin levels increase and the sex steroids normally associated with the gonads (e.g. testosterone and oestradiol) begin to appear in the plasma in significant amounts (Collu and Ducharme 1978); they continue to increase throughout the pubertal period until adult levels ($\sim 150\,\mu g/100$ ml) are reached by 16–18 years of age (Fig. 8.14) (Korth-Schutz et al.

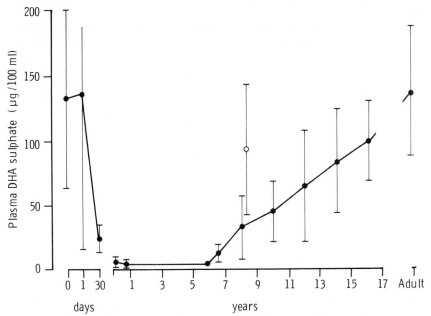

Fig. 8.14. Levels of DHA sulphate during development (*closed circles*, from the data of Peretti and Forest 1978) and in cases of precocious 'adrenarche' (*open circle*, from the data of Reiter et al. 1977), $\pm$ SD (*bars*).

1976b; Reiter et al. 1977). Other adrenal C_{19} steroids such as 11β-hydroxyandrostenedione do not show such a pronounced pubertal rise although they do increase relative to cortisol (Parker et al. 1978; Franckson et al. 1980). These changes are collectively referred to as the 'adrenarche' after Albright (1947) and are reflected in increased urinary 17-ketosteroids. Histological changes in the human cortex at this time have been described elsewhere and are thought to involve increased prominence of the zona reticularis (p. 52).

The adrenarche does not, however, occur in all primates (Cutler et al. 1978). There is, furthermore, little evidence that adrenal androgens, or the adrenarche as a whole, play any qualitatively important or limiting role in normal puberty. Their role in the adolescent growth spurt is, at best, equivocal (Sklar et al. 1980), and at least some patients with Addison's disease also proceed normally through puberty (Urban et al. 1980) when given glucocorticoid replacement therapy.

In so-called 'precocious adrenarche' or 'precocious pubarche' as it is sometimes termed, there is a premature appearance of sexual hair without the concurrent development of other secondary sex characteristics, such as breast development in the female children in whom this condition is more frequently seen. Levels of various androgenic and potentially androgenic steroids such as DHA and DHA sulphate are raised in cases of precocious pubarche (Fig. 8.14) (Sizonenko 1975; Doberne et al. 1975; Korth-Schutz et al. 1976a; Warne et al. 1978). 17α-Hydroxyprogesterone and most other C_{21} steroids are not raised in this benign condition (August et al. 1975) (c.f. late onset congenital adrenal hyperplasia). However, despite the changes in C_{19} steroids the pubertal process is completed normally in these cases and they experience menarche at the usual time (Grumbach et al. 1978). 'Premature adrenarche' may simply reflect a variant of normal development.

Several hypotheses have been proposed to explain the rise in adrenal androgens during normal puberty. They include effects of gonadotrophins, prolactin, oestradiol and the hypothetical 'adrenal androgen stimulating hormone'. There is, however, no more evidence to support a role for any of these factors in puberty than in adult steroidogenesis.

Albright's original suggestion that pituitary gonadotrophins are involved is refuted by studies of direct administration of these hormones to children (Lee et al. 1975) and the fact that plasma concentrations of adrenal androgens (DHA and DHA-S) are normal for chronological age in hypogonadotrophic hypogonadism (Copeland et al. 1977; Sklar et al. 1980). Prolactin levels in adolescence are actually declining (Aubert et al. 1974) when adrenal androgen levels are still rising, thus apparently eliminating this hormone as a candidate (Grumbach et al. 1978).

At high concentrations oestradiol-17β will inhibit the 3β-hydroxysteroid dehydrogenase enzyme that is necessary to produce glucocorticoids, but not Δ^5-C_{19} steroids such as DHA (Fig. 8.4) (Yates and Deshpande 1975). However, no changes in adrenal androgen levels have been observed with physiological (<30 μg/day) oestrogen therapy in either gonadectomised women (Anderson and Yen 1976) or hypogonadal children (Rosenfield and Fang 1974). Thus while long-term treatment with pharmacological levels of oestrogens (1 mg/day) may enhance 'adrenal' androgen levels in man (Sobrinho et al. 1971; Abraham and Maroulis 1975) it seems improbable that the oestrogen levels in normal puberty, or in premature pubarche, could enhance C_{19} steroid formation by this mechanism, particularly since direct effects of oestrogen (e.g. breast development) postdate the adrenarche.

Several workers, notably Grumbach (Grumbach et al. 1978; Sklar et al. 1980) have attempted to overcome this problem by postulating the existence of a separate 'adrenal androgen stimulating hormone' or AASH (see p. 90). The major argument against this hypothesis is the lack of relevant pathophysiological syndromes (such as AASH-secreting pituitary tumours) and the fact that no such hormone has yet been isolated. Is it indeed necessary to postulate its existence? We, together with Anderson (1980), suggest that it is not, and would propose as an alternative that changes in C_{21}/C_{19} steroid ratios stem from intra-adrenal responses of the cortical cells to both ACTH and their own products. We believe that such effects are, furthermore, of crucial importance in determining the functional zonation of the gland (see p. 108). Culture studies (Neville and O'Hare 1978; O'Hare et al. 1978; O'Hare et al. 1980a) have shown that the relative levels of different steroids produced by the human adrenal cells can vary quite independently of specific hormonal stimuli, and that proportional changes may take place in response to a single stimulus, ACTH (Fig. 8.7). We therefore conclude that similar changes observed in vivo do not predicate the existence of further, unidentified, hormones as their cause, but merely illustrate the subtlety of the responses of the adrenal cell to its cortical microenvironment, and a single major stimulus to function, ACTH.

Hormonogenesis by the Prenatal Adrenal Cortex

Pathways of Steroidogenesis

Qualitatively the prenatal cortex expresses essentially the same steroidogenic repertoire as the adult gland synthesising the hormones from acetate and/or cholesterol (Teledgy et al. 1970; Carr et al. 1980a,d; Fig. 8.3). Quantitatively, however, there are considerable differences in the proportions of the secreted steroids (Table 8.7)

Table 8.7. Concentrations of representative steroids in mid-term fetal (12–17 week), neonatal and adult human adrenal glands[a]

Steroid	Concentration ($\mu g/100$ g)		
	Fetal	Neonate	Adult
Pregnenolone sulphate	558	442	45
Pregnenolone	160	315	82
DHA sulphate	133	130	25
DHA	<20	58	31
16α-OH-DHA sulphate	63	<5	<5
16α-OH-DHA	<20	13	<5
Cortisol	<20	344	416

[a]From the data of Matsumoto et al. 1968; Huhtaniemi et al. 1970; Huhtaniemi 1973.

which arise for three main reasons, namely, the higher levels of (i) sulphotransferase and (ii) 16-hydroxylase and (iii) the relatively lower level of 3β-hydroxysteroid dehydrogenase activity in the prenatal cortex as compared with the adult gland.

Fetal adrenal sulphotransferase activity at mid-term is 4–5 times as high as the adult cortex (Böstrom et al. 1964) and higher than in the fetal liver (Villee and Loring 1969). Not only are C_{19} steroids such as DHA secreted predominantly as sulphate esters (as in the adult gland) but there is also, unlike the adult cortex, significant sulpho-conjugation of C_{21} steroids including cortisol, cortisone, corticosterone and 6β-hydroxycortisol (Klein and Giroud 1967). At least half of these steroids (and their reduced metabolites) appear as sulphate esters in fetal blood (Eberlein 1965) and also in the urine of neonates (Ducharme et al. 1970).

Kinetic experiments (Cooke et al. 1970) indicate that most steroid sulphates are formed from individual free steroid precursors, although minor routes involving interconversions of the sulphates themselves may also operate (Huhtaniemi 1974). Although the very earliest stage at which steroid-metabolising activities occur in the fetal gland has not been defined precisely, sulphotransferase activity is already detectable at 6–8 weeks when the glands weigh 3–4 mg (Cooke et al. 1968).

Adrenocortical sulphotransferase activity is of particular significance in the fetal economy. Not only does it act to limit the effective biological concentration of a wide variety of circulating steroids in prenatal life, but it also substitutes for inactivation through hepatic glucuronide formation. This enzymatic process is dependent on glucocorticoids for its induction (Ducharme et al. 1970) and does not occur in significant amounts until after birth (Brown and Zuelzer 1958).

Adrenal 16-hydroxylation is a feature of higher primate fetuses only. In man it is present in both the liver and the adrenal (Matsumoto et al. 1968) as a microsomal enzyme (Yamasaki and Shimuzu 1973) and 16α-hydroxysteroids and their sulphate esters (e.g. 16-OH-DHA-S) provide the main substrates for placental oestriol formation by the so-called 'neutral' pathway (Fig. 8.15) (Easterling et al. 1966; Kirshner et al. 1966).

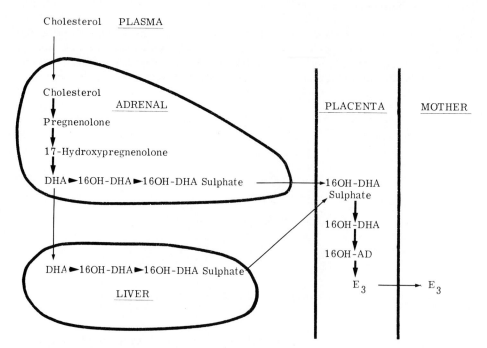

Fig. 8.15. Steroid metabolism by the adrenal cortex, liver and placenta in the human fetus. Major pathways of estriol (E_3) formation by the so-called 'neutral' pathway are shown; analogous reactions convert adrenal DHA sulphate into estrone by the 'phenolic' pathway with 19-hydroxyandrostenedione as an intermediate in the placental aromatisation of androstenedione (AD).

Most of the hydroxylating enzymes involved in glucocorticoid synthesis (Fig. 8.4) are present from an early stage of gestation (8–10 weeks) (Bloch and Benirschke 1959; Ville et al. 1959, 1961; Solomon et al. 1967). The formation of glucocorticoids from endogenous precursors is, however, limited by the low levels of effective 3β-hydroxysteroid dehydrogenase activity in the gland as a whole during the 1st and 2nd trimesters (Bloch and Benirschke 1959; Villee et al. 1959, 1961). In the mid-term fetus, the adrenal levels of this enzyme are one or even two orders of magnitude lower than the testis (Payne and Jaffe 1972) and it exhibits a substrate preference for DHA as opposed to pregnenolone (Serra et al. 1971) so that while some androstenedione can be formed, (Bloch and Benirschke 1962; Taylor and Hamilton 1973) there is relatively little synthesis of progesterone and glucocorticoids such as cortisol and corticosterone (Fig. 8.4).

Further insight into fetal adrenal hormonogenesis has been afforded by studies of its functional zonation. Using the Glick microbore method, Cooke and his colleagues (Shirley and Cooke 1969; Cooke and Taylor 1971) found that the fetal zone contains the higher levels of steroid sulphotransferase activity. Studies on anencephalic fetuses, in which the inner fetal zone is absent or much reduced (p. 272), have shown that the fetal zone as well as being the source of steroid sulphates must also be responsible for the synthesis of the majority of the 3β-hydroxy-5-ene steroids such as DHA (Eberlein 1965) and of the 16-hydroxysteroids (Easterling et al. 1966). Thus, most 16-hydroxysteroids have disappeared from the urine of normal infants by 6 months of age (Mitchell and Shackleton 1969) when involution of the fetal zone is complete.

There is good evidence that the definitive zone of the fetal cortex is responsible for such glucocorticoid (and other 4-ene-3-oxosteroid) synthesis as occurs in the prenatal gland. Bloch and Benirschke (1962) showed that the separated fetal zone was less capable of forming C_{21} steroids of this type than the entire gland, and histochemical studies (Goldman et al. 1966) revealed that 3β-hydroxysteroid dehydrogenase activity was effectively confined to the definitive zone, where it appears at 12–14 weeks, in contrast to the placenta and testis, where it is detectable by the 6th week.

Histochemical studies of the cortex in anencephalics (Goldman et al. 1966) have shown that the definitive zone cells of which it is largely composed also possess an active 3β-hydroxysteroid dehydrogenase, and in vitro studies have demonstrated their capacity to synthesise glucocorticoids (Cooke et al. 1971; Carr et al. 1980b). The normal definitive zone is therefore almost certainly the source of the majority of endogenously synthesised fetal glucocorticoids during prenatal life, although the fetal zone may not be totally devoid of this capability (Hillman et al. 1962). By birth in the normal infant the cortisol content of the cortex is approaching adult levels as the outer zone matures, although both C_{19} compounds and sulphate esters are still present in high levels prior to the postnatal involution of the fetal zone tissue (Table 8.7).

The relative proportions of different glucocorticoids in the blood at birth differs significantly from the adult, there being higher levels of cortisone compared to cortisol (Murphy and D'Aux 1972) and corticosterone to cortisol (Villee and Loring 1965). The difference in cortisol/cortisone ratios stems in part from the prior influx of maternal glucocorticoids and the metabolic interconversion of this pair of 11-hydroxy/11-dehydro-steroids by fetal organs and extraembryonic structures such as the chorionic membrane.

The Feto-Placental Unit

The inter-conversion of steroids produced by the fetal adrenals and the placenta has been the subject of much investigation (Diczfalusy et al. 1965; Solomon et al. 1967). To understand the relationship between fetal adrenal function and the excretion of the metabolic products of such adrenal steroids in the maternal urine, the latter being a useful index of fetal well-being, it is necessary only to note that several steroid-metabolising enzyme activities show a reciprocal relationship in the cortex and the placenta (Table 8.8). As a consequence a substantial proportion of these fetal adrenal

Table 8.8. Steroid-metabolising enzyme activities in the mid-term fetus

Enzyme	Adrenal	Placenta
Cholesterol side-chain cleavage	Present	Present
Δ^5-3β-hydroxysteroid dehydrogenase	Low	High
17-Hydroxylase	High	Low
$C_{17\ 20}$ Lyase	High	Low
16α-Hydroxylase	High	Low
Sulphotransferase	High	Low
Sulphatase	Low	High
Aromatase	Low	High

(See fig. 8.15 for pathways).

steroids ultimately appear in the maternal urine as oestriol, by the pathways illustrated in Fig. 8.15. In cases where the output of C_{19} 16-hydroxylated and sulphated steroids is low (e.g. anencephalia), the maternal oestriol levels are correspondingly low (Frandsen and Stakemann 1964).

Functions of Fetal Adrenal Steroids

Despite the size of the fetal adrenal and the magnitude of its steroid output ($<$ 100 mg/ day in late pregnancy) the functional role of many of these compounds in the embryo is not clear. Insofar as fetal adrenal C_{19} steroids and their metabolites are concerned, it seems that most, if not all, of them can be dispensed with for most of the later part of fetal life. Anencephalia, with its reduced fetal zone and low C_{19} steroid output and correspondingly low oestriol levels does not curtail either pregnancy or, apparently, the development of the fetus itself. Indeed, if any role can be ascribed to the fetal zone in later stages of pregnancy it is that of ensuring, by sulphoconjugation, that active steroids are inactivated and excreted via placental oestriol formation. Its development must also reflect some specialised feature of higher primate development and maternal fetoplacental relationships because many other mammals do not possess a recognisable fetal zone as such, or show the complex steroid interconversions seen in the human fetoplacental unit. The role, if any, of fetal zone steroids in the early stages of gestation remains unknown.

Late in gestation glucocorticoids advance lung maturation in several mammals and may also do so in man. Thus, there is some evidence that the number of surfactant granules in the tissue may be reduced in anencephalics (Naeye et al. 1971), and there is an inverse correlation between blood cortisol levels at term and the respiratory distress syndrome (hyaline membrane disease) (Murphy 1974).

There is also evidence that fetal adrenal glucocorticoids may play a role in the initiation of parturition in man as they do in ruminants (Liggins 1976). Fetal cortisol levels increase substantially ($\sim$ 10-fold) in the 3rd trimester in man (Murphy 1973). Cortisol and corticosterone sulphates are good markers of fetal adrenal function at term (Murphy et al. 1980) and Fencl et al. (1980) using these indices found a sharp rise in fetal glucocorticoid secretion in the week immediately prior to birth. Although studies of various related pituitary peptides (Silman et al. 1976) have shown a gradual shift towards intact ACTH, compared with smaller peptides such as CLIP (p. 80) as gestation proceeds, evidence for a corresponding rise in fetal ACTH at term in man is not as convincing (Winters et al. 1974). Nevertheless, the tendency of human gestation to be significantly prolonged in anencephaly (Anderson et al. 1969) and congenital adrenal hypoplasia (Roberts and Cawdery 1970) where fetal blood cortisol levels are depressed (Fencl et al. 1976) provides further circumstantial evidence of at least a contributory role of the prenatal adrenal cortex via glucocorticoid secretion in initiating parturition.

Mineralocorticoid secretion by the prenatal gland does not appear to have any obvious role in fetal economy. Nevertheless, aldosterone can be detected in amniotic fluid by nine weeks (Blankstein et al. 1980a) and it can be formed by the gland at 16 weeks (Pasqualini et al. 1966; Dufau and Villee 1969) and, by term, blood levels have reached maternal levels (Katz et al. 1974) with up to 80% of the aldosterone in the fetal blood originating from the fetal adrenal (Bayard et al. 1970).

Control of Prenatal Hormonogenesis

There is, in our opinion, no compelling evidence that prenatal hormonogenesis by the human adrenal gland is controlled by any polypeptide hormone other than ACTH. Thus, although growth hormone and chorionic somatomammotrophin (Isherwood and Oakey 1976), prolactin (Glickman et al. 1979) and notably HCG (Lauritzen and Lehmann 1965, 1967; Lehmann and Lauritzen 1975; Jaffe et al. 1977; Strecker et al. 1977; Dell'Acqua et al. 1978; Seron-Ferré et al. 1978) have all been implicated in the control of fetal steroidogenesis in various studies, the evidence for their involvement is, as yet, far from conclusive.

In most cases large, non-physiological doses of hormones have been used and the possibility of their contamination by pituitary ACTH, or the more recently discovered placental ACTH-like peptides (Rees et al. 1975a) has not been excluded. The reported responses have been small and dose-response relationships have not been convincingly established (e.g. Glickman et al. 1979). Other studies with both HCG (Honnebier et al. 1974; Voutilainen et al. 1979) and prolactin (Winter et al. 1980) have failed to demonstrate any effects in vivo or in vitro, and bromocryptine-induced hyper-prolactinaemia does not enhance fetal adrenal steroid output (Pozo et al. 1980). Furthermore, in vivo studies have relied on DHA and DHA sulphate (or steroids such as oestriol derived therefrom) as indices of fetal adrenal function (Strecker et al. 1977; Dell'Acqua et al. 1978). This is probably not realistic in all cases because the fetal testis (like the adult testis) may make a small but significant contribution to these steroids (Jaffe and Payne 1971; Huhtaniemi 1977). This may account for some of the reported effects of prolactin and HCG; and it should be noted that in no case has concurrent alteration in ACTH due to stress been excluded in these experiments.

By contrast to these equivocal results, there is substantial evidence of functional responses to ACTH by the human adrenal gland from an early stage of gestation. This hormone is detectable in the fetal pituitary by the 9th–10th weeks (Pavlova et al. 1968) and most circulating ACTH in the fetus is of embryonic rather than maternal origin (Berson and Yalow 1968). ACTH-induced steroidogenic responses can be elicited in vitro with glands from 10-week-old fetuses (Seron-Ferré et al. 1978), and high endogenous levels of cortisol have been found in 8-week fetuses (Murphy and D'Aux 1972). When the hormone has been infused into the mid-term fetus in utero occasional responses have been noted (Strecker et al. 1977), while responses have invariably been obtained with abortuses infused ex utero (e.g. MacNaughton et al. 1977), and with material of this age in short-term in vitro studies (Bloch and Benirschke 1962; Lehmann and Lauritzen 1975; Isherwood and Oakey 1976) and a large number of cell culture experiments (Kahri et al. 1976; Goodyer et al. 1977; Branchaud et al. 1978; Voutilainen et al. 1979; Winter et al. 1980). Second trimester fetal adrenal cells also show ultrastructural responses to ACTH after perfusion in utero (Johannisson 1968) and when cultured in vitro show the same retraction response that we have observed with adult cortical cells. By the end of the third trimester responses to acute ACTH infusion can be readily obtained in vivo (Dell'Acqua et al. 1978) and after birth in normally delivered infants there is a substantial response to the hormone (Jaffe et al. 1977). This body of data clearly demonstrates the capacity of even the youngest material to respond to long-term ACTH stimulation, although there remains the possibility that the glands may, at the earlier stages, be relatively refractory to a single acute exposure to the hormone.

As already mentioned, Silman et al. (1976) have reported marked changes in the relative proportions of ACTH-related peptides (Fig. 8.8) in the fetal human pituitary. On the basis of these observations and some animal experiments (Challis and Torosis 1977) the hypothesis has been proposed that it is αMSH rather than $ACTH_{1-39}$ that sustains the fetal adrenal gland in the younger embryo. However, the evidence that αMSH stimulates the fetal human gland is at present restricted to a single study (Glickman et al. 1979) in which ACTH proved the more active peptide. Cell culture studies have failed to elicit responses to αMSH, CLIP, β-LPH or β-endorphin (Winter et al. 1980) and although a caveat must be noted in respect of whether the cell culture conditions were appropriate for the maintenance of hormone receptor levels, it cannot yet be claimed that hypothesis of pro-opiocortin-derived ACTH-related peptides as adrenotrophic stimuli in the fetus has been proved.

The distinctive morphological and functional properties of the fetal zone of the prenatal gland (pp. 41 and 95) raise the possibility that it might be under separate control. However, the studies of Seron-Ferré et al. (1978) and Carr et al. (1980c) on separated definitive zone and fetal zone cells show, however, that ACTH as well as stimulating cortisol secretion by the former, as might be expected, also stimulates DHA sulphate secretion from the fetal zone.

Collectively, therefore, these observations can only be interpreted as demonstrating a dominant, and possibly exclusive role for ACTH in the control of prenatal steroidogenesis by the human adrenal gland.

Chapter 9
Regulation of Growth of the Adrenal Cortex

Many experiments in animals, and pathological observations in man, have demonstrated an association between physiologically, pharmacologically and pathologically elevated levels of ACTH and enhanced protein synthesis, cellular hypertrophy, and eventually hyperplasia or conversely varying degrees of atrophy in the absence of ACTH (see Gill 1976 for review). It is clear, therefore, that ACTH, or some closely related factor, plays an important role in the regulation of growth of the human adrenal cortex. However, the simplistic view that growth takes place by the same mechanism as stimulation of steroidogenesis, i.e. with cyclic AMP as an intracellular effector, has been seriously challenged by recent observations on cultured adrenocortical cells.

The growth of the human adrenal cortex can be divided for convenience into three phases. These are (1) the rapid prenatal growth phase terminated by the dramatic involution of the gland at birth, (2) the slower postnatal growth of the gland to its adult dimensions, and (3) adult homeostasis when normal tissue mass is sustained, restored during regeneration, and enhanced in response to functional demand. Absolute and relative adrenal weights during prenatal and postnatal life have been illustrated in Figs. 3.2 and 3.3.

The Prenatal Gland

Growth

The fetal pituitary undoubtedly plays a major role in regulating the later stages of prenatal adrenal growth (Jost 1975). Thus, in anencephalia, and other conditions in which normal hypothalamo-pituitary relationships are disturbed, the cortex fails to enlarge beyond the size that it normally attains by about the 20th week of gestation (~ 1 g) (Fig. 9.1). Complete absence of the anterior pituitary results in even smaller gland weights (<0.2 g) (see e.g. Brewer 1957), although they are seldom if ever completely absent in this condition, or in cases of congenital ACTH unresponsiveness (p. 268).

The initial stages of adrenal growth and differentiation must, therefore, be relatively independent of pituitary control. It is during the first trimester that the greatest relative increase in adrenal weight (Fig. 3.3) and the most prominent mitotic activity takes place. Hence no direct quantitative relationship appears to exist between levels of circulating ACTH in the fetus, and proliferative activity in the embryonic adrenal cortex.

In later fetal life, there is circumstantial evidence that pituitary ACTH, or some closely related material, influences cortical growth (Lanman 1962). The biosynthetic relationship of ACTH to other polypeptides (Fig. 8.8) has provoked the suggestion that some of the latter may act as specific adrenotropic factors during fetal life (Silman et al. 1977). Some may even antagonise the effects of ACTH (Jones and Roebuck 1980); their involvement in adrenal growth, however, remains speculative.

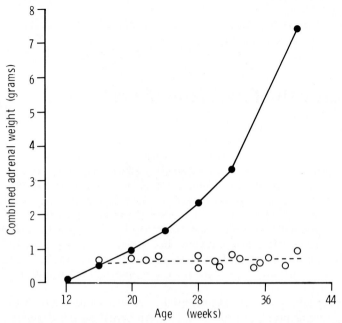

Fig. 9.1. Adrenal growth. The weights of adrenal glands from anencephalic fetuses (*open circles*) are shown in comparison with normal adrenal weights during development. (After Jost 1975)

Prolactin has also been proposed as an adrenal growth-regulating hormone, as it alone of the pituitary hormones rises steadily during all phases of fetal life (Winters et al. 1975). As it is subject to inhibitory rather than stimulatory hypothalamic control, its levels reportedly continue to rise in anencephalics (Honnebier et al. 1974) most of which retain some adenohypophyseal tissue, but in which the size of the pituitary remnant is not correlated with adrenal size (Angevine 1938). It seems unlikely, therefore, that prolactin is involved in the regulation of the later stages of adrenal growth. The specific effects of other pituitary hormones, such as growth hormone, are not known, but there appears to be no evidence of any disproportionate adrenal 'dwarfing' in cases of isolated GH deficiency.

Another potential source of prenatal 'adrenotropins' is the placenta. Corticotrophin-like materials (Rees et al. 1975a) are synthesised in the placenta (Liotta et al. 1977) but their concentrations are only 10^{-6} that of the pituitary and it seems unlikely that they play a major role.

HCG can be rejected as a putative adrenotropin. Chester Jones (1955), after Rotter (1949), suggested a role for this placental hormone on purely hypothetical and speculative grounds but there is no direct experimental evidence to sustain this hypothesis. While continuous or repeated administration of ACTH causes some enlargement of the adrenal cortex in anencephalic fetuses and newborn (Lanman 1961, 1962; Honnebier et al. 1974), HCG does not (Lanman 1956). Furthermore, HCG can hardly be held responsible for the enlargement and maintainance of the fetal zone of the prenatal cortex, as it is precisely this zone that is deficient in anencephalics (p. 272). Moreover, HCG (and LH) levels are actually declining during the later stages of pregnancy (Reyes et al. 1974).

Involution

There is, as yet, no completely convincing explanation of adrenal involution.

Withdrawal of HCG after birth cannot be responsible as there is no evidence that HCG supports the fetal zone (vide supra). Moreover, infusion of ACTH does not preserve it after birth (Lanman 1956), although there is some evidence that pituitary hormones may be involved at least indirectly. Whereas fetal zone involution proceeds normally in cases of congenital adrenal hyperlasia with elevated levels of ACTH (p. 163) we have observed apparently delayed involution in some cases of congenital Cushing's syndrome in which ACTH levels are low or undetectable (p. 132).

It seems more probable, however, that involution is primarily triggered by changes in steroid rather than polypeptide hormone levels following detachment of the placenta. Thus, a notable feature of the fetus is the high level (200–400 ng/100 ml) of circulating oestrogens (Reyes et al. 1974). If these steroids in some way protect the inner zones of the prenatal cortex then their withdrawal at birth may initiate involution. One plausible mechanism that has recently received some experimental verification is the inhibition of adrenal Δ^5-3β-hydroxysteroid dehydrogenase-isomerase activity by oestrogens. Winter et al. (1980) have shown that C_{18} steroid levels comparable to those found in the fetus and compatible with cell viability will suppress cortisol and enhance DHA secretion by cultures of human fetal adrenocortical cells. Such a mechanism creates a positive feedback situation because the increased adrenal secretion of C_{19} steroids, such as DHA, act as further precursors for placental aromatisation (Fig. 8.15). As a possible corollary, partial suppression of glucocorticoid secretion will tend to cause compensatory (ACTH-dependent?) hypertrophy and perhaps account for the size of the fetal adrenal cortex.

Why withdrawal of placental oestrogens should provoke involution must remain speculative, but perhaps relief of the partial inhibition of Δ^5-3β-hydroxysteroid-dehydrogenase-isomerase activity temporarily raises the intra-adrenal concentrations of Δ^4-3-oxosteroids to levels that exceed the limits of viability of the innermost cells exposed to the highest steroid concentrations, triggering autolysis and involution. Circumstances in which the gland is not exposed to perinatal ACTH stimulation (e.g. congenital Cushing's syndrome) might delay this process to some extent by limiting the rise in intracellular steroid concentrations. Changes in vascular dynamics due to the cessation of umbilical circulation and the establishment of the pulmonary oxygenation circuit may also modify the intra-adrenal environment in such a way as to favour involution; certainly hyperaemia, vascular stasis and altered capillary permeability with extravasation within the fetal zone are notable features of the immediate postnatal cortex.

The Postnatal Gland

Unfortunately, we know even less about the regulation of adrenal growth in man during the postnatal period than we do about prenatal growth, except that it coincides more or less with the pubertal growth spurt with adrenal weights remaining relatively constant relative to total body weight (Fig. 3.3). The specific involvement of individual pituitary hormones, or other trophic stimuli in the process remains a matter for speculation.

Adult Tissue Homeostasis and Regenerative Growth

The development of cell culture techniques for the maintenance of adult adrenocortical cells in vitro (O'Hare and Neville 1973a,b; O'Hare et al. 1978; Neville and O'Hare 1978), and the fact that such cortical cells will under some circumstances proliferate actively in vitro (O'Hare and Neville 1973c; Ramachandran and Suyama 1975; Hornsby and Gill 1977) has opened an entirely new avenue for the experimental study of adrenal growth. Results obtained with these systems have, however, challenged a number of commonly held assumptions about the proliferogenic role of ACTH in vivo.

In monolayer cell culture $ACTH_{1-24}$ or $ACTH_{1-39}$, far from stimulating cortical proliferation, inhibits it in a specific and dose-dependent manner (O'Hare and Neville 1973c; Ramachandran and Suyama 1975; Hornsby and Gill 1977). This effect is mediated not by secreted steroids as suggested by Saez et al. (1977) but by intracellular cyclic AMP generated in response to the hormone (Fig. 8.9). Thus aminoglutethimide inhibits steroidogenesis in vitro without abolishing the inhibitory effect of ACTH on growth (O'Hare et al. 1978).

Evidence that this paradoxical response to ACTH is not an 'artifact' of culture has come from the studies of Rao et al. (1978) who have shown that administration of anti-ACTH antibodies in vivo will inhibit steroidogenesis without preventing the postnatal growth of the gland in the rat. Furthermore, Dallman et al. (1980) have recently shown that ACTH will inhibit, at least in the short-term, the compensatory adrenal growth that occurs in this species after unilateral adrenalectomy.

It has not, unfortunately, been possible to reproduce all of these observations made with rodent and bovine adult cells in culture using human tissue because the adult human cells show little or no tendency to divide in culture (Fig. 9.2). This situation is in marked contrast to the behaviour of adult bovine adrenocortical cells which proliferate sufficiently rapidly, extensively and persistently to enable clonal cell strains to be established (Simonian et al. 1979). Factors such as fibroblast growth factor (Hornsby and Gill 1977) and angiotensin II (Gill et al. 1977) which are both potent mitogens for the bovine cells have, in our hands, proved ineffective when applied to adult human cultures (Fig. 9.2). We have, furthermore, been unable to confirm, despite extensive studies, one report claiming a stimulatory effect of $ACTH_{1-24}$ on the growth of adult human adrenocortical cells (Armato et al. 1977). Fetal human adrenocortical cells from the definitive cortex, which do proliferate actively in culture, are nevertheless inhibited rather than stimulated to divide by ACTH (Simonian and Gill, 1981) and we, therefore, have no reason to doubt that ACTH in vitro is not mitogenic for human cells.

These observations can be interpreted in one of two ways. They can be taken as evidence favouring the old, but unsubstantiated concept of a separate 'adrenal weight-maintaining factor' which is not ACTH (Nichols and Gourley 1963). Alternatively they can be interpreted as evidence that ACTH plays an indirect rather than a direct proliferogenic role in vivo and that its weight-maintaining and enhancing properties are crucially dependent on the tissue structure of the gland as a whole.

It is noteworthy that among the effects of ACTH in vivo are hyperaemia and increased blood flow (Grant et al. 1957a). We suggest that the resultant increase in the supply of oxygen and/or nutrients may well be an important factor stimulating the proliferation of the cortical cells. Such cellular hyperplasia would evidently, on the basis of the in vitro studies, take place in the face of an immediate and powerful inhibition of proliferation in the form of increased intracellular cyclic AMP levels. It would, however, probably be facilitated in the longer term by a gradual desensitisation

Fig. 9.2. Adrenal growth in culture. Monolayer cell cultures of (A) adult bovine, and (B) adult human ▷ adrenocortical cells. Both cultures were maintained with fibroblast growth factor (100ng/ml) in the culture medium. Note the rapid proliferation of the bovine cells after (1) 4 days (2) 8 days and (3) 12 days culture, in contrast to the human cortical cells (C) which remain proliferatively quiescent after (1) 4 days, (2) 9 days and (3) 16 days culture with the mitogen, although small groups of endothelial cells (E) have divided. Mitotic cells are indicated with *arrows*. (PC × 50)

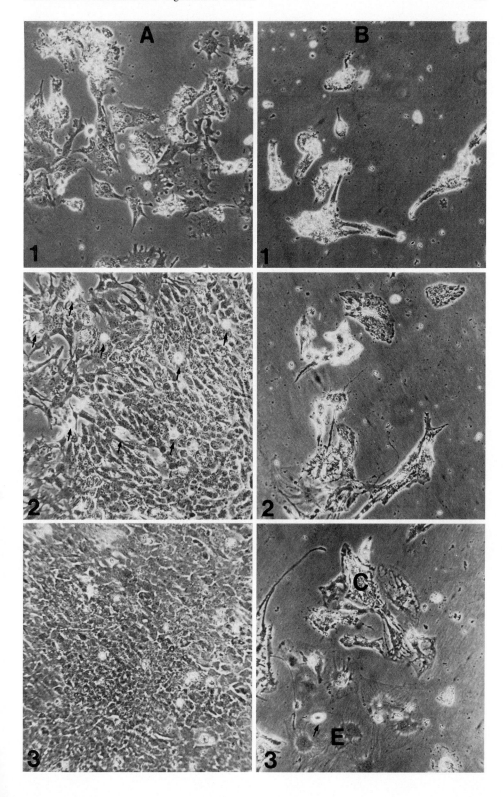

of the cortical cells to the effects of the hormone, as takes place when bovine cortical cells are cultured with ACTH in vitro (Hornsby and Gill 1977).

What sort of time course of proliferation might be anticipated in man? The normal adult cortex contains only about one mitosis per 10,000 cells (Carr 1959), and in glands removed from patients treated with 'crude' ACTH for several weeks prior to adrenalectomy, this rises by a factor of 3–4 times. Mitoses are seen only in compact-type cells, and are thus confined in the normal gland to the zona reticularis, in marked contrast to the peripheral distribution of dividing cells in most animal glands, and in the embryonic human gland (p. 13). On the basis of these findings, and the considerations outlined above, we would expect the regenerative growth of the adult human gland to be particularly slow. This accords with the prolonged period of time that has been observed to elapse between subtotal bilateral adrenalectomy for Cushing's disease and the recurrence of hypercortisolism (Egdahl and Melby 1967). Moreover, successful autotransplants of the human cortex do not seem to cause hypercortisolism or regenerate to a significant degree for at least several years, despite elevated ACTH levels (Barzilai et al. 1980).

If hyperaemia and increased adrenal blood flow are crucial to hyperplasia in man then how are they caused by ACTH? A relatively simple mechanism seems to be available. The propensity of the cortical cells to utilise cholesterol arachidonate for steroidogenesis means that ACTH also enhances intra-glandular prostaglandin synthesis via increases in free arachidonic acid, a sequence of events that has been directly observed in experimental animals (Laychock et al. 1977). Despite the fact that these compounds will, in varying degrees depending on their precise type, stimulate or inhibit human adrenal steroidogenesis (Honn and Chavin 1976, 1977) there is no convincing evidence that they play an obligatory role as intermediates in hormone action (Saruta and Kaplan 1972; Gallant and Brownie 1973). However, their effects on vascular tone are well known, and their release and that of the even more potent vasodilator, prostacyclin, could well cause increased blood flow and hyperaemia, as originally envisaged by Maeir and Staehelin (1968a, b).

Innervation of the cortical vasculature, a neglected topic in man, may also play a role. Thus, there is evidence from animal studies that compensatory adrenal growth after unilateral adrenalectomy can be prevented by hypothalamic lesions (Engeland and Dallman 1975) and neither ACTH nor corticosteroids appear to play a direct role in this regenerative process (Engeland et al. 1975; Dallman et al. 1980).

In summary therefore, it appears that while ACTH does play an important role in regulating at least some aspects of adrenocortical growth, it probably has both inhibitory and stimulatory as well as direct and indirect effects, with the final outcome in terms of cellular hyperplasia versus cellular hypertrophy being the result of a fine balance between these processes.

Whether angiotensin directly regulates the proliferation of zona glomerulosa cells in man remains unknown. It is, however, worth noting that in the bovine cortex in vitro it will also stimulate the proliferation of inner zone cells (Gill et al. 1977). Glands we have seen from cases of secondary aldosteronism with high renin (p. 229) have tended to be large (18–20 g) and one is tempted to speculate whether this peptide may not have some general adrenotropic properties in man as well.

Chapter 10
Functional Zonation of the Adrenal Cortex

The concept of functional zonation of the adrenal cortex, and the mechanisms of intraglandular regulation of steroidogenesis that underlie it, are important both for an understanding of the normal gland, and to explain certain hitherto puzzling or paradoxical aspects of its pathology. We believe that functional zonation stems, in part at least, from different steroid concentration gradients across the cortex, and have proposed that it is the responses of the individual cortical cells to this aspect of their local microenvironment that creates and sustains some zonal differences in their steroidogenic functions (Hornsby and O'Hare 1977; O'Hare et al. 1978; Neville and O'Hare 1979).

Zonal Functions of the Cortex

All three classical zones of the adrenal cortex viz.: glomerulosa, fasciculata and reticularis, are active in steroid secretion. The exclusive origin of aldosterone from the outermost layers of the cortex was first demonstrated in man by Ayres et al. (1958) confirming previous results obtained with experimental animals, and consistent with the enlargement of this zone reported in patients with low plasma sodium (Nichols 1956). It is generally assumed, furthermore, that the human aldosterone-secreting cells do not synthesise cortisol, although this has not been formally proved. However, both the steroid content of pathological aldosterone-containing tissues (p. 233) and the responses of plasma steroids to the glomerulotrophic stimulus of angiotensin II (p. 84) provide strong evidence that they form little or no cortisol.

18-Hydroxycorticosterone is another major product of the aldosterone-secreting cells formed in approximately equal quantities by normal cells (Appendix A and Fig. 8.4). Corticosterone, deoxycorticosterone and 18-hydroxydeoxycorticosterone are, on the basis of their responses to angiotensin II, also synthesised by the zona glomerulosa, but the greater part of these steroids are, however, produced by inner zone cells and under ACTH control (see e.g. Tan and Mulrow 1975). One caveat should, nevertheless, be noted. Neither the steroids themselves, nor the specific enzymes involved in their biosynthesis have as yet been localised to individual cortical cell types. The belief that aldosterone is formed specifically and exclusively by the small focal aggregates of zona glomerulosa-type cells in the normal human cortex is therefore based essentially on circumstantial evidence. The fasciculata-type cells which reach the capsule in many areas of the normal gland (Fig. 4.5) probably secrete cortisol as this steroid is also formed, together with aldosterone, by preparations of isolated subcapsular cells from the human gland (Williams and Braley 1977). With regard to the specific functional attributes of the compact-type cells appearing under the zona glomerulosa after certain forms of stress (p. 39) and in some other conditions (p. 228) we unfortunately know nothing.

The zona fasciculata (clear cells) and zona reticularis (compact cells) are undoubtedly collectively responsible for the bulk of both glucocorticoid and adrenal

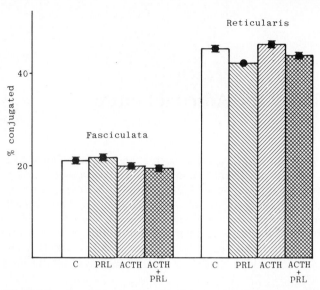

Fig. 10.1 Functional zonation. Steroid sulphonconjugation in freshly isolated adult human zona fasciculata and zona reticularis cells. Neither ACTH (0.1 μg/ml) nor ovine prolactin (1 μg/ml) singly or in combination, significantly influenced the percentage of sulphoconjugated metabolites formed from (^{3}H) pregnenolone, although marked differences between the two zones were noted (O'Hare et al. 1980a). Reproduced by kind permission of Raven Press

sex steroid (mainly DHA) production (Table 8.1). Their precise individual contributions have, however, been uncertain and the old inference (Blackman 1946) that the reticularis is the sole source of adrenal 'androgens' certainly cannot be sustained. It was specifically disproved by the studies of Grant and Griffiths (1962) who showed that individual slices of compact and clear cells both could secrete C_{21} steroids such as cortisol and contained similar levels of 11β-hydroxylase activity. These, and further experiments using radioactive steroid precursors (Ward and Grant 1963) showed a general similarity of steroidogenesis by zona fasciculata and zona reticularis cells and it was concluded (Griffiths et al. 1963) that their functions in man may be the same. Studies in organ culture (Jones et al. 1970) also showed cortisol production by both zones.

Two significant differences emerged from these studies. One was the substantially higher levels of steroid sulphoconjugation in the zona reticularis compared with zona fasciculata (Cameron et al. 1969). Furthermore, the cells of the zona fasciculata were more responsive to ACTH in short-term in vitro experiments than those of the zona reticularis (Grant and Griffiths 1962; Grant et al. 1968). This latter result seemed clearly at variance with the hypothesis of Symington (1962) that the zona fasciculata is a 'reserve' zone of steroidogenically quiescent cells activated only by prolonged stress or ACTH treatment, with the bulk of the glucocorticoids emanating from the compact cells of the zona reticularis.

We have recently re-examined the problem of inner zone functions using more sophisticated techniques of analysis including high-performance liquid chromatography (HPLC) (O'Hare et al. 1976; O'Hare and Nice 1981) which was not available to earlier workers. Our results (O'Hare et al. 1980a) confirm the high steroid sulphotransferase activity of the zona reticularis (Fig. 10.1) and show, in addition, that while steroid profiles of freshly isolated zona fasciculata and reticularis cells are similar, there are distinct differences. These are illustrated in Fig. 10.2.

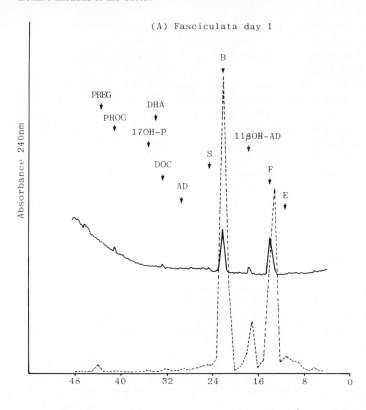

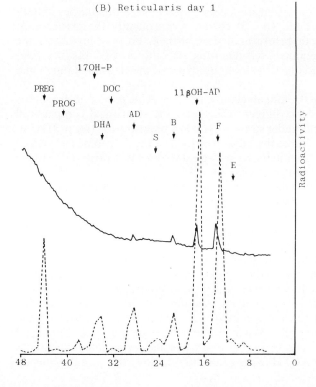

Fig. 10.2. Functional zonation. Patterns of endogenous steroid production (*solid lines*) and radiometabolites (*dotted lines*) produced by freshly isolated adult human zona fasciculata (**A**) and zona reticularis (**B**) cells. From O'Hare et al. (1980a). Reproduced by kind permission of Raven Press

While both zones secrete cortisol in approximately equal amounts it is evident that the clear cells produce relatively more 17-deoxysteroids such as corticosterone, while the compact cells produce more C_{19} steroids such as 11β-hydroxyandrostenedione as well as slightly more 11-deoxysteroids including androstenedione and deoxycorticosterone. Higher relative levels of 11-deoxysteroids have also been noted in purified preparations of zona reticularis compared with zona fasciculata cells from the rat (Bell et al. 1978) and this may well, therefore, be a general phenomenon in other mammals. It is consequently true that to a certain extent the reticularis is the source of relatively greater quantities of potentially androgenic C_{19} steroids than the outer zones, but the difference is evidently quantitative rather than qualitative. This conclusion is further substantiated by recent studies of the steroid content of the different zones of the human cortex (Maroulis and Abraham 1980).

The zonal distribution of aromatase activity and C_{18} steroid secretion by the adrenal cortex, such as it is, remains unknown at present.

Mechanisms of Functional Zonation

A concept of dynamic alterations in steroidogenesis by local microenvironmental conditions has been suggested by our results with cell cultures of both human and animal adrenocortical cells. It enables both the 'escalator' theory of adrenocortical cell migration and the evidence of functional zonation, long held to be mutually incompatible, to be reconciled.

Embryological evidence (p. 13) indicates that all cells of both the prenatal and postnatal cortex have a common origin. As a corollary it might be expected that they would form a functional continuum. In fact, the discontinuities seen as zonal boundaries with the light microscope may be more apparent than real. Thus, ultrastructural studies clearly show transitional cell types at such boundaries in both the prenatal (p. 48) and the adult (p. 25) cortex. Consequently the existence of functionally distinct zones both before and after birth in no way predicates the existence of discrete, self-contained, self-renewing or ontologically distinct populations of cortical cells. Instead one must look to a dynamic mechanism of functional zonation.

Histological observations on the human gland already provide good evidence of the potential interconvertibility of the different cell types; the centrifugal compact-cell conversion of the outer clear cells under stress or ACTH administration (see p. 31) is an example in point. Cell culture studies described shortly indicate that some and indeed possibly all the specific functional differences between the zones are attributable to the local microenvironment within the cortex.

The unique vasculature of the gland with its centripetal blood-flow through the concentrically arranged zones of the cortex, together with the absence of a significant direct arterial supply to the innermost layers of the parenchyma (Fig. 4.14) must result in marked arteriovenous gradients across the cortex, diagrammatised in Fig. 10.3. Such gradients include secreted steroids (Maroulis and Abraham 1980).

The first clues that the adrenal steroids themselves directly modulate the functions of adrenocortical cells came from the studies of rat zona glomerulosa cells in culture (Hornsby et al. 1974). These cells continued to secrete aldosterone in vitro for only a short time. While ACTH initially stimulated its secretion it ultimately suppressed it, a biphasic response very similar to that seen in vivo in man (p. 84). Furthermore, the ACTH-stimulated glomerulosa cells assumed the ultrastructural and functional attributes of zona fasciculata cells. A similar effect has also been noted when fetal adrenal cells are cultured with ACTH (Kahri et al. 1970). However, we subsequently

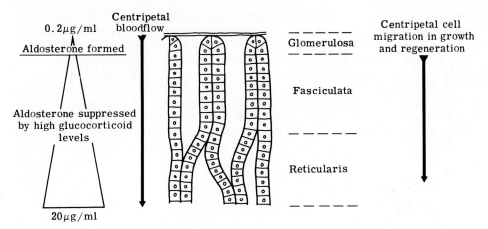

Fig. 10.3. Functional zonation. Postulated role of adrenal steroids in functional zonation of the cortex. See Nicolis et al. (1972) and Maroulis and Abraham (1980) for steroid levels in adrenal venous effluent and in the cortex itself.

extended our observations to the direct effects of exogenous steroids on glomerulosa function in vitro and found (Hornsby and O'Hare 1977) that aldosterone (and 18-hydroxycorticosterone) synthesis was suppressed by glucocorticoids, such as cortisol. The concentrations used (10 μg/ml) were not greatly dissimilar to those found in the adrenal venous effluent, or in the gland itself (Maroulis and Abraham 1980).

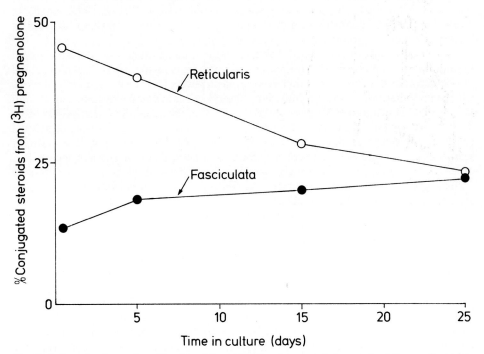

Fig. 10.4. Functional zonation. Steroid sulphoconjugation by separated normal adult zona fasciculata (*closed rings*) and zona reticularis (*open rings*) cells in monolayer culture. Note that marked differences at the outset declined with time until the steroid-metabolising activities of the cultures became identical. A similar convergence in the pattern of secreted UV-absorbing steroids was also noted. Reproduced by kind permission of Raven Press

A logical conclusion from these results is that aldosterone synthesis may well be impossible in the inner zones of the cortex because of this suppressive effect of glucocorticoids, which appear to act on the later stages of aldosterone biosynthesis (Hornsby and O'Hare 1977). As a corollary therefore it is not surprising that zona glomerulosa-type cells are found only in the vicinity of fresh arterial blood either immediately beneath the capsule or near the arteriae comitantes in the wall of the central vein in the cortical cuff (p. 29). Experiments carried out with zona fasciculata and reticularis cells by Kahri et al. (1979) have indicated that a similar steroid-dependent mechanism may dictate functional zonation within the inner layers of the cortex as well. Thus, corticosterone at high concentrations suppresses cortisol and enhances DHA secretion by cultured human fetal adrenocortical cells. Perhaps therefore the synthesis of C_{19} steroids by human adult zona reticularis preparations is a consequence of the prior synthesis of corticosterone by the clear cells of the overlying zona fasciculata (Fig. 10.2). While it is entirely possible that other microenvironmental factors within the cortex may also modulate zonal steroidogenesis the experiments described above, and their results provide a plausible mechanism to account for several major facets of functional zonation in man.

Further compelling evidence for the role of local factors dictating zonal differences in steroidogenic functions comes from our studies of the behaviour of long-term cultures prepared from separated human fasciculata and reticularis tissue. Marked differences observed at the outset, in for example sulphoconjugation, (Fig. 10.1) disappeared with time until the cultures showed identical patterns of steroidogenesis (Fig. 10.4). This failure of the cells to sustain zonal attributes has been observed by us in repeated experiments utilising separated tissue from different glands. After 7–10 days culture both types of cell show an equivalent response to ACTH (not illustrated), in marked contrast to their differing responses immediately after isolation (vide supra), confirming their capability of behaving as a functional unit.

Under conditions of functional demand and trophic stimulation, therefore, zonal boundaries may change by recruitment of adjacent cells further up or down the zonal gradient, rather than by expansion by hyperplasia per se. It is less immediately obvious why zonal boundaries, however indistinct, should exist at all and why functions should not vary as a continuum. However, not only may the steroid gradient across the cortex itself be non-linear (Maroulis and Abraham 1980), but the capacity of the individual cells also to secrete products that may alter their own functions as well as those of subadjacent cells makes it quite conceivable that positive feed-back effects operate (i.e. mineralocorticoid switching to glucocorticoid synthesis itself further suppressing aldosterone). Rapid shifts in function over quite short distances from one metastable state to another may, therfore, occur.

The concept of functional interactions between outer and inner zones due to direct effects of steroids on adjacent cells has also been formulated, albeit in a mechanistically different form, by Vinson and Whitehouse (1976). The scheme that we have proposed here enables the concepts of an 'escalator' migration of adrenal cells inwards to be reconciled with evidence of functional zonation. It follows that wherever they originate, when cells come to lie deeper in the cortex by, for example, accretionary growth processes, their functions will change as a response to the local microenvironment. This synthesis is particularly relevant in the case of the human prenatal cortex where embryological studies (p. 13) leave little doubt that cells originating in what is termed the definitive cortex must ultimately come to reside in the fetal cortex zone. We would suggest that local steroid gradients may also be responsible for the manifestations of functional zonation in the prenatal cortex. Direct evidence for the validity of this concept has come from recent studies on the ultimate convergence of the functional attributes of definitive and fetal zone human tissue maintained in cell culture in a uniform environment with ACTH (Simonian and Gill 1981).

A final conclusion that may be drawn from these considerations is that both quantitative and qualitative aspects of steroidogenesis may well change quite rapidly once the cells are withdrawn from the intact cortical circulation. Old microchemical studies demonstrating local high levels of steroidogenic enzyme activities (and possibly high levels of endogenous steroid secretion) at, for example, the boundary of the zona fasciculata and zona reticularis in man (Symington 1962) may well be more important than they are generally given credit for at present. Certainly they correspond well with certain ultrastructural features of zonation (p. 25) and details of cortical zonation may well be more subtle than can be revealed by in vitro experiments on mechanically separated zones.

Part B
HYPERCORTICALISM

Chapter 11

General Incidence and Pathological Changes

Hyperfunction of the adrenal cortex (hypercorticalism) may be associated with either hyperplasia, or benign or malignant neoplasms. Hyperplasia is in our experience always bilateral, neoplasia almost always unilateral.

There are three principal forms of hypercorticalism, namely Cushing's syndrome (excess production of glucocorticoid hormones, characteristically cortisol), Conn's syndrome (excess production of aldosterone or less commonly, related salt-active steroid hormones) and the adrenogenital syndrome which takes the form of either virilism or feminisation and is due to an excess of circulating androgenic or oestrogenic hormones. Each syndrome may either occur as a clearly distinct entity (i.e. in pure form) or, as is often the case with carcinomas, admixed signs and symptoms may be present.

We have had the opportunity over the past two decades of studying the adrenal changes in hypercorticalism in over 400 patients. Many of these cases in the decade to 1970 were referred to the Glasgow group and have been the subject of several previous reports (Neville and Symington 1966, 1967, 1972; Ferriss et al. 1970).

The relative frequency with which these disorders are encountered at a clinical level is, however, different from that shown in Table 11.1 which summarises those cases we

Table 11.1. Adrenocortical hyperfunction: the pathology of the adrenal cortex in 401 patients

Disease	No. of patients	Adrenal lesion		
		Bilateral hyperplasia	Adenoma	Carcinoma
Cushing's syndrome	202 (50%)	157	26	19
Hyperaldosteronism with low plasma renin (Conn's syndrome)	153 (38%)	28	120	5
Adrenogenital syndrome				
Virilism	41 ⎱(12%)	20	8	13
Feminisation	5 ⎰	–	–	5
Total	401 (100%)	205	154	42

have examined histologically. Many cases of hyperplasia in e.g. Conn's syndrome or the congenital virilising form of the adrenogenital syndrome do not now come to surgery due to improvements in diagnostic technique and they are, therefore, seldom found in the histopathologist's province. Moreover, our extensive experience of the adrenal tumours in Conn's syndrome has arisen from our close liaison with the MRC Blood Pressure Unit at the Western Infirmary, Glasgow, to whom many examples of Conn's syndrome are referred from throughout the United Kingdom, and this has undoubtedly weighted our series in favour of this syndrome.

With these provisos the following account is, nevertheless, based largely on this personal series, and on our functional and tissue culture studies of a number of these lesions carried out during the past decade (Neville and MacKay 1972; Neville 1978; Neville and O'Hare 1978; Neville and O'Hare 1979; O'Hare et al. 1978, 1979). The latter studies have aimed at clarifying the reasons for the structural and functional pathological changes in these and related disorders, and at using functional criteria for improving the discrimination between benign and malignant neoplasms.

Factors Predisposing to Hypercorticalism

Genetic changes appear to be the cause of several forms of hypercorticalism associated with hyperplasia, notably congenital adrenocortical hyperplasia (CAH) (p. 155). In so far as neoplasia is concerned, most cortical tumours, whose overall incidence in a malignant form is about 2 persons/million of population/year, cannot be linked with known predisposing factors of either genetic or environmental types. However, the left gland is the site of carcinoma somewhat more frequently than the right. There are, furthermore, some other exceptions.

Thus, malignant adrenocortical tumours are among the manifestations of the so-called 'cancer family syndrome' first reported by Bottomley and Condit (1968) and defined as a specific clinico-pathological entity by Li and Fraumeni (1969). This tumour complex has an incidence consistent with a rare autosomal dominant mutation, and comprises a familial cancer aggregation comprising sarcomas, brain tumours, leukaemias, and carcinomas of the breast, larynx, lung and adrenal cortex (the SBLA complex). Adrenocortical carcinomas have also been recorded in adults with the Gardner syndrome and the Werner syndrome (Schimke 1978), and in children with trisomy D (Nevin et al. 1972).

Congenital hemihypertrophy (CH) is probably the most significant predisposing factor to adrenal neoplasia in children. Thus 2/62 cases of adrenal tumours in children examined by Fraumeni and Miller (1967) were CH cases, and further cases of the association have since been reported (Haicken et al. 1973), with both Cushing's and the adrenogenital syndrome among the presenting features. A high risk of Wilm's tumour and hepatoblastoma has also been noted in CH and similar associations have been noted in the Beckwith-Weidemann syndrome. Histological adrenal changes in these syndromes are described on p. 289. Congenital adrenocortical tumours causing virilism have also been noted in otherwise normal sibs (Mahloudji et al. 1971; Artigas et al. 1976) and may have arisen from fetal zone tissue.

In the majority of cases, however, adrenocortical tumours are not associated with detectable chromosomal aberrations, or known hereditary syndromes.

Chapter 12
Cushing's Syndrome

Cushing's syndrome is due to chronically increased levels of circulating glucocorticoid hormones, and manifests itself, as Cushing himself described it in 1932, as truncal obesity, amenorrhea, hirsutism, hypertension, abdominal striae, polyphagia, polydipsia, polycythaemia and susceptibility to infections.

For the definitive diagnosis of the syndrome it is generally considered that urinary free cortisol should exceed 100 μg/day, mean plasma cortisol 20 μg/100 ml (700 nmols/ 1) or the cortisol excretion rate should be >20 mg/g creatinine. No single test is, however, completely reliable and diagnostic procedures can be complicated and time-consuming. A detailed review of the clinical tests used for the diagnosis of Cushing's syndrome has recently been published by West and Meikle (1980), and its clinical features have been summarised by Nelson (1980), and by Jeffcoate and Edwards (1979).

While this chapter is devoted to the adrenal changes which occur as a result of intrinsic hypothalamo-pituitary-adrenocortical disorders associated with the syndrome, it is nevertheless important to remember that Cushing's syndrome is more frequently encountered as an iatrogenic disorder resulting from the therapeutic administration of excessive amounts of glucocorticoids (or ACTH) for diseases such as rheumatoid arthritis or asthma. Similar symptoms are also encountered in chronic alcoholism when they are termed pseudo-Cushing's syndrome, the cause of which remains obscure (Rees et al. 1977). Because of its protean characteristics, which in their milder and intermittent forms often elude diagnosis, the overall incidence of non-iatrogenic Cushing's syndrome is difficult to ascertain; it is, however, rare in comparison with some other endocrine disorders, and rarer in children, where it may be associated with growth retardation.

Cushing's syndrome, and all attendant forms of adrenal change may be found at any age. It is commoner in adults and affects females two to three times more frequently than males. If all age groups are considered together, about 75 % of cases are associated with bilateral adrenocortical hyperplasia with the remainder due to adrenocortical neoplasms, approximately half of which are malignant (Table 12.1). However, the incidence of the various adrenal changes in adults and children is significantly different (Table 12.2). From personal analysis of the reported cases of Cushing's syndrome in children, it may be seen that tumours, particularly carcinomas, are more frequent in children ($\sim$60%) than bilateral adrenocortical hyperplasia, which tends to occur around puberty (Table 12.3).

Bilateral adrenocortical hyperplasia is associated with an increased effective stimulation of the adrenals by ACTH and is often referred to as 'Cushing's disease'. Originally, Cushing (1932) postulated that this disorder was caused by a basophil adenoma of the pituitary gland. Subsequent studies found a predominance of pituitary chromophobe adenomas considered at the time to be 'non-functioning' lesions. The primary role of the pituitary in causing hyperplasia was therefore called into question particularly as only a minority of patients with pituitary-dependent Cushing's disease had demonstrable radiological fossa abnormalities (<20%) (McErlean and Doyle

Table 12.1. Cushing's syndrome: incidence of adrenal changes at all ages

Authors	No. of patients	Adrenal changes		
		Bilateral hyperplasia	Adenoma	Carcinoma
Plotz et al. (1952)	94	67	11	16
Sprague et al. (1955)	88	69	14	5
Soffer et al. (1961)	45	24	8	13
Personal series[a]	202	157	26	19
Total	429	317	59	53
Incidence	–	74%	14%	12%

[a]These cases include previously published data by Neville and Symington (1967); Symington (1969); Neville and O'Hare (1979).

Table 12.2. Incidence of adrenal lesions in Cushing's syndrome as a function of age

Adrenal lesion	Incidence (%)	
	Adults[a]	Children[b]
Hyperplasia	78	42
Adenoma	13	12
Carcinoma	9	46

[a]Personal series (Table 12.1).
[b]Review of paediatric Cushing's syndrome (Table 12.3).

Table 12.3. Age distribution of the adrenal lesions in 197 children with Cushing's syndrome: 73 boys and 120 girls[a]

Adrenal lesions	Number of patients with syndrome					
	Males aged			Females aged		
	<1 yr	1–8 yr	9–15 yr	<1 yr	1–8 yr	9–15 yr
Hyperplasia						
simple	1	3	18	0	3	13
with pituitary tumours	0	1	7	0	1	3
with 'non-endocrine' tumours	1	3	3	1	1	3
nodular	2[b]	1	2	9[b]	2	3
Tumours						
adenoma	2	3	2	9	7	1
carcinoma	4	13	7	10	42	12

[a]The sex of four children, two with hyperplasia and two with carcinoma in the reviewed literature series was not stated.
[b]Both males and six females were three months of age or less (Table 12.5).

1976). The hypothalamus and hypothetical disorders of the as yet unidentified corticotrophin-releasing factor (CRF) have, therefore, been implicated as the site of the primary pathological lesion in recent years, notably by Krieger et al. (1975). More recently attention has been redirected towards the role of the pituitary, largely because of the successful treatment of Cushing's disease by selective removal of pituitary microadenomas by the method of Hardy (1971), leaving other pituitary functions intact (Salassa et al. 1978). In recent studies of Cushing's disease with adrenal hyperfunction (and presumably hyperplasia) ACTH-secreting microadenomas not visible by surface inspection or associated with sellar changes were present in nearly half the cases, and their removal was followed by regression of the Cushing's syndrome in 80% of patients (Tyrell et al. 1978). The aetiology of the microadenomas remains, however, a matter for debate (Daughaday 1978) and it is doubtful if most represent autonomous neoplasms; the hypothalamus may consequently regain its status as the ultimate cause of the disease, although changes within the pituitary itself (e.g. micro-vascular accidents) may provide an equally plausible explanation. It is indeed possible that no single cause may account for all cases.

Whatever its original cause, in the 'pituitary-dependent' form of the disease the aetiological abnormality results in over-secretion of ACTH, with loss of regular nycthemeral rhythmicity although irregular episodic secretion may still occur, and $ACTH_{1-39}$ is the predominant molecular form of the hormone found in the circulation in most cases (Yalow and Berson 1973). By contrast, in Cushing's syndrome due to the production of ACTH by so-called 'non-endocrine' tumours (the 'ectopic ACTH' syndrome so named by Liddle et al. 1965), the circulating form of ACTH is mostly 'big' ACTH, a form of precursor molecule or molecules (Yalow and Berson 1971; Gewirtz and Yalow 1974; Ratter et al. 1977; see also Fig. 8.8).

In the majority, but not all instances of pituitary-dependent Cushing's syndrome, $ACTH_{1-39}$ is detected in raised amounts in the plasma, typically 200–500 pg/ml compared with normal levels of 10–50 pg/ml (Besser and Landon 1968) but in nearly half the cases single measurements of the hormone do not reveal substantial increases (Jeffcoate and Edwards 1979). For this reason ACTH measurements are not always reliable in the primary diagnosis of Cushing's disease. There is a close correlation between immunoreactive and bioactive ACTH levels (Ratter et al. 1977) and between these and plasma cortisol levels (Susuki 1976) although in some patients occasional peaks of ACTH not associated with a commensurate rise in cortisol levels can be detected (Krieger and Allen 1975). The great majority of patients with Cushing's disease show a 40% plus suppression of corticosteroids after high-dose dexamethasone (2 mg every 6 h for 48 h) (Liddle 1960), whereas suppression of ACTH does not occur in the ectopic ACTH syndrome in the majority of cases.

In the remaining quarter of patients, the cause of Cushing's syndrome is an adrenal neoplasm, about half of which are carcinomas (Tables 11.1 and 12.1). In children, however, the incidence of tumours as the cause, particularly carcinomas, is much higher (Table 12.2). Rarely, Cushing's syndrome is caused by tumours arising from adrenal rests outside the gland proper (p. 283). Cortisol (or other glucocorticoid) production by tumours causing Cushing's syndrome is generally regarded as autonomous, although it probably reflects as much the increased mass of steroidogenic tissue as any abnormalities of functional responses (p. 199). Plasma ACTH levels are reduced to <10 pg/ml in most such cases, levels which are generally considered pathognomonic of adrenocortical tumours in Cushing's syndrome (Jeffcoate and Edwards 1979). Occasionally suppression with high-dose dexamethasone is seen in patients with adrenocortical tumours (Kendall and Sloop 1968; Rayfield et al. 1971).

Bilateral Adrenocortical Hyperplasia

On the basis of the weight and the gross and histological features of the adrenal gland, it is possible to subdivide adrenocortical hyperplasia into one of three morphological forms: simple (or diffuse) hyperplasia, nodular hyperplasia and hyperplasia with 'non-endocrine' tumours ('ectopic ACTH' syndrome). Their relative incidence in adults and children is shown in Table 12.4.

Table 12.4. The relative incidence of different pathologies in bilateral adrenocortical hyperplasia in Cushing's syndrome

Pathology	Adults			Children		
	%	Age (years)	Sex (F:M)	%	Age (years)	Sex (F:M)
Simple hyperplasia	62	20–40	3:1	62	9–15	2:3
Nodular hyperplasia	20	40–50	3:1	23	<1	3:1
Hyperplasia with 'ectopic ACTH' syndrome	18	40–60	1:3	15	Any	1:1

Simple (or Diffuse) Hyperplasia

This is the commonest form of adrenal hyperplasia in both adults and children. In the latter overt pituitary tumours are often found and the disorder is commoner in males than females and tends to occur predominantly around puberty (Table 12.4) (Kracht 1971; Neville and Symington 1972). In adults, females are more frequently affected, particularly between the ages of 20 and 40 years (Table 12.4).

Gross appearance Almost all the adult adrenal glands showing this pathological change are enlarged. At operation, each gland typically weighs between 6 and 12 g (Fig. 12.1) while at autopsy, weights in excess of 12 g are the rule. In children,

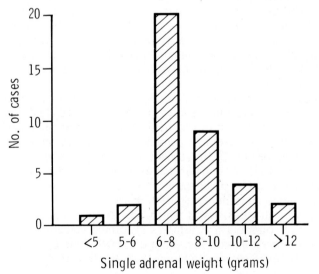

Fig. 12.1. Cushing's syndrome. The weights of a personal series of single adrenal glands removed at operation and showing bilateral diffuse (simple) hyperplasia.

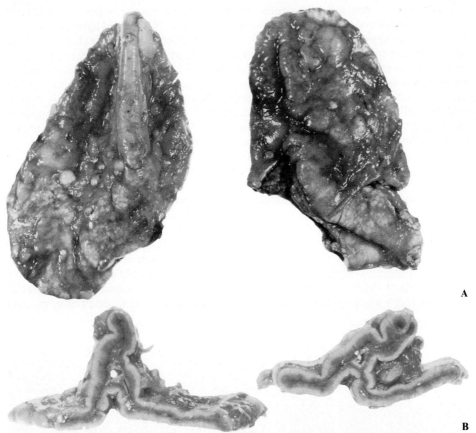

Fig. 12.2. Cushing's syndrome. Bilateral diffuse hyperplasia. The glands removed at surgery are enlarged, heavier than normal (**A**, 6.0 g; 6.1 g) and have rounded contours. On section (**B**), the cortex is broadened and has an inner brown layer corresponding to the zona reticularis which is more prominent than normal (see fig. 4.2. and 4.3. for comparison).

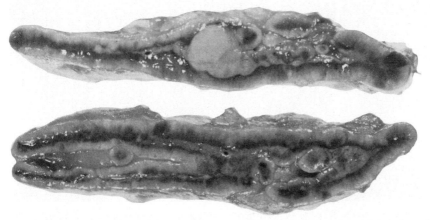

Fig. 12.3. Cushing's syndrome. Bilateral diffuse hyperplasia (operation specimen; 7.4 g). A small nodule is noted within the substance of the hyperplastic gland. Its size is, however, not sufficient to warrant inclusion in the category of nodular hyperplasia.

depending upon their age, the glands are also commensurately heavier than normal although not always strikingly so (McArthur et al. 1972; Neville and Symington 1972). Each gland appears yellow/brown in colour and has rounded contours (Fig. 12.2), and on section the cortex is seen to be broadened, and, in glands removed at operation, consists of an inner brown layer occupying one half to one third of the cortex and an outer yellow layer. In glands examined from autopsy material, this distinction is lost and the cortex has a diffuse brown colour. Not infrequently, small (<0.25 mm) nodules, yellow in colour, may also be noted in the cortex (Fig. 12.3) or in relation to the central vein emphasising the essential continuity of this condition with the nodular hyperplastic form with large, macroscopic nodules. The presence of small nodules in otherwise diffusely hyperplastic glands is particularly notable in glands removed from children around puberty (Neville and Symington 1972).

Microscopic appearance   Microscopically, in conventionally prepared paraffin-embedded material from surgically removed glands, the inner brown zone corresponds to a broadened compact cell zona reticularis while the outer yellow area consists of the clear lipid-laden cells of the zona fasciculata (Fig. 12.4). The zona reticularis comprises one-third to one-half of the total cortical width and is separated by an undulating boundary from the outer zona fasciculata (Fig. 12.4). The zona glomerulosa is usually within normal limits, maintaining its focal peripheral distribution. However, occasionally in adults and more commonly in children, it is more prominent than

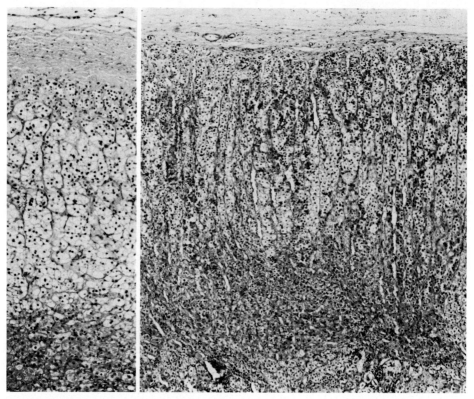

Fig. 12.4. Cushing's syndrome. Bilateral diffuse hyperplasia (operation specimen; 6.6 g). On the *right* is the Cushing's gland where the cortex is wider than normal and has a broadened zona reticularis, which has an undulating border with the zona fasciculata. On the *left* a normal gland removed at operation is shown for comparison. (H + E × 55 [normal × 90])

normal, although the normal variation in zonal distribution is less well documented in children than in adults.

The cells themselves in each zone are usually normal in appearance and size. At the ultrastructural level, the organelles of the cells in the broadened zona reticularis are similar to those found in the normal zona reticularis (p. 27) although the relative proportion of the cytoplasm occupied by for example mitochondria and SER may be altered (Tannenbaum 1973). The cells of the zona fasciculata and zona glomerulosa in diffuse hyperplasia possess for the most part ultrastructural features characteristic of cells in normal glands (MacKay 1969; Urushibata 1971; Neville and MacKay 1972).

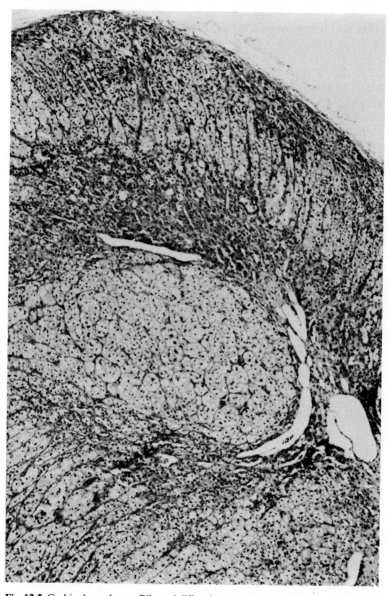

Fig. 12.5. Cushing's syndrome. Bilateral diffuse hyperplasia. A small clear cell micronodule in relation to the central vein is seen. The overlying cortex shows diffuse hyperplasia. (H + E × 55)

Collectively the morphological appearances in diffuse hyperplasia are those anticipated in view of the elevated levels of plasma ACTH in this form of hypercortisolism, together with the known effects of ACTH on the morphology and functional zonation of the human adrenal cortex (p. 31).

Rarely adults with biochemically proved Cushing's syndrome are found to have at operation adrenal glands within the normal weight (Fig. 12.1) with a normal cortical width. Morphologically, however, these glands show a broadened compact cell zona reticularis, although its overall breadth is not as great as that which occurs in the classical hyperplastic gland.

The autopsy adrenal from subjects with Cushing's syndrome and bilateral adrenocortical hyperplasia has a different appearance to the surgically removed gland. The differences are explicable on the basis, first, of the raised plasma ACTH causing the primary disorder and, second, what is probably an even greater elevation of ACTH caused by the stress of dying. These pathophysiological changes usually result in a cortex which consists almost exclusively of compact-type cells extending out to the capsule, or the underlying zona glomerulosa, where present (Symington 1969).

Three other types of microscopic changes may also be noted in simple bilateral hyperplasia with Cushing's syndrome. Despite its nature, small micronodules are seen not infrequently in the cortex, usually around the periphery of the gland or in relation to the central vein (Fig. 12.5). Generally they consist of clear lipid-laden cells similar to those of the zona fasciculata, although occasionally, they may comprise compact cells,

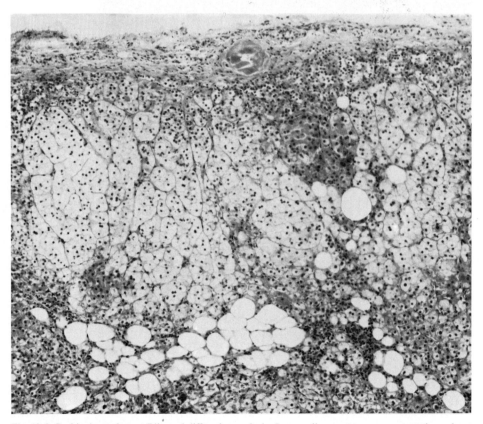

Fig. 12.6. Cushing's syndrome. Bilateral diffuse hyperplasia. Large adipose spaces are present throughout the hyperplastic cortex, but particularly in the zona reticularis. (H + E × 90)

a feature occurring particularly but not exclusively in autopsy glands. Intimal proliferation and hyaline arteriosclerosis (Fig. 6.16). of the capsular arteries may also be seen in such micronodule-containing glands.

Second, large adipose spaces (fat cells) may be present in the zona reticularis, replacing, or displacing, some of the innermost compact cells (Fig. 12.6).

Finally, in a limited number of cases adrenal cell hypertrophy may be superimposed on the hyperplasia, with enlarged cells in both the zona fasciculata and zona reticularis. Nuclear pleomorphism may also be prominent and these appearances may also involve micronodules when these are present. Such features are most often found in glands weighing in excess of 12–14 g each, and in our experience, generally occur with overt pituitary tumours and may reflect prolonged excess ACTH stimulation. However, they can also occur in the absence of an overt pituitary lesion. We have illustrated similar features which occur in the 'ectopic ACTH' syndrome (Fig. 12.10).

Several spontaneous remissions have been recorded in Cushing's syndrome in association with bilateral adrenocortical hyperplasia (e.g. Pasqualini and Gurevich 1956; Hayslett and Cohn 1967; Symington 1969; Mornex et al. 1972; Putnam et al. 1972) and a recent report has detailed complete clinical and biochemical remission but persistent defects in the functioning of the hypothalamic-pituitary axis (Scott et al. 1979). Cyclical hormone secretion in Cushing's syndrome with 'ectopic ACTH' syndrome has also been recorded with temporary remission of symptoms (Chajek and Romanoff 1976).

Adrenal venography and the administration of ACTH have also been reported to induce occasionally remission of Cushing's syndrome with hyperplasia (and adenomas) probably due to haemorrhage and subsequent necrosis (Fellerman et al. 1970; Melby 1972; Pratt et al. 1974).

Bilateral Nodular Hyperplasia

Bilateral nodular hyperplasia accounts for about 20 % of all examples of hyperplasia in adults and 23 % in children (Tables 12.3, 12.4 and 12.5). While microscopic clear cell nodules occur in many glands in pituitary-dependent Cushing's syndrome, the term nodular hyperplasia is generally restricted to describe the presence of one or more prominent yellow nodules (>0.5 cm) with brown foci, often visible to the naked eye and often 2–2.5 cm in diameter (Fig. 12.7). These occur in glands in which the remaining cortex is clearly hyperplastic. In children, bilateral nodular hyperplasia is encountered most commonly in the first year of life while in adults it tends to affect a somewhat older age group than that showing bilateral simple hyperplasia (Tables 12.3 and 12.4). In adults, nodular hyperplasia may simply be a reflection of a greater degree of vascular damage to the capsular arteries and further growth with time of the micronodules noted in simple hyperplasia (see p. 56 for discussion of the aetiology of nodules).

Gross appearance   The weight and size of the glands showing nodular hyperplasia is in general greater that the weight of most cases of diffuse hyperplasia. There is also a marked difference, often greater than 2 g, between the weight of both glands, a feature seldom found in diffuse hyperplasia where right and left gland weights are usually closely comparable (Neville and Symington 1967).

In nodular hyperplasia, nodules are almost always found in both glands, and they are frequently multiple, either projecting from one pole of the gland or occurring within its substance compressing the related cortex and are only detected when the gland is sectioned.

Table 12.5. Bilateral nodular hyperplasia in 21 children with Cushing's syndrome: adrenal glands removed at operation

Case no.	Age (yr)	Sex	Weight of adrenal glands (g) Left		Right	Reference
1	8/52	F	d		d	O'Bryan et al. 1964
2[a]	10/52	M	–		–	Donaldson et al. 1981
3[a]	10/52	F		9.0[e]		Donaldson et al. 1981
4	11/52	M	–		–	Lightwood 1932
5	12/52	F	6.0		35.0	Powell et al. 1955
6	3/12	F	2.5[f]		12.0	Marks et al. 1940
7[b]	3/12	M	4.7		4.3	Klevit et al. 1966
8	3/12	F	1.0		3.0	Neville and Symington 1967; Aarskog and Tverteraas 1968
9[b]	3/12	F	1.0		1.5	Loridan and Senior 1969
10	4.5/12	F	3.5		2.7	Perlmutter et al. 1962
11	6/12	F	3.5		1.7	Danon et al. 1975
12	7/12	F	2.5[f]		3.0[f]	Loridan and Senior 1969
13[b]	1	F	–		–	Goldblatt and Snaith 1958
14	3	M	7.1		6.7	Loridan and Senior 1969
15	8	F	4.7		5.3	Chute *et al.* 1949
16	10	M	(1 cm diam)		–	Peterman 1957
17[bc]	14	F	5.5		4.0	Meador et al. 1967
18	15	F		16.2[e]		Mosier et al. 1960
19	7	F	10.5		10.5	Najjar et al. 1964
20[a]	13	M	7.0		7.0	Arce et al. 1978
21[a]	15	F	6.0		–	Arce et al. 1978

[a]Cases 2/3 and 20/21 were sibs in two different families.
[b]Slight or no response to ACTH infusion; no suppression with dexamethasone or 9α-fluorohydrocortisone.
[c]Plasma ACTH <0.12 m.units per 100 ml (bioassay; normal 0.1–0.3 m.units per 100 ml).
[d]Gland weight stated to be normal (see Fig. 3.2 for normal weight in infancy).
[e]Weight of both glands.
[f]Gland weight at necropsy.

Microscopic appearance Nodules in Cushing's syndrome with bilateral hyperplasia consist mainly of clear cells arranged in nests and cords contiguous with the compressed related cortex (Fig. 12.8). The latter also shows the typical histological features of diffuse (simple) adrenocortical hyperplasia (Fig. 12.4). Small foci of compact cells are also present within the nodules and correspond to the brown foci noted macroscopically. The capsular arteries frequently show arteriopathic changes.

The only striking ultrastructural feature of nodular hyperplasia is the increased perivascular collagen and basement membrane material separating the endothelium and the cells of the nodules, both of which result in a broadening of the perivascular space (Neville and MacKay 1972). Most nodule cells themselves show similar features to normal zona fasciculata cells (MacKay 1969) although the SER may be somewhat more prominent (Urushibata 1971; Tannenbaum 1973).

Cellular hypertrophy and pleomorphism may occur in some nodules in Cushing's disease and sometimes has been interpreted as evidence of functional autonomy and possibly preneoplasia (Kay 1976; Anderson et al. 1978). This has, however, not been the authors' personal experience, as such changes appear to be too frequently observed to enable a causal relationship with neoplasia to be convincingly established. Cushing's syndrome with nodular hyperplasia is frequently diagnosed as bilateral adenomas or as a simple solitary adenoma when only one adrenal gland is available for study. This is

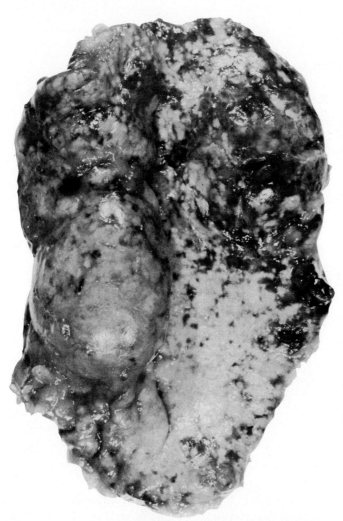

Fig. 12.7. Cushing's syndrome. Bilateral nodular hyperplasia; (21 g). The enlarged adrenal gland exhibits rounded full contours together with a large 2.5 cm nodule (*left*). Several further 1–2 cm nodules were found on sectioning the gland. (× 2.0)

perhaps not surprising when it is appreciated that the morphology of the nodule itself with Cushing's syndrome is virtually identical to that of the so-called 'non-functioning' adrenal nodules (Fig. 6.15) and the true adenomas of Cushing's syndrome (Fig. 12.15). It is important to note that clear-cut histopathological differentiation of these entities can be achieved only by examining the attached cortex, which is of normal width and appearance with 'non-functioning' nodules, clearly atrophic with cortisol (or corticosterone) producing adenomas (Fig. 12.25) and always hyperplastic in nodular hyperplasia (Fig. 12.4 and 12.8).

Relationships   Debate and dispute continue with regard to the genesis of nodular hyperplasia, whether for example it is a preneoplastic lesion in certain cases and whether such nodules possess functional autonomy in vivo (Kirschner et al. 1964; Choi et al. 1970). In all the examples of nodular hyperplasia that we have seen (Neville and

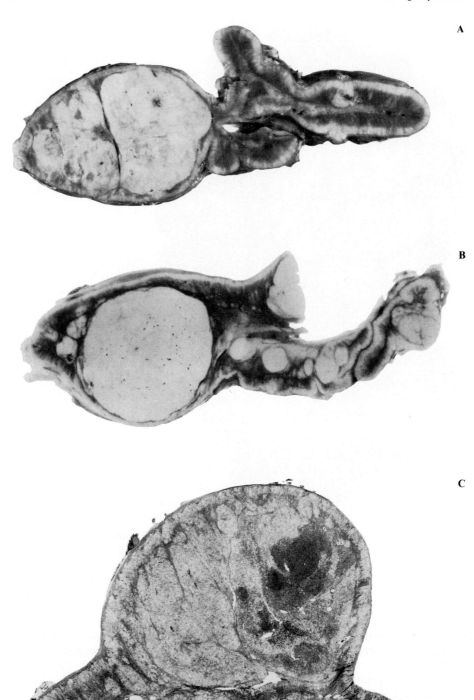

Symington 1967; Neville and O'Hare 1979) the attached cortex has exhibited the features of simple (diffuse) hyperplasia (Figs. 12.4 and 12.8), the changes have been bilateral, and the Cushing's syndrome has never been cured until both adrenal glands have been removed, as was also recently recorded by Arce et al. (1978). Suzuki (1976) found hyperresponsiveness to exogenously administered ACTH in both simple and nodular hyperplasia and also that the steroid levels correlated with the endogenous ACTH values. Thus, we regard the entity as an ACTH-dependent form of simple hyperplasia with the coincident occurrence of nodules, probably because of vascular changes, with the nodules contributing no more, and possibly even less than the rest of the cortex to the circulating cortisol levels. Nevertheless, several groups have failed to detect ACTH in patients with what has been described as nodular hyperplasia (e.g. Raux et al. 1975). However, a careful review of a further case reported in the literature (Josse et al. 1980), where unilateral 'nodular hyperplasia' was diagnosed histologically in the presence of low plasma ACTH levels, has shown that the data and histology indicate that the correct diagnosis should, in fact, have been an adenoma with for example typical loss of compact cells in the attached gland. This emphasises yet again the necessity for a careful examination of attached and contralateral glands in such cases, and recognition of the histological features of the atrophic gland. It may be that some other reported cases with low ACTH levels were also adenomas and not nodules, although intermittent ACTH secretion in Cushing's disease proper may have resulted in sampling during a trough, emphasising the necessity for serial measurements.

We can therefore find no compelling reason to doubt the original conclusions reached by Neville and Symington (1967) who distinguish histologically between simple and nodular hyperplasia but regard them as different morphological aspects of a single disease process, in the vast majority of cases.

Hyperplasia and the 'Ectopic ACTH' Syndrome

In our own and the reviewed paediatric series, the ectopic ACTH syndrome accounts for about 15–18% of all examples of Cushing's syndrome associated with adrenocortical hyperplasia (Tables 12.3 and 12.4).

In children, where there is an approximately equal sex incidence, the source of the 'ectopic' ACTH is most frequently noted with tumours which are relatively common in this age group e.g. paragangliomas, phaeochromocytomas, neuroblastomas, ganglioneuroblastomas, thymic and islet cell tumours (Kracht 1971). In adults, the commonest source of 'ectopic' ACTH is an oat cell bronchial carcinoma although other tumours including those of the thymus, adrenal medulla, islets of Langerhans, ovary, and carcinoid tumours at various sites may also be implicated (Rees and Ratcliffe 1974).

Gross appearance The adrenal glands in this instance are much enlarged compared with other forms of bilateral hyperplasia, having a mean weight between 14 and 16 g

◁ **Fig. 12.8.** Cushing's syndrome. Bilateral nodular hyperplasia. In gland **A** (21 g) and in gland **B** (12 g), there are large yellow nodules 2 × 1.5 cm (**A**) and 2.5 × 1.5 cm (**B**) at one pole of the gland, compressing the surrounding cortices. Note the numerous smaller nodules especially in gland **B** in the attached cortex which shows the characteristic appearances of bilateral hyperplasia with inner brown and outer yellow layers of approximately equal width. In gland **C** (18 g) the nodule (1.5 cm diameter) on the superior surface of the gland is seen to be composed mainly of clear cells with foci of compact cells. The attached cortex shows diffuse hyperplasia and contains numerous clear-celled micronodules. **Figs. 12.8A and C** reproduced by kind permission of authors and publisher, Neville and Symington 1967. **Fig. 12.8B** reproduced by kind permission of author and publisher, Neville and MacKay 1972. (H + E × 2.5 [**A**]; × 2.5 [**B**]; × 3.8 [**C**])

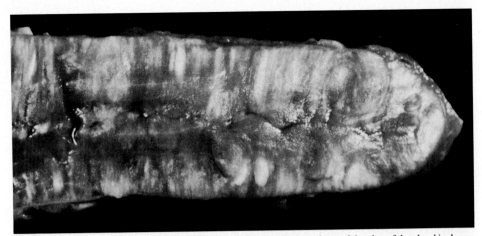

Fig. 12.9. Cushing's syndrome. 'Ectopic ACTH' syndrome. A portion of one of the alae of the gland is shown in which the cortex is broadened. It consists of a wide inner brown zone with brown columns extending out to the capsule between which are foci of yellow tissue. (× 6)

although weights in excess of 20 g are not unusual (Neville and Symington 1967). The cut surface of the greatly broadened cortex (Fig. 12.9) reveals a diffuse brown colour.

Microscopic appearance   Columns of compact cells extend from the medulla up to or almost up to the zona glomerulosa or capsule (Fig. 12.10). Foci of clear cells may remain as isolated islands or be situated subcapsularly, capping the compact-cell columns. Usually the compact and clear cells show hypertrophy and may also exhibit nuclear pleomorphism (Fig. 12.10). These marked cellular features resemble the adrenal changes caused by the preoperative administration of large amounts of 'crude' ACTH preparations (p. 31 and Fig. 4.13) and are consistent with the very high levels of plasma ACTH found in association with some such 'non-endocrine' tumours (~ 10 000 pg/ml, Ratcliffe et al. 1972). The severity of the consequent hypercorticalism often leads to the rapid demise of the patient in these cases, although many cases of ectopic ACTH syndrome show much lower levels of bioactive hormone.

Metastatic deposits of tumour are detected not infrequently in the cortex or medulla.

Congenital and Familial 'Idiopathic' Cushing's Syndrome with Hyperplasia

Infantile Onset

During the past decade, an increasing number of neonates and infants have been diagnosed as having Cushing's syndrome. Whilst the earliest reported cases were due to adrenal tumours, bilateral nodular (or so-called micronodular) hyperplasia has been recognised with increasing frequency as an alternative cause and a number of these patients have now been recorded in which ACTH levels were unexpectedly low or undetectable. Most such cases are detected within the first three months of life (Table 12.5), and seem commoner in females than males. We have personally had the opportunity of seeing three cases of bilateral nodular hyperplasia in infancy (cases 2, 3 and 8, Table 12.5) of which cases 2 and 3 are familial examples. The Cushing's syndrome and adrenal hyperplasia probably commence prenatally. Some cases may be associated with other inherited defects including Albright's disease (Danon et al. 1975) and dysmorphism (cases 2 and 3, Table 12.5).

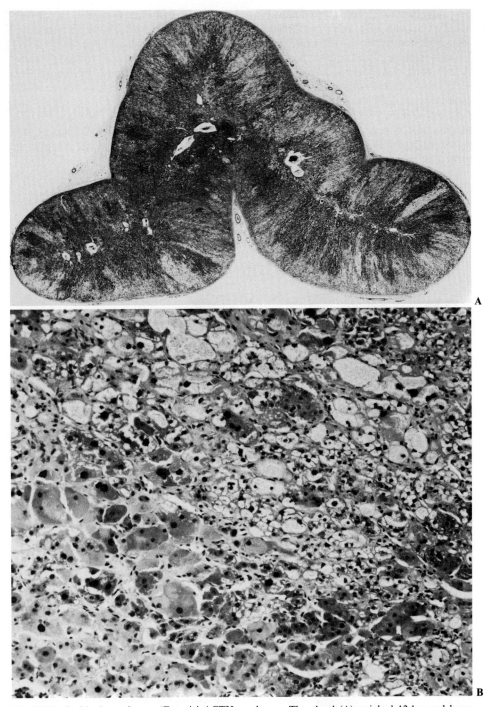

Fig. 12.10. Cushing's syndrome. 'Ectopic' ACTH syndrome. The gland (**A**) weighed 12.1 g and has a rounded outline. The broadened cortex consists of a prominent inner zona reticularis with columns of compact cells extending out reaching the capsule in some areas while in others these columns are capped by clear cells. Many of the clear and compact cells (**B**) in such glands show nuclear and cellular pleomorphism and hypertrophy. (H + E × 6 [**A**]; × 150 [**B**])

Gross appearance   The adrenal glands are enlarged and heavier than normal for their age (Fig. 3.2 and 3.3). Thus, combined weights of between 6 and 9 g have been recorded for glands removed at operation from infants less than 3 months of age (Table 12.5). The adrenals have full, rounded contours and, on section, may be seen to have an outer yellow zone clearly demarcated and separate from an inner broad red/brown area (Fig. 12.11). Numerous small yellow nodular excrescences are readily noted on the outer aspect of the cut surface of these glands.

Microscopic appearance   The outer yellow zone corresponds microscopically to a broadened definitive cortex with small lipid-filled cells with a high nuclear:cytoplasmic ratio arrayed in arched cords (Fig. 12.12).

On its inner aspect, compact lipid-sparse cells may be present forming a diffuse zone

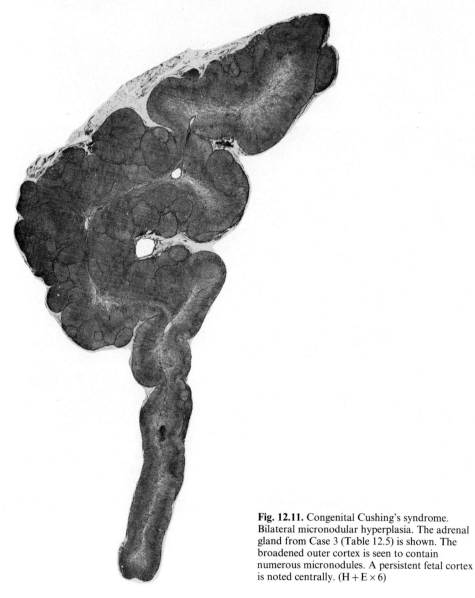

Fig. 12.11. Congenital Cushing's syndrome. Bilateral micronodular hyperplasia. The adrenal gland from Case 3 (Table 12.5) is shown. The broadened outer cortex is seen to contain numerous micronodules. A persistent fetal cortex is noted centrally. (H + E × 6)

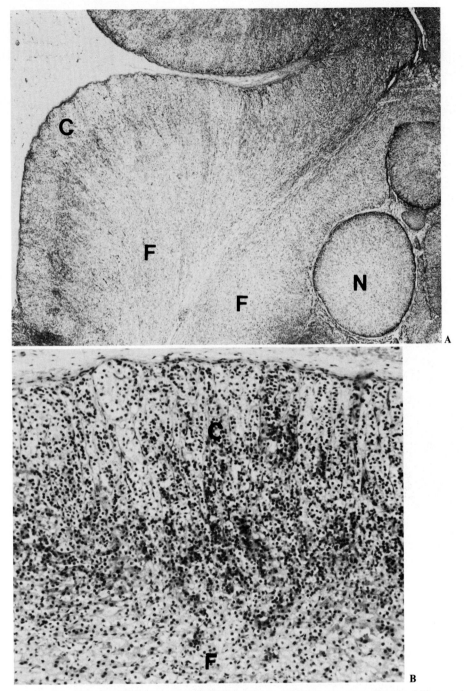

Fig. 12.12. Congenital Cushing's syndrome. Bilateral micronodular hyperplasia. The gland illustrated in Fig. 12.11 is shown at higher magnifications. The outer cortex (C) is broader than normal (**A**) and may be seen to consist of lipid-laden cells towards the periphery, with compact cells on its inner aspect (**B**). Compact cell columns extend out toward the capsule (**A**). The fetal cortex (F) is present and is seen to occur together with the outer zone cells in the nodules (N). A small nodule is also seen on the outermost aspect of the cortex. (H + E × 15 [**A**]; × 175 [**B**])

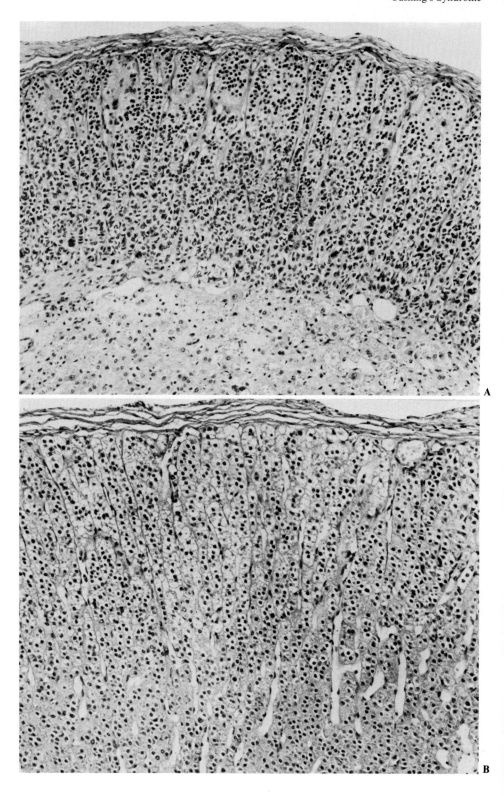

A

B

or arranged in columns which extend out towards the capsule (Figs. 12.12 and 12.13). The outer cortex, thus, is similar to that of the normal neonate except for increased cellularity (breadth) and the presence of compact cells.

However, the inner dark red/brown zone corresponds to a persistent fetal zone which shows only minimal, and in most areas, no evidence of involution even when examined ultrastructurally (Fig. 12.14). It is the persistence of this zone (e.g. Klevit et al. 1966) which presumably accounts for the high levels of Δ^5-steroids detected in such cases (Donaldson et al. 1981). Cytomegaly, pleomorphism and cellular hypertrophy were not observed in any of our cases.

The nodules consist usually of both outer and inner cortical tissue (Fig. 12.12) and thus represent extrusions rather than true nodules. Small intracortical nodules of outer zone cells can also be noted (Fig. 12.12).

Aetiology As this lesion is bilateral and involves an increase in cortical growth with folding of the cortex to form nodular extrusions it would not be unreasonable to assume that increased ACTH secretion was involved. However, when plasma levels have been assayed, they have been found to be low or undetectable (Danon et al. 1975; Donaldson et al. 1981). This, together with other in vivo functional tests, has led to the suggestion that such lesions may possess functional autonomy. However, our tissue culture studies on one such case (3; Table 12.5) have shown that the cells can respond to ACTH, as indeed they do in vivo (Danon et al. 1975), and that they produce cortisol in amounts similar (on a per cell basis) to normal adult adrenal cells without evidence of hyperresponsiveness to the hormone. Neither enzyme defects nor inappropriate responses to other trophic hormones such as FSH, LH, TSH and prolactin seem able to account for the high dexamethasone non-suppressible C_{21} and C_{19} steroid production. Although no pituitary abnormalities have been recorded in those cases coming to autopsy, it is possible that the primary cause may be extra-adrenal. In the case examined, however, the patient's serum did not stimulate steroidogenesis by normal human adrenal cells. The aetiology of this condition must therefore remain an enigma for the present. It does, however, seem to be a disorder of cortical growth rather than function (p. 99).

Pubertal/Adult Onset

Several late-onset cases of bilateral micronodular hyperplasia have also been recorded (Meador et al. 1967; Ruder et al. 1974; Arce et al. 1978; Schweizer-Cagianut et al. 1980; Table 12.5); their aetiological relationship to the cases described in infancy is uncertain, but some are also familial (Schweizer-Cagianut et al. 1980). Early cases of this type have been reviewed by Meador et al. (1967). Some have been associated with depressed plasma ACTH levels (Arce et al. 1978), so that functional autonomy has again been proposed (Meador et al. 1967) and some of these patients seem unresponsive or hyporesponsive to exogenous ACTH. Their morphological features are different to those of nodular hyperplasia with CAH. Thus, intraglandular nodules are often composed of hypertrophied compact cells (Meador et al. 1967; Arce et al. 1978) and are associated with myelolipomatous changes in some cases (Schweizer-Cagianut et al. 1980). Atrophy of the attached cortex is stated not to be present. Such

---

◁ **Fig. 12.13.** Congenital Cushing's syndrome. Bilateral micronodular hyperplasia. These are illustrations of the glands removed from Case 8 (Table 12.5). The outer zone is broadened and has a diffuse inner compact cell area (**B**) although in other parts it is of normal width and contains only clear lipid-laden type cells (**A**). The fetal cortex is still present in this 3-month-old gland. (H + E × 90 [**A** and **B**])

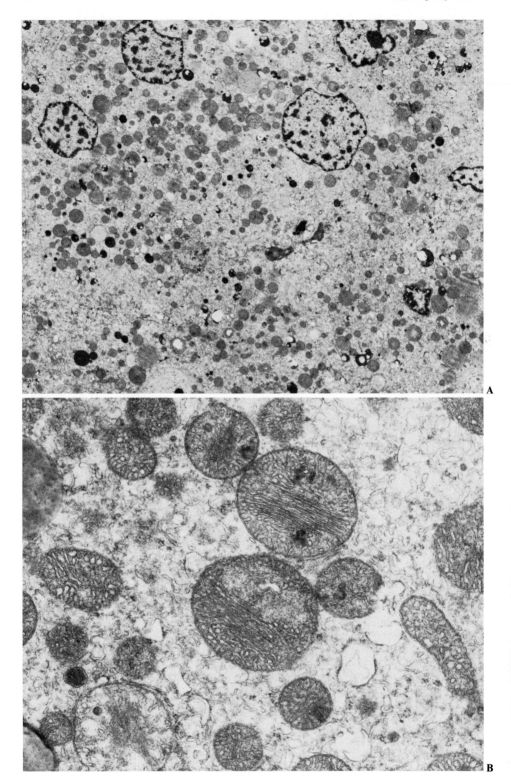

features are very reminiscent of the effects of ACTH as seen in the 'ectopic ACTH' syndrome.

Further study of such cases with particular respect to the possibility of abnormal forms of non-dexamethasone-suppressible ACTH being produced might be helpful. In some cases (e.g. Schweizer-Cagianut et al. 1980) lymphocytic infiltration has been observed. While the obvious explanation of their presence is myelolipomatous change (p. 290) it is worth bearing in mind the possibility that autoimmune stimulation of the adrenal cortex may conceivably occur in some instances in a manner analogous to Graves disease, and such a condition would simulate 'idiopathic' Cushing's syndrome with low ACTH. Antiadrenal auto-antibodies have, for example, been detected in Cushing's syndrome in some instances (Andrada et al. 1979), with in one case (Wegienka et al. 1966) lymphocytic infiltration and hyperplasia.

Adrenocortical Tumours

Adrenocortical tumours account for about one quarter of all cases of Cushing's syndrome (Table 12.1). The incidence of tumours, especially carcinomas, is higher in children (Table 12.2) particularly girls. In our own series, which consists predominantly of adults and part of which has been published previously (Neville and Symington 1967) (Table 12.3), both adenomas and carcinomas occur more frequently in females and are particularly prevalent between the ages of 30 and 60 years (Tables 12.6, 12.7, 12.8). Adenomas are generally associated with the 'pure' form of the syndrome in adults. On occasion, especially in children, there may, however, also be

Table 12.6. Age, sex and site incidence of adrenal tumours in Cushing's syndrome (Personal series)

	Adenoma	Carcinoma
Age (years)[a]		
0–10	1	2
11–30	2	3
31–50	17	9
51–60	1	4
61–70	1	–
Sex (M:F)	7:19	2:16
Site (L:R adrenal)	12:9[b]	7:6[c]

[a]Not stated in four cases, only adult.
[b]Not stated in five cases.
[c]Not stated in five cases.

virilism (Stewart et al. 1974). Carcinomas on the other hand in addition to stigmata of hypercorticalism are frequently associated with degrees of virilism and hypertension not found in hyperplasia causing Cushing's disease. There does not appear to be a side predilection (Table 12.8). In young children, adrenocortical carcinomas are sometimes associated with other anomalies or neoplasms (p. 116).

◁ **Fig. 12.14.** Congenital Cushing's syndrome. The ultrastructure of the fetal zone in the gland illustrated in Fig. 12.11 and 12.12. The cells in this zone show no evidence of involution at 10 weeks of age (**A**) and a higher power (**B**) show typical features of this zone in the fetus, viz.: large mitochondria with prominent, mainly tubulo-vesicular cristae, and extensive smooth endoplasmic reticulum and few liposomes. (**A** × 3500; **B** × 27 000)

Table 12.7. Personal series of adrenocortical adenomas in Cushing's syndrome

Case no.	Age (yrs)	Sex	Side	Weights (g)
1	5	M	L	33
2	37	F	L	24
3	39	F	R	10
4	40	F	L	18
5	Adult	F	–	35
6	Adult	F	L	15
7	31	M	L	250
8	Adult	F	–	71
9	35	F	L	13
10	46	F	L	24
11	15	F	–	5
12	36	M	L	13[a]
13	34	M	–	–
14	54	F	R	–
15	32	F	R	5
16	42	F	L	–
17	49	F	L	48
18	38	F	R	7
19	62	F	R	66
20	50	F	R	–
21	39	M	L	10[a]
22	40	F	R	14[a]
23	31	F	–	5[a]
24	24	M	R	9
25	Adult	M	L	15
26	39	M	R	37

[a]Black adenomas.

Table 12.8. Personal series of adrenocortical carcinomas in Cushing's syndrome

Case no.	Age (yr)	Sex	Side	Weights (g)
1	15	F	R	139
2	19	M	R	–
3	29	F	L	4040
4	49	F	R	386
5	55	F	R	125
6	58	F	L	1250
7	59	F	L	3000
8	32	F	L	420
9	42	F	R	1143
10	1	M	–	165
11	35	F	–	119
12	59	F	–	230
13	50	F	L	170
14	48	F	L	90
15	34	F	R	650
16	35	F	–	67
17	52	F	–	Massive
18	9	F	L	270

Adenomas

The benign adrenocortical tumour associated with Cushing's syndrome is, in the main, a highly characteristic unilateral lesion. Bilateral examples have only rarely been recorded (Loridan and Senior 1969). If bilateral or multiple, one should consider carefully whether the lesions are examples of nodular hyperplasia rather than neoplasia. The appearance of the attached gland is the clue to the correct diagnosis (p. 152).

Gross appearance   Generally, they are small, circumscribed, rounded and apparently encapsulated growths with a yellow cut surface in which dark red or brown foci may be noted (Plate A, facing p. 146). Necrosis and haemorrhage are uncommon except in larger lesions. Very rarely, the cut surface presents a homogeneous dark brown to black appearance (the so-called 'black adenoma') (Plate A). This was noted in four of our cases (cases 12, 21, 22 and 23, Table 12.7). The presence of microscopic lipofucsin does not justify the inclusion of a tumour in this category unless the colour of the cut surface is correspondingly dark (Plate A).

The weights of adenomas at surgery tend to be < 50 g and often < 30 g (Table 12.7). It is rare to find an adenoma weighing > 70 g although we have seen one tumour of 250 g which has subsequently pursued a benign course (case 7, Table 12.7).

Microscopic appearance   On microscopic examination, a tenuous capsule surrounds the lesion. The yellow areas visible macroscopically correspond to lipid-laden clear cells, morphologically similar to the cells of the zona fasciculata of the normal adrenal cortex (Fig. 12.15). The brown areas consist of compact cells with eosinophilic lipid-poor granular cytoplasm and are similar to the cells of the zona reticularis of the normal adrenal cortex. The relative proportion of clear and compact cells varies from one tumour to another and between different areas of one tumour. Usually clear cells predominate but compact cells as the sole component can be found (vide infra). The tumour cells are arranged in small cords or alveoli. Nuclear or cellular pleomorphism is generally uncommon, but may be evident focally (Fig. 12.15). The associated and contralateral adrenal cortex associated with adenomas is always atrophic (Fig. 12.26).

Ultrastructurally, these small adenomas contain clear and compact cells which, in general, show similar features to their normal cellular counterparts (MacKay 1969; Tannenbaum 1973; O'Hare et al. 1979). Although there is considerable variation in the structure and proportion of different organelles, characteristic features such as mitochondria with fasciculata-like or reticularis-like internal structure (i.e. vesicular and tubulo-vesicular cristae), discrete stacks or short strands of rough endoplasmic reticulum and extensively developed SER are commonly present (Figs. 12.16 and 12.17). Junctional complexes are rare.

Black adenomas associated with Cushing's syndrome present a different pattern and consist exclusively, or almost so, of compact eosinophilic lipid-sparse cells similar to those of the zona reticularis. In the cytoplasm, abundant lipofuscin granules are present (Fig. 12.18). Ultrastructurally their abundant cytoplasm contains only small amounts of RER, extensively developed SER, many lipofuscin granules and mitochondria with occasional vesicular cristae (Bahu et al. 1974; Kovacs et al. 1976). Only four such tumours have been recorded previously (Symington 1969; Bahu et al. 1974; Visser et al. 1974; Kovacs et al. 1976). Together with our own present four cases, they have all behaved in a benign fashion with complete regression of the Cushing's syndrome after removal.

True black adenomas (i.e. tumours) are, however, not unique to Cushing's syndrome and can cause other forms of hypercorticalism such as hyperaldosteronism

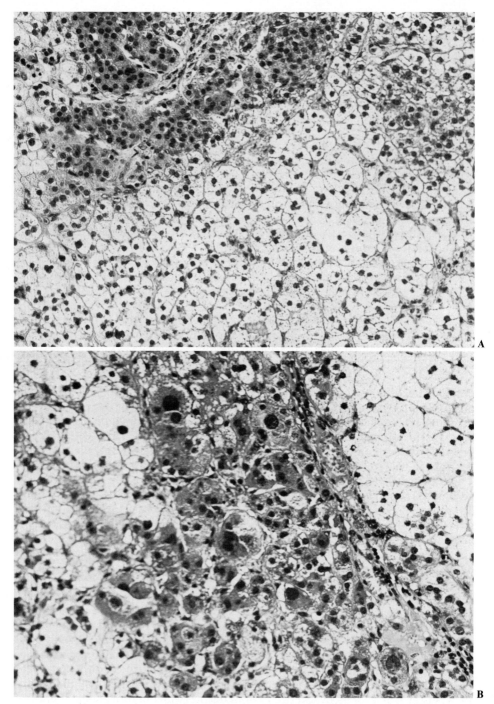

Fig. 12.15. Cushing's syndrome. Adrenocortical adenoma. The tumour shown in (**A**) weighed 5 g and was removed from a 15-year-old girl. It consists predominantly of clear cells of the zona fasciculata-type arranged in cords interspersed with foci of compact zona reticularis-type cells. Little pleomorphism is present whereas the tumour (**B**), removed from a 39-year-old woman and weighing 10 g, shows, in some areas, prominent nuclear and cellular pleomorphism. (H + E × 240 [**A** and **B**])

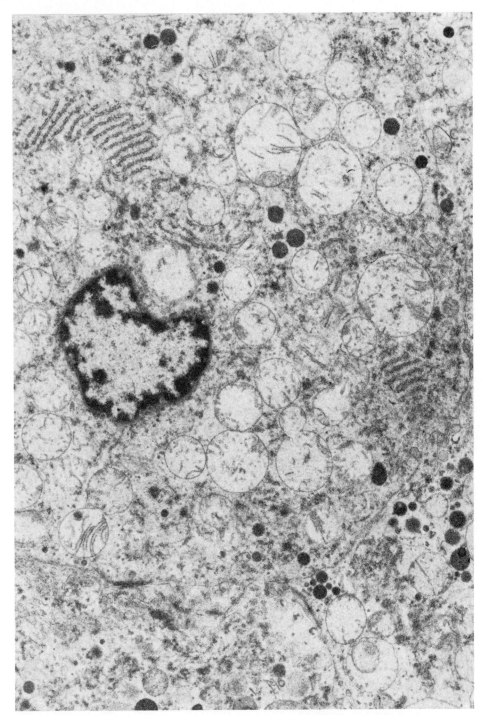

Fig. 12.16. Ultrastructure of typical compact cells from a 15 g adenoma causing Cushing's syndrome. The mitochondria are relatively rarified with a few lamellar or tubulo-lamellar cristae. Stacks of RER are prominent as are microbodies (lipofuscin granules); occasional desmosomes can be seen (cf. Fig. 4.10). (× 10 500)

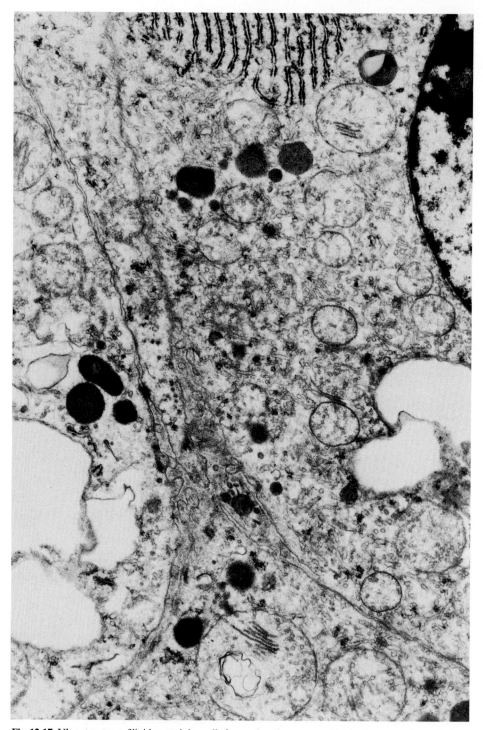

Fig. 12.17. Ultrastructure of lipid-containing cells from a 5 g adenoma causing Cushing's syndrome showing extensive smooth endoplasmic reticulum and mitochondria with tubulo-vesicular cristae (cf. Fig. 12.16 and see also Kano and Sato 1977). (× 21 000)

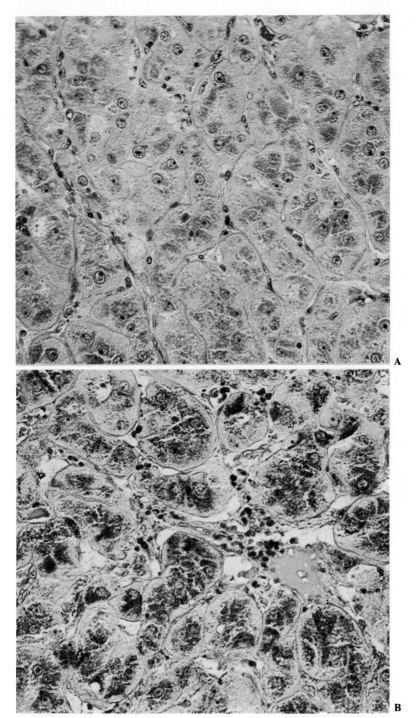

Fig. 12.18. Cushing's syndrome. Adrenocortical 'black' adenoma (15 g). The 'black' adenoma, one of four that we have seen (Table 12.7) was removed from a 39-year-old man. It contained only compact-type cells in which abundant lipofuscin granules are present (**A**). These granules can be made to appear more prominent by the use of a Giemsa stain (**B**). (H + E × 380 [**A**]; Giemsa × 380 [**B**])

or virilisation (p. 211). Occasionally, nodules may present a diffuse brown colour but without evidence of cortical hyperfunction (p. 60). Such nodules appear to evolve in the same way as do the commoner clear cell-containing yellow nodules so frequent in autopsy glands. The appearance of the attached cortex will give the clue to its identity and enable distinction from a black adenoma to be made.

Spontaneous remission of Cushing's syndrome in association with adrenal adenomas has been recorded (Øvlisen and Anderson 1966; Blau et al. 1975). In one case, the tumour was calcified; in the other, the adenoma appeared normal without haemorrhage or infarction. In this latter case, periodic hormonogenesis, which has been reported in association with adrenal adenomas causing Cushing's syndrome (as well as other endocrine or paraendocrine tumours) (Bailey 1971; Brown et al. 1973; Green and Van't Hoff 1975), may have been responsible for the temporary remission of the disease.

Carcinomas

Adrenocortical carcinomas causing Cushing's syndrome tend to be large lesions, most weighing in excess of 100 g. This may be related on a per cell basis to their relatively ineffective production of cortisol (p. 199). However, not all carcinomas are large (cases 14 and 16; Table 12.8) so that weight alone cannot be used rigidly to assist in the differentiation of benign and malignant lesions.

Gross appearance   Carcinomas tend to affect the right more often than the left gland for reasons that remain obscure, and are usually encapsulated, soft in consistency, often with a pink lobulated cut surface although yellow areas may be seen (Plate B, facing p. 147). Areas of necrosis, haemorrhage, cystic change and calcification are not uncommon and increase in frequency as the lesions rise in size and weight. In larger tumours, there may be obvious macroscopic evidence of capsular penetration with infiltration of the related neighbouring tissues including the ipsilateral adrenal, kidney, liver, diaphragm and venous system. Satellite tumour nodules may be also be present.

Microscopic appearance   Typically the larger carcinomas consist solely of compact-type cells with eosinophilic, granular, lipid-poor cytoplasm, grouped in large alveoli, sheets or trabeculae separated by a fine fibrovascular stroma (Fig. 12.19); in some cases viable tumour cells form cords or tubules surrounding vessels in carcinomas (Fig. 12.19). Characteristically, the tumour cells exhibit pleomorphism and marked nuclear vesicularity (Fig. 12.20) with one or more prominent nucleoli. They often form diffuse sheets in which cell cohesion is poor. Extensive areas of necrosis may be present. In rare instances, and particularly the smaller tumours, the cells and nuclei may be relatively uniform in size. However, the latter tend to be larger and more vesicular than normal (Fig 12.21). Smaller carcinomas may contain foci of lipid-laden clear cells (Fig. 12.20), although such appearances are uncommon and disappear with increasing size and weight.

Bizarre and giant cellular forms may be present in some lesions while others exhibit little nuclear atypicality (Fig. 12.21); occasionally the same tumours may show contiguous areas with markedly different appearances (Fig. 12.22). Vascular invasion through the walls of blood vessels is uncommon, although tumour cells may be observed within vessels or thrombi containing cells may be present in the tumour sinusoids or main adrenal vein.

Metastases when they evolve are generally detected in the draining lymph nodes, mediastinal nodes, bones, contralateral adrenal gland and particularly the lungs and liver (Bennett et al. 1971) (Fig. 12.23).

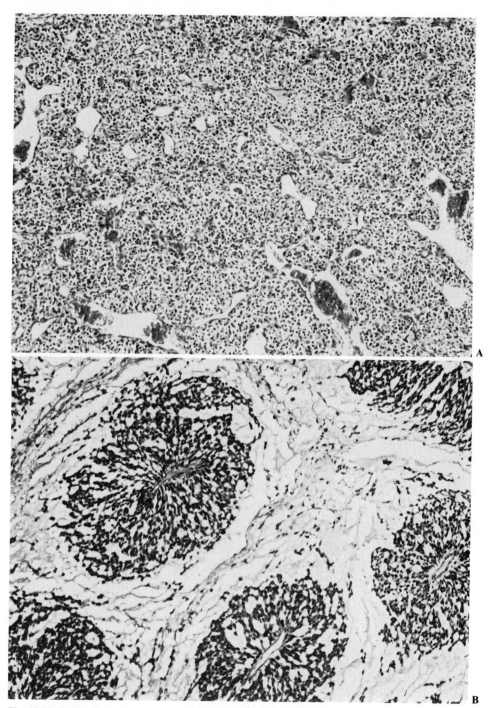

Fig. 12.19. Cushing's syndrome. Adrenocortical carcinoma. Two different cellular patterns which may be found in adrenocortical carcinomas are illustrated. In **A**, a tumour which weighed 71 g, the cells form broad trabeculae and sheets punctuated by numerous vascular sinusoids whereas in **B**, the cells form cords or tubules which surround blood vessels and between which are areas of necrosis and oedematous fibrovascular tissue. (H + E × 100 [**A**]; × 100 [**B**])

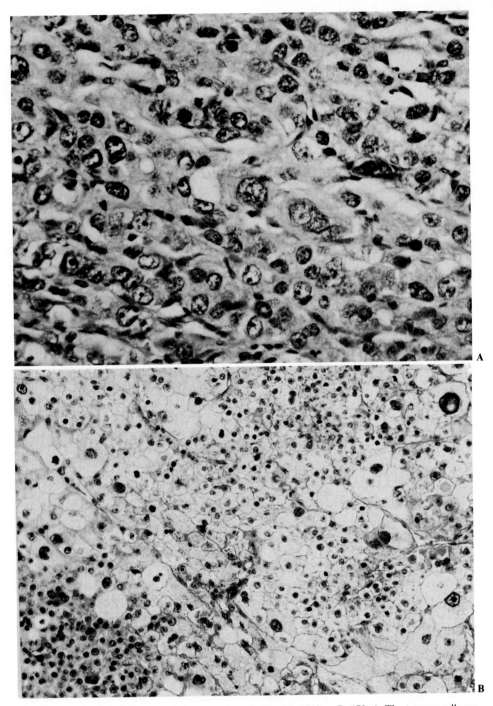

Fig. 12.20. Cushing's syndrome. Adrenocortical carcinoma (**A**, 1250 g; **B**, 170 g). The tumour cells are usually enlarged and compact in type (**A**) with eosinophilic lipid-sparse cytoplasm. The nuclei are characteristically pleomorphic and vesicular with one or more prominent nucleoli. Mitotic activity may or may not be obvious. In some small lesions foci may be present of enlarged lipid-laden cells (**B**) which often show marked nuclear and cellular pleomorphism. (H + E × 350 [**A**]; × 240 [**B**])

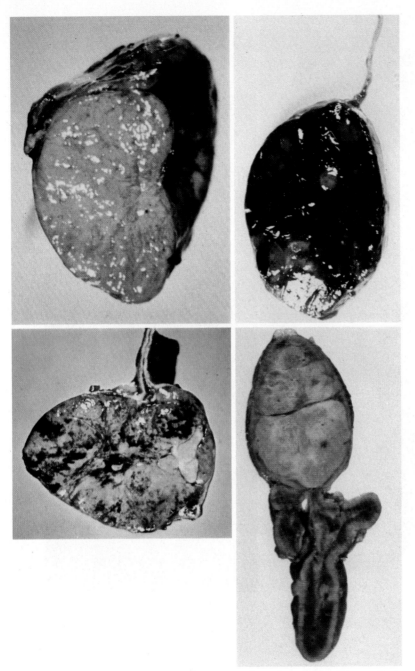

Plate A. The characteristic golden yellow cut surface of a small adenoma (5 g) causing hyper-aldosteronism with low plasma renin (Conn's syndrome) is shown (*above left*). The compressed cortex is seen attached at one side. Below (*left*) is a classical 20 g adenoma which caused Cushing's syndrome with its typical yellow-coloured cut surface in which brown foci may be noted. The attached cortex is thinned and atrophic. Below (*right*) for comparison is an example of bilateral nodular hyperplasia (21 g) with a 2.0 × 1.5 cm nodule. Note the attached cortex is hyperplastic, broader than usual and with a prominent inner brown zone. Above (*right*) is a 'black' adenoma (10 g) which caused Cushing's syndrome. Again note the atrophic attached cortex.

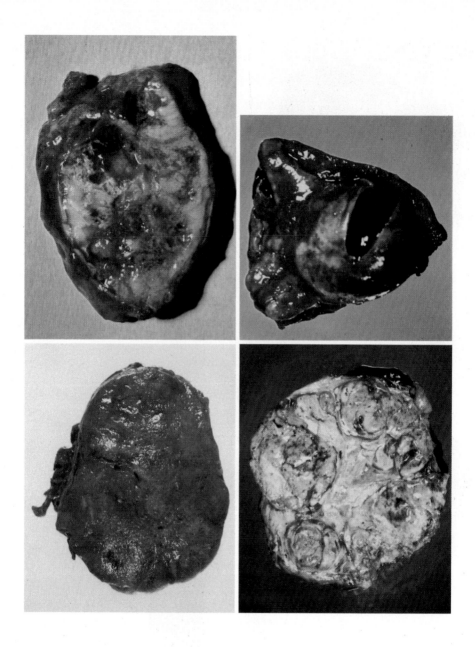

Plate B. Below (*left*) is a 228 g virilising adenoma removed from an eight-year-old boy. The cut surface is homogeneous and brown in colour. Above (*right*) is a 4 g virilising adenoma where the cut surface is darker. In contrast are two carcinomas, the one on the left caused Cushing's syndrome and weighed approximately 90 g. The one on the right was a non-hormonal tumour weighing 700 g, both show areas of haemorrhage and necrosis.

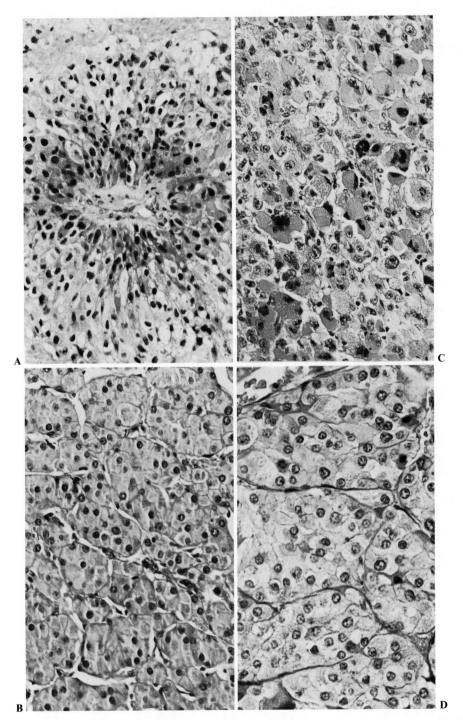

Fig. 12.21. Cushing's syndrome. Adrenocortical carcinoma (**A**, 170 g; **B**, 230 g; **C**, 1143 g and **D**, 386 g). Various different cellular patterns together with cell types, degrees of nuclear and cellular pleomorphism and atypia are illustrated. Note in **A** the large area of necrosis at the top with viable cells only around the blood vessel. (H + E × 150 [**A**]; × 240 [**B**]; × 180 [**C**]; × 240 [**D**])

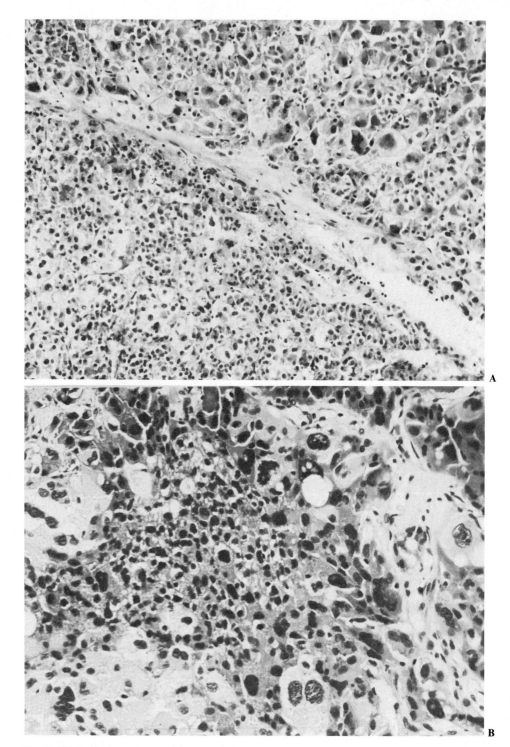

Fig. 12.22. Cushing's syndrome. Adrenocortical carcinoma (**A**, 71 g; **B**, 92 g). Both these rather small malignant tumours exhibit markedly different appearances in contiguous areas. (H + E × 180 [**A**]; × 240 [**B**])

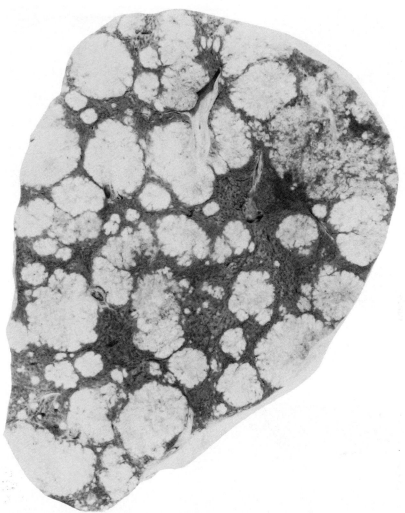

Fig. 12.23. Cushing's syndrome. Hepatic metastases. Numerous irregularly rounded metastatic foci from a primary adrenocortical carcinoma are illustrated. (× 0.5)

Ultrastructure   Ultrastructural features of functioning adrenocortical carcinomas, including those associated with Cushing's syndrome, include most of the characteristics of the normal steroid-secreting cell represented in individual tumours to varying degrees. Thus, they may contain abundant mitochondria, with or without overtly specialised internal structure, and extensive SER in many cases, either organised in the form of lamellae or showing a disorganised tubulo-saccular appearance (Fig. 12.24), or it may be poorly developed (MacKay 1969). Complex interdigitating processes between adjacent cells and microvilli have been reported as common in carcinomas (Tannenbaum 1973) and we have seen them in some examples that we have recently studied (Fig. 12.25). There may also be marked variability in the distribution of organelles in different cells of the tumour (Theile 1974).
     The question may be posed whether ultrastructural studies provide additional discriminants to assist in the diagnosis of benign and malignant tumours, in addition to

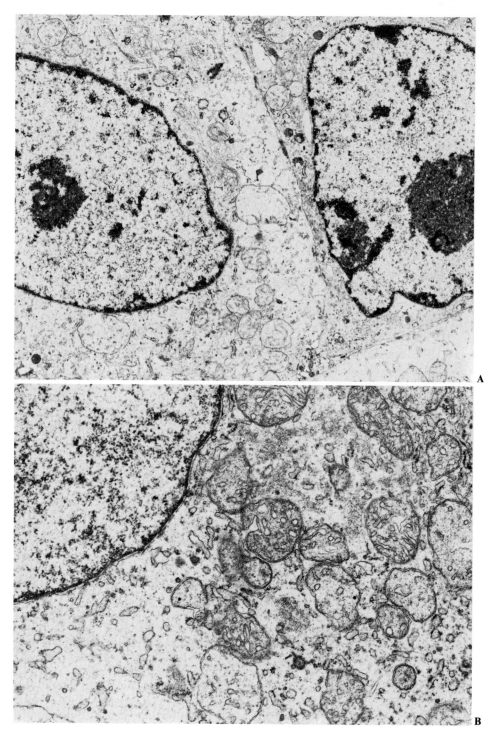

Fig. 12.24. Ultrastructure of a 650 g carcinoma causing Cushing's syndrome. The light-microscopical appearance of this lesion is illustrated in Fig. 15.11. Some disorganisation of cytoplasmic organelles is notable but mitochondria show typical steroidogenic features (**B**). (**A** × 9900; **B** × 21 000)

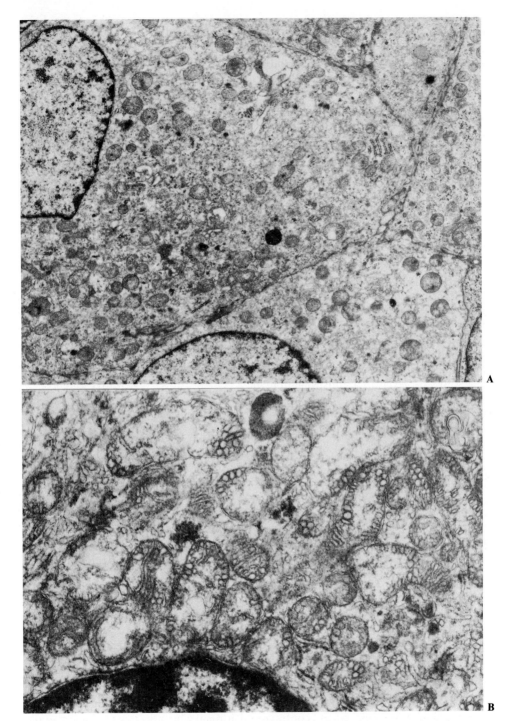

Fig. 12.25. Ultrastructure of a 92 g carcinoma causing Cushing's syndrome with virilisation. Note the well organised cells with extensive interdigitations of the adjacent cell membranes (**A**). At higher power (**B**) the mitochondria show well developed tubulo-vesicular cristae. The relatively regular appearance of this tumour at the ultrastructural level did not indicate its aggressively malignant nature. (**A** × 7500; **B** × 27 400)

features of gross cellular pleomorphism and nuclear atypia visible at the light microscopical level. Both MacKay (1969) and Tannenbaum (1973) suggest that disruption of basement membrane material around the tumour cells may provide one such discriminant. Such basement membrane material does not, however, enclose each individual cortical cell, but merely outlines large clusters thereof. It is our experience that under these circumstances the extent to which it is truly disorganised is extremely difficult to judge without examining many low-power fields (Tannenbaum 1973). We doubt, therefore, whether such criteria can usefully be applied to the 'borderline' lesions of 50–150 g weight where histological discriminants may be ambiguous.

Mitschke et al. (1973) have studied 4 adenomas and 1 carcinoma associated with Cushing's syndrome at the EM level; they concluded that only differences in degree existed between the two types of tumour, a conclusion with which we would concur. Some carcinomas undoubtedly show highly differentiated organelles (Fig. 12.25), and whilst some degree of progressive disorganisation and loss of specialisation may be encountered in the larger examples, smaller tumours of this type may present a highly organised structure, indeed more so than some adenomas (Fig. 12.17). Such specialised features may enable metastatic deposits to be identified as steroidogenic in type (Gyorkey et al. 1975).

Our experience of ultrastructural studies of smaller 'borderline' tumours is that no unique EM features enable the distinction between benign and malignant to be made with confidence. Likewise, the nature of the syndrome of hormone excess cannot be reliably deduced from ultrastructural (or for that matter light microscopical) criteria.

There is, thus, a wide spectrum of cellular change in tumours proved subsequently to be carcinomas by their ability to metastasise. The usual histological criteria of malignancy (mitoses, vascular and capsular invasion) are, however, frequently absent and some can occur in lesions which pursue a benign course. A tentative diagnosis is possible if large areas of necrosis are present and if enlarged, vesicular pleomorphic nuclei with one or more prominent nucleoli are noted (Figs. 12.20 and 12.21). However, additional criteria are undoubtedly needed to assist the histologist in determining the prognosis.

As mentioned before, weight can be a helpful, but not absolute, criterion. Thus, Schteingart et al. (1968) found that malignant tumours causing Cushing's syndrome weighed >100 g while benign tumours were <27 g. King and Lack (1979), on the other hand, found benign tumours weighing up to 155 g. In our own series most benign tumours were <70 g although there were occasional exceptions (Tables 12.7 and 12.8), while most malignant tumours weighed >100 g. With this significant overlap and the frequent absence of definitive histological and ultrastructural criteria, we have examined the functional characteristics of various neoplasms in vitro and the results and diagnostic significance of these studies is discussed later (p. 186).

The range of cellular appearances of carcinomas causing Cushing's syndrome are, in our experience, indistinguishable from carcinomas causing other forms of hyper-corticalism such as the adrenogenital syndrome and from so-called non-functioning carcinomas.

The Attached and Contralateral Adrenal Gland

The histological distinction of each entity may, however, be reached by histological examination of the attached and contralateral adrenal when this is available for study. The attached and contralateral adrenal cortex found with benign and malignant functioning adrenal tumours in Cushing's syndrome is always small and atrophic. The cortex consists of clear cells only and is surrounded by a thickened oedematous capsule

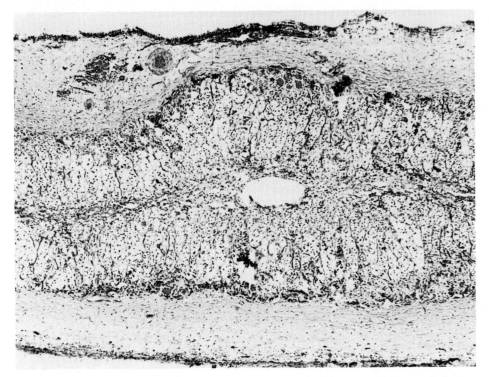

Fig. 12.26. Tumorous Cushing's syndrome. Attached or contralateral adrenal gland. The adrenal cortex is atrophic, narrower than normal and is surrounded by a thickened oedematous capsule. The cortex is composed solely of clear cells of the zona fasciculata-type typical of steroid-induced atrophy. Reproduced by kind permission of the authors and publisher, Neville and Symington 1967. (H + E × 50)

(Fig. 12.26). Occasionally zona glomerulosa cells are noted between the clear cells and the capsule. This is the appearance expected in view of the generally undetectable or very low levels of peripheral plasma ACTH (<10 pg/ml) resulting from the excessive neoplastic production of cortisol. These atrophic changes are a most important guide to the diagnosis of corticosteroid-secreting neoplasms and we would reiterate that they are the only reliable means of distinguishing between certain cases of nodular hyperplasia and true tumours (Figs. 12.8 and 12.15).

Prognosis

Untreated Cushing's disease carries a high mortality. Following diagnosis and treatment by total ablation of the adrenal glands, total hypophysectomy or removal of pituitary microadenomas, or more rarely by medical adrenalectomy effected by aminoglutethimide or o,p′-DDD, steroid replacement therapy will maintain most patients with erstwhile Cushing's disease more or less indefinitely (Welbourn et al. 1971). In a minority of cases ($<10\%$) treated by adrenalectomy there is progressive sellar enlargement and high levels of circulating ACTH, followed by intense cutaneous pigmentation. This is Nelson's syndrome (Nelson et al. 1960) and while most pituitary tumours found in this condition are of the benign variety, occasional carcinomas have been described, and in all cases hypophysectomy is ultimately required to preserve optic nerve function. Steroid replacement therapy in treated Cushing's disease will restore most normal physiological functions, although osteoporosis is seldom reversed. In the 'ectopic ACTH' syndrome adrenalectomy is of only palliative value.

With benign cortical neoplasms causing Cushing's syndrome surgical removal will effect complete cure. Temporary hypocortisolism ensues, however, and replacement therapy may be required initially, to be tapered off when the erstwhile quiescent contralateral normal gland has re-established normal pituitary-adrenal relationships. In malignant tumours, survival is seldom prolonged beyond three years, even when 'complete' removal of the primary lesion is feasible. Even in relatively recent cases overall survival rates of 13 % at five years have been reported, and although staging has been attempted (Bradley 1975), the overall prognosis is pessimistic. Carcinomas with signs of Cushing's syndrome seem particularly aggressive and the number of authenticated cures remains very small (Lipsett et al. 1963; Hutter and Kayhoe 1966a).

In addition to the classical symptoms of hypercorticalism, some adrenocortical tumours have been noted to cause a form of paroxysmal hypoglycaemia that is also associated with a variety of other unrelated abdominal malignancies (Kahn 1980). In one case a non-suppressible insulin-like activity (NSILA) was extracted from such an adrenal tumour (Hyodo et al. 1977); it is not known, however, whether it represents the cause of such symptoms in all cases, or indeed whether it reflects a capability of normal human adrenocortical cells to synthesise and secrete such peptides, in addition to their normal repertoire of steroid hormones. Alternatively, the hypoglycaemia may stem from imbalance in catabolic and anabolic steroid levels (Eymontt et al. 1965).

Chapter 13

The Adrenogenital Syndrome and Related Conditions

The adrenogenital syndrome is associated with abnormal levels of circulating sex steroid hormones and encompasses all cases of sexual precocity and heterosexual abnormalities due to adrenocortical dysfunction. The adrenal changes may take the form of congenital adrenocortical hyperplasia or neoplasia, both benign and malignant.

Incidence In our own series, the adrenogenital syndrome accounted for only 12% of all examples of hypercorticalism examined histologically (Table 11.1). In terms of clinical incidence this figure is too low and is due to the fact that its commonest cause, congenital adrenocortical hyperplasia, is now readily diagnosed and effectively treated by steroid therapy, and such cases seldom present in a pathological practice. Tumours causing the disease are most often detected before the age of twelve years (Symington 1969; Benaily et al. 1975).

Congenital Adrenocortical Hyperplasia (CAH)

Congenital adrenocortical hyperplasia is the most important cause of the adrenogenital syndrome in infancy and childhood (see New and Levine 1973 and Mininberg et al. 1979 for reviews) and in one form or another it appears in about one in 80 000 live births (Childs et al. 1956), although regional differences exist with about one in 5000 infants affected in Switzerland (Prader 1958), and one in 500 in Eskimos (Hirschfeld and Fleshman 1969). The frequency of the disease is the same in both sexes. It may also, rarely, become manifest during adult life (Riddick and Hammond 1975; Blankstein et al. 1980b) and may be expressed in varying degrees of severity (Migeon et al. 1980). It is a classic example of an 'inborn error of metabolism'; the clinical manifestations of most examples being due to hereditary defects in the biosynthesis of cortisol, resulting in increased levels of ACTH secretion and consequent hyperplasia of the gland, often with the production of excessive quantities of other adrenal steroids.

CAH With Virilism

Three enzyme defects may be associated with virilism or sexual ambiguity, a loss of 21-hydroxylase, less commonly reduced 11β-hydroxylase activity, and, even more rarely, deficient Δ^5-3β-hydroxysteroid dehydrogenase-isomerase, in which a more limited degree of virilisation may be noted (Table 13.1).

Table 13.1. Clinical and laboratory features of various forms of congenital adrenal hyperplasia*

Enzyme deficiency	Clinical features					Laboratory features				
	Newborn with sexual ambiguity		Salt wasting	Hyper-tension	Postnatal virili-sation	Urinary excretion				Plasma
	Female	Male				17-Ketosteroids	17-Hydroxy-steroids	Pregnane-triol	Aldo-sterone	Testosterone
1) 21-Hydroxylase										
w/o salt loss	+	0	0	0	+	↑↑	N or ↓	↑↑	N	↑
with salt loss	+	0	+	0	+	↑↑	↓[c]	↑↑	↓→	↑
2) 11β-Hydroxylase	+	0	0	+	+	↑[b]	↑↑	↑↑	↓→	↑
3) Δ5-3β-HSD-I[a]	+	+	+	0	0	↑↓	↑↑	↑	↓→	↑
4) 17-Hydroxylase	0	+	0	+	0	↓↓	↓↓	↓↓	↓→	↓↓
5) Cholesterol side-chain cleavage	0	+	+	0	0	↓↓	↓↓	↓↓	↓↓	↓↓
6) Corticosterone methyl oxidase type I	0	0	+	0	0	N	N	N	↓↓	—
7) Corticosterone methyl oxidase type II	0	0	+	0	0	N	↑[d]	N	↓→	—

*From the data of New and Levine (1973) by permission.
N = Normal.
[a] The values presented apply to the infant and very young child.
[b] Mostly Δ5-17-ketosteroids.
[c] Mostly THS.
[d] Largely 18-hydroxy THA, which gives a Porter-Silber reaction.

21-Hydroxylase Deficiency

This is the commonest enzyme defect associated with CAH, accounting in its several clinical forms for about 90% of all recorded examples (see Migeon 1980 for review).

21-Hydroxylase defect, which is partial in nature in ~70% of cases, results in a lowered cortisol output (Fig. 13.1). Because of the negative feedback system, increased

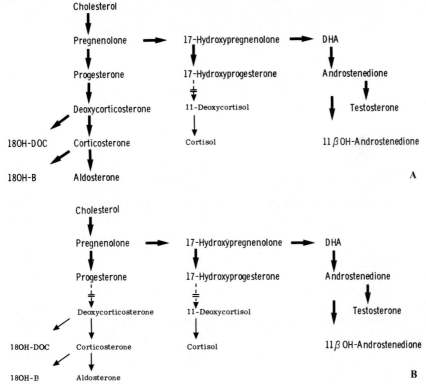

Fig. 13.1. Congenital adrenocortical hyperplasia. Pathways of steroidogenesis in 21-hydroxylase deficiency associated with (**A**) simple virilism and (**B**) virilism with salt loss.

amounts of ACTH are produced resulting in adrenal hyperplasia and a 'normal' cortisol output may then be achieved. However, this is only attained at the expense of the accumulation of cortisol precursors such as 17α-hydroxyprogesterone and their subsequent conversion to sex steroids (Fig. 13.1) notably those with androgenic activity. 17α-Hydroxyprogesterone is characteristically found in elevated amounts (up to 100-fold) in the blood (Loriaux et al. 1974) and as its metabolite pregnanetriol and 11-ketopregnanetriol in the urine (Finkelstein and Goldberg 1957) where the 11-deoxy to 11-oxy-17-ketosteroid ratio is nearly 1:1, compared with 1:4 in normal subjects. Oestrogenic steroids are also elevated (Wajchenberg et al. 1980) as is testosterone, their immediate precursor (Solomon and Schoen 1975) and 21-deoxycortisol (Loriaux et al. 1974).

Virilisation commences in utero (Pang et al. 1980) as significant adrenal biosynthesis begins at about the second month of intra-uterine life (p. 93). The result is pseudohermaphroditism in females with clitoral enlargement and labioscrotal fusion evident at birth. In extreme cases, even a penile urethra may be present. However, such females retain a uterus and Fallopian tubes. In later life progressive virilisation with hirsutism occurs in untreated cases. At birth, most males, by contrast, appear normal but isosexual precocity rapidly develops with early epiphyseal fusion and eventually a shortened stature. This is the simple virilising form of the syndrome, in which hydromineral regulation is unaffected.

In about 30 % of the patients with 21-hydroxylation defect a salt-losing syndrome is also present and is due to reduced aldosterone secretion. In these patients 21-hydroxylase is almost completely lost (Eberlein and Bongiovanni 1958). This variant becomes manifest most often about 10–15 days after birth as an acute adrenal crisis and is life-threatening, particularly in males in whom no other symptoms or signs are visible.

Patients with the two variants of the 21-hydroxylation defect, with and without salt loss, are apparently of different genotypes. The sparing of the aldosterone secretion in the common form suggests that there are two 21-hydroxylase enzymes, one effective in the pathway to corticosterone and aldosterone in the zona glomerulosa and another for the cortisol pathway in the zona fasciculata (Fig. 13.1), and also that these two putative enzymes are under different genetic control (Bartter et al. 1968). Thus in the 'compensated' form with normal aldosterone levels, the 21-hydroxylase responsible for converting progesterone to deoxycorticosterone (DOC) would appear to be unaffected, at least in the zona glomerulosa. This explanation also accords with the fact that in any one family the compensated or salt-losing varieties breed true (Prader et al. 1962). An alternative explanation is that the difference between the two forms of 21-hydroxylase deficiency is one of degree and that only one enzyme is involved (Eberlein and Bongiovanni 1958; Ulick et al. 1980). Recent evidence (West et al. 1979) tends however to favour the multiple enzyme theory, although it is not completely conclusive (Ulick et al. 1980).

Other congenital defects have been rarely recorded in association with the 21-hydroxylase form of CAH and comprise forms of congenital asymmetry (Hirano and Seeler 1978) and the Saethre-Chotzen syndrome (Escobar et al. 1977). The incidence of upper urinary tract anomalies is also enhanced in CAH cases (Kirkland et al. 1972).

11β-Hydroxylase Deficiency

The 11β-hydroxylase defect is much less common (<5 % of cases). It too results in virilism but may additionally be associated with moderate hypertension. It is relatively more frequent in Jews of North African origin (Porter et al. 1977). Gynaecomastia has

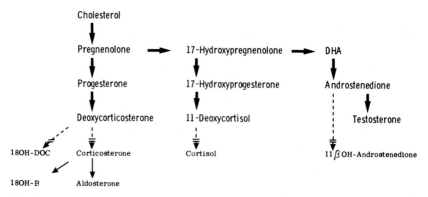

Fig. 13.2. Congenital adrenocortical hyperplasia. Pathways of steroidogenesis in an 11β-hydroxylase deficiency with hypertension and virilism.

also been reported (MacLaren et al. 1975; Zachmann and Prader 1975). Several late-onset examples of the syndrome have been described (Cathelineau et al. 1980).

The 11β-hydroxylation defect first described by Eberlein and Bongiovanni (1955) results in raised deoxycorticosterone (DOC) levels (Fig. 13.2) which have been invoked to explain the hypertension, as well as increases in relatively inactive 11-deoxysteroids such as 11-deoxycortisol which, together with its reduced metabolites in the urine (e.g. THS), has provided another marker of the disease. However, there is circumstantial evidence to suggest the possible existence of more than one 11β-hydroxylase enzyme system (Levine et al. 1980b) and that different degrees of effect on the cortisol or aldosterone-corticosterone pathways can exist with, for example, elevation of S but not DOC (Zachmann et al. 1971; Zachmann and Prader 1975) and vice versa (Gregory and Gardner 1976). 18-Hydroxylase activity in the zona fasciculata is also reduced in cases of 11β-hydroxylase deficiency (Levine et al. 1980b) providing further evidence of the close linkage between these two activities in this zone (Ulick 1976a).

Δ^5-3β-Hydroxysteroid Dehydrogenase-Isomerase Deficiency

This is a rare defect with only about twenty cases having been recorded, and seems to be commoner in females than in males. This defect results in low aldosterone, low cortisol and low androgen (except DHA) production (Bongiovanni 1961, 1962) (Fig. 13.3) and correspondingly enhanced Δ^5-3β-hydroxysteroids. Severe adreno-cortical deficiency usually ensues with marked salt loss often proving fatal although, recently, patients with partial defects and milder degrees of electrolyte disturbance have been recorded and survival achieved with replacement therapy (Kenny et al. 1971; Rosenfield et al. 1980).

In males, the sexual presentation is one of incomplete male differentiation and results from the enzyme defect, usually, but not invariably, involving the testis to the same degree (Schneider et al. 1975). In females, mild clitoral enlargement may be present due to the high level of dehydroepiandrosterone (DHA) but often virilisation proper is considered to be absent, although it may occur in late-onset cases (Rosenfield et al. 1980).

In some males, breast development may occur at puberty in accord with the concept of a fetal testosterone deficiency and hence the lack of inhibition of primitive breast duct development by androgens (Parks et al. 1971).

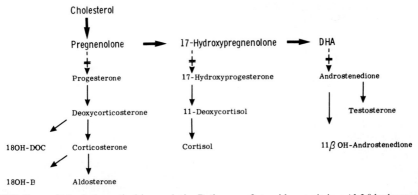

Fig. 13.3. Congenital adrenocortical hyperplasia. Pathways of steroidogenesis in a Δ^5-3β-hydroxysteroid dehydrogenase-isomerase deficiency.

Pathology of CAH With Virilism

All the adrenocortical changes seen in CAH with virilism are explicable on the basis of the effects of markedly elevated levels of ACTH, and the precise nature of the enzyme defect.

The average weight of a single autopsy adrenal of untreated affected children (neonates to twelve years of age) is 15 g compared to normal figures of 1–4 g depending on age (Fig. 3.2). However, weights up to 32 g and 37 g have been recorded in twelve- and six-year-old children respectively. In cases in adults which have been personally examined each gland has weighed around 30–35 g, or nearly ten times the normal weight (Symington 1969).

The glands present macroscopically a characteristic cerebriform convoluted appearance and their cut surface is diffusely brown in colour (Fig. 13.4).

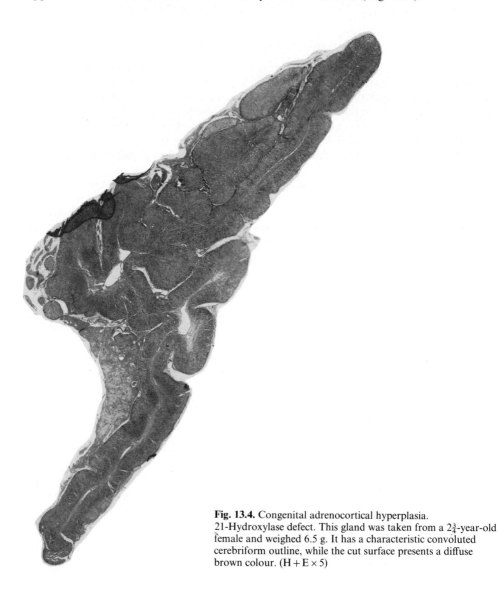

Fig. 13.4. Congenital adrenocortical hyperplasia. 21-Hydroxylase defect. This gland was taken from a 2¾-year-old female and weighed 6.5 g. It has a characteristic convoluted cerebriform outline, while the cut surface presents a diffuse brown colour. (H + E × 5)

Histologically, the appearances are also characteristic but will depend upon the age of the patient. In older children and adults, the cortex is broadened and consists of compact cells, often with lipofuscin granules, often extending out from the medulla to reach the zona glomerulosa (Fig. 13.5). Such compact cell columns are frequently separated from the zona glomerulosa by a thin layer of clear lipid-laden cells which constitute the outer aspect of a residual zona fasciculata. Occasionally, small compact cell nodules are present in the cortex or as extra-capsular extensions (Fig. 13.4). These are the predicted changes knowing the effects of ACTH upon adrenal morphology and weight (p. 31).

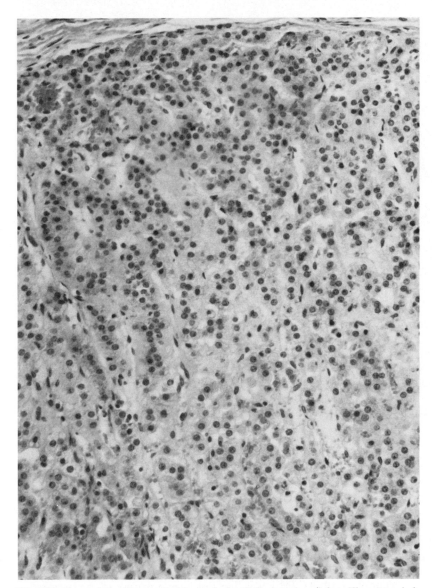

Fig. 13.5. Congenital adrenocortical hyperplasia. 21-Hydroxylase defect. The cortex is broadened and consists exclusively of compact cells of the zona reticularis type which extend out to reach the capsule. The zona glomerulosa is not obvious in this part of the cortex. (H + E × 180)

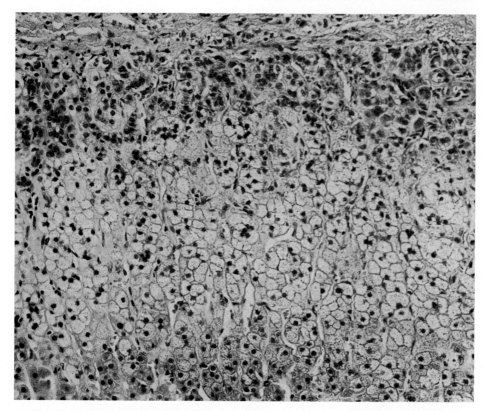

Fig. 13.6. Congenital adrenocortical hyperplasia. 21-Hydroxylase defect. A prominent zona glomerulosa is seen under the capsule together with a zone of clear cells separating the zona glomerulosa from the broadened compact cell zona reticularis (*below*). (H + E × 100)

In the personally examined cases of this syndrome (21-hydroxylase deficiency) in children, the zona glomerulosa has always been hyperplastic (Fig. 13.6). This is anticipated where the enzyme defects result in reduced aldosterone secretion with compensatory hyperplasia probably being induced by activation of the renin-angiotensin system. However, with the more recent recognition that certain 21-hydroxylase deficiencies may spare the pathway to aldosterone (Fig. 13.1), such changes need not necessarily be anticipated in all cases. Indeed, certain examples have been previously recorded where the zona glomerulosa was stated to be within normal morphological limits (Blackman 1946; Lewis et al. 1950; Marie et al. 1952).

A hyperplastic zona glomerulosa would not be anticipated in most cases of 11β-hydroxylase deficiency due to the excessive secretion of DOC and consequent hypertension, although the remainder of the gland will be enlarged, with compact cell conversion.

In glands obtained from neonates and infants, although there is degeneration and involution of the fetal zone, the definitive zone by contrast is hyperplastic, consisting exclusively of compact cells with eosinophilic lipid-sparse cytoplasm (Fig. 13.7). These cells extend from the degenerating fetal zone to the capsule. An identifiable zona glomerulosa has not been noted in the glands available for study (Fig. 13.8). Cellular hypertrophy, despite the high ACTH levels, has not been a feature of the personally examined cases. Nodules consisting of compact cells are frequently present also at this early stage as they are later in life.

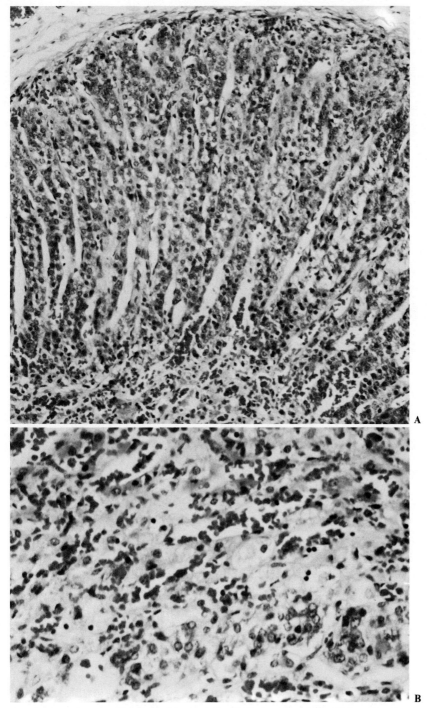

Fig. 13.7. Congenital adrenocortical hyperplasia. 21-Hydroxylase defect. This neonatal example shows a broadened outer cortex composed solely of compact cell columns (**A**) by prominent sinusoids. The fetal cortex, shown at a higher power (**B**) is congested and undergoing degeneration. Compare with congenital hyperplasia causing Cushing's syndrome. (H + E × 180 [**A**]; × 330 [**B**])

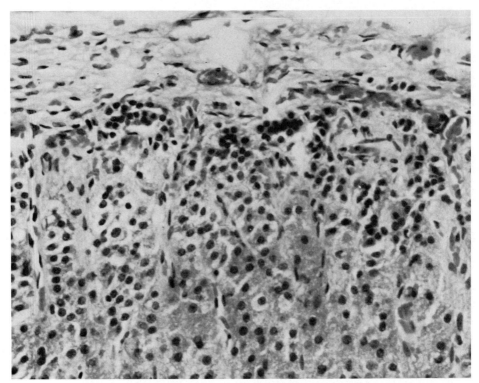

Fig. 13.8. Congenital adrenocortical hyperplasia. Δ^5-3β-Hydroxysteroid dehydrogenase-isomerase defect. The outer part of the cortex from a neonatal gland is illustrated. No identifiable zona glomerulosa is seen. (H+E × 330)

Bilateral testicular tumours varying from microscopic to <200 g in weight may be found in subjects with virilising congenital adrenal hyperplasia. For further discussion of their aetiology and significance, see p. 283. In untreating virilising CAH of the milder form, the increased adrenal androgen output will suppress pituitary gonadotrophins and in some cases spermatogenic arrest and infertility have been observed (Gabrilove 1958).

The prognosis for children presenting with the 21- and 11β-hydroxylase defects is now good provided diagnosis is made early and effective therapy is instituted promptly. Growth and development can be normal and the cosmetic results of plastic recon-structive surgery, when needed, are also satisfactory. Until recently, the Δ^5-3β-hydroxysteroid dehydrogenase-isomerase defect has usually proved fatal but with early detection or a lesser degree of defect, a satisfactory outcome has been recorded. Thus, hopefully, even fewer of these cases will come to autopsy as methods of prediction of genetic risks (see below), and prenatal diagnosis are developed.

Non-Virilising CAH Syndromes and Related Defects

All of these defects are extremely rare; in most instances only a handful of cases have been described. A precis of some of their clinical and laboratory features is shown in Table 13.1.

17-Hydroxylase Deficiency

This defect, which has been described in about a dozen cases, most of them adults, reduces the output of cortisol and of sex steroids and results in increased mineralocorticoid production with hypertension and hyperkalaemia (Fig. 13.9). It was

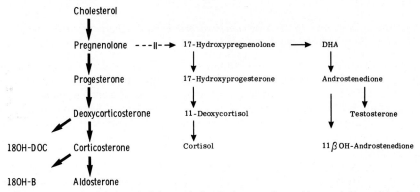

Fig. 13.9. Congenital adrenocortical hyperplasia. Pathways of steroidogenesis in a 17α-hydroxylase deficiency.

first recognised by Biglieri et al. (1966) and seems to be more frequent in females. Urinary metabolites of progesterone (e.g. pregnanediol) are much increased. Aldosterone production is reduced because of the effects of the deoxycorticosterone levels on renin secretion (Rovner et al. 1979). This defect also affects the gonads and reduces their sex steroid output. Females affected have sexual infantilism while male children, because of a lack of testosterone production in utero, present with complete female external genitalia or male pseudohermaphroditism with ambiguous genitalia (c.f. testicular feminisation). Such males lack a uterus because of the continued production of the Mullerian inhibitory factor by the primitive gonads in utero. Breast development will occur in untreated boys at puberty (New 1970). One case of chromosomal abnormality (Xq-) has been detected in this condition (Check et al. 1977).

A combined 17α- and 18-hydroxylase deficiency (vide infra) has been reported in a male (Waldhausl et al. 1978).

Defective Cholesterol Utilisation

This rare form of CAH, first described in detail by Prader and Gurtner (1955) is associated with defective utilisation of cholesterol which, therefore, results in a reduction in the formation of all forms of adrenal steroids. Salt loss occurs due to defective aldosterone secretion and, in males, there is incomplete masculinisation due to the enzyme defect also affecting testosterone production by the fetal testis. The disease, therefore, has severe metabolic effects, and, in the past, has been uniformly fatal although several patients recently have been recognised sufficiently speedily for therapy to be instituted and long term survival achieved. Occasionally, milder forms of the disorder have been reported (e.g. Camacho et al. 1968). Cases reported seem equally distributed between the sexes.

Recent studies have demonstrated that the impaired utilisation of cholesterol may arise from a defect in the cholesterol side-chain cleavage system following Prader and Ander's (1962) original suggestion of a 20.22-desmolase defect. Examples of purportedly defective 20α-hydroxylase have also been described (Degenhart et al.

1972; Kirkland et al. 1973). It is, however, unlikely that these moeities exist as separated entities (Burstein et al. 1970); cytochrome P-450$_{scc}$ levels are correspondingly reduced (Koizumi et al. 1977). The result is that cholesterol and its esters accumulate in the adrenal cortex, plasma ACTH levels rise and result in adrenocortical hyperplasia. The term congenital 'lipoid' hyperplasia is applied to this entity (vide infra).

Defective Aldosterone and 18-Hydroxycorticosterone Biosynthesis (Corticosterone methyl oxidase Type I and Type II deficiencies)

These are inordinately rare congenital familial defects. They have been found in infants who fail to thrive, have intermittent fever, but in whom no sex defects or detectable abnormalities of cortisol metabolism are present. Salt insufficiency appears to occur (e.g. Milla et al. 1977) and the disease is not, therefore, lethal. Selective aldosterone deficiency has also been described in adults (Vagnucci 1969) but whether congenital or acquired, or due to enzymatic deficiencies or lack of trophic factors is not known in most cases (Brown et al. 1973).

With 18-hydroxylase defect (corticosterone methyl oxidase Type I) the symptoms are due to low aldosterone, but 18-hydroxycorticosterone production is also reduced (Jean et al. 1969) (Fig. 13.10). In the 18-dehydrogenase defect or corticosterone methyl

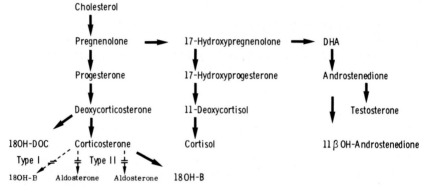

Fig. 13.10. Congenital adrenocortical hyperplasia. Pathways of steroidogenesis in corticosterone methyl oxidase deficiences (Type I and Type II), equivalent to '18-hydroxylase' and '18-dehydrogenase' defects respectively.

oxidase type II deficiency as it is now sometimes known (Veldhuis et al. 1980) there is also low aldosterone production but corticosterone, DOC and 18-hydroxycortico-sterone are elevated (Fig. 13.10) (Ulick et al. 1964; David et al. 1968; Rappaport et al. 1968; Milla et al. 1977); the rise in DOC and B must in this instance be insufficient to prevent salt loss. 18-Hydroxycorticosterone is not a potent mineralocorticoid (Fraser and Lantos 1978). The 18-dehydrogenase defect is relatively frequent in certain Iranian Jewish groups (Rösler et al. 1977).

C_{17-20} Desmolase (Lyase) Deficiency

To complete the pattern of congenital abnormalities of adrenal steroid metabolising enzyme activities a deficiency of C_{17-20} desmolase (lyase) activity has recently been reported in several children (Forest et al. 1980). This manifests itself as male pseudohermaphroditism due to deficient testicular steroidogenesis, but basal levels of DHA sulphate may be reduced, suggesting that this defect probably also involves the adrenal cortex; cortisol secretion is not, of course, reduced, and no adrenogenital syndrome ensues.

Pathology of CAH Without Virilism

The adrenal changes in 17α-hydroxylase deficiency remain to be described as no reported cases have come to autopsy, but changes similar to those of the 21-hydroxylase defect could be anticipated.

Due to high circulating ACTH levels in individuals with congenital lipoid hyperplasia (cholesterol side-chain cleavage deficiency) the adrenal glands are heavier than normal, individual weights of between 3.0 and 12 g having been reported in neonates and in children. If death occurs very shortly after birth the dominant changes

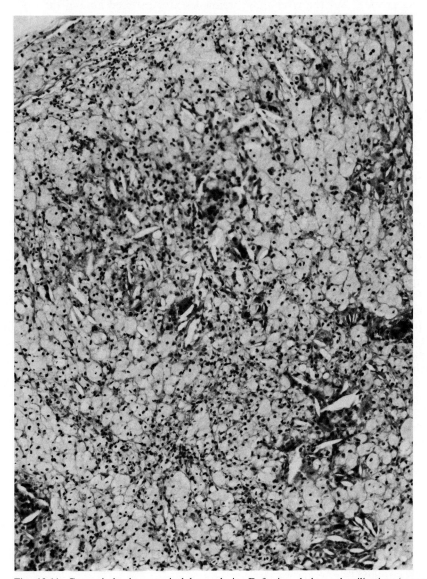

Fig. 13.11. Congenital adrenocortical hyperplasia. Defective cholesterol utilisation (congenital lipoid hyperplasia). The cortex consists exclusively of lipid-laden clear cells extending from the capsule (*above left*) to the medulla (not shown). Numerous cholesterol clefts together with associated foreign-body giant cells are also present. (H + E × 140)

will be seen in the fetal cortex although similar features will also be present in the definitive cortex (Moragas and Ballabriga 1969). More often, death is delayed for a month or two, when the definitive cortex will be dominant and the lipoid changes well established in this part of the gland.

On sectioning, the cortex is seen to be nodular and to have a diffuse yellow to white colour. Microscopically, all the adrenal cells appear as clear lipid-laden cells which occupy the entire cortex (Fig. 13.11). In addition, foci of cholesterol crystals or 'clefts' and associated foreign body-type giant cells are common. Ultrastructurally, the adrenal cells are distended with lipid and appear as 'spongiocytes' in which mitochondria are few and the remaining organelles are scattered among the lipid vacuoles (Tsutsui et al. 1970).

The adrenal changes in corticosterone methyl oxidase deficiency have not been adequately described so far; in one case of the '18-hydroxylase' defect the glands were of normal weight for their age with the outer layer of the cortex having 'a tubular and loose' aspect with 'adenomatous' change (Visser and Cost 1964).

Genetics of CAH

The 21-hydroxylase deficiency is inherited as an autosomal recessive trait affecting males and females equally within sibships (Childs et al. 1956). The gene frequency in the population varies from between 1:11 and 1:128, depending on the racial group involved (p. 155). In Great Britain, for example, heterozygotes occur in the normal population with a frequency of 1 in 40. For the purposes primarily of genetic counselling considerable effort has been devoted to the detection of heterozygotes, the great majority of whom show no overt clinical abnormalities. A proportionately greater response of 17α-hydroxyprogesterone to ACTH has been observed under some conditions in known heterozygotes, but similar effects have been noted in a minority of otherwise apparently normal subjects (Child et al. 1979); detection cannot therefore be considered entirely reliable at the present using solely endocrine parameters.

Recent studies have, however, clearly located the recessive gene in the vicinity of the HLA complex (Dupont et al. 1977) with close linkage to HLA-B (Levine et al. 1978). HLA haplotyping can, therefore, be used to identify heterozygotes in families with an affected member, albeit retrospectively rather than prospectively (Lorenzen et al. 1980). Allelic forms of 21-hydroxylase have been detected in late-onset, attenuated and cryptic forms of the disease (Levine et al. 1980a; Migeon et al. 1980) and other studies (Morillo and Gardner 1979; New et al. 1979) have reported that some so-called 'acquired' forms of virilising CAH may represent an entirely separate disorder.

11β-Hydroxylase, 17α-hydroxylase and corticosterone methyl oxidase deficiencies are also probably transmitted as autosomal recessive traits (Cohen et al. 1977), although owing to their infrequency, reliable genetic studies remain to be reported in some cases. There is, however, apparently no linkage between either the 11β-hydroxylase gene (Brautbar et al. 1979) or 17-hydroxylase (Mantero et al. 1980) and the HLA complex.

Virilising Adrenocortical Tumours

Incidence and Symptoms

Whereas much is known about the aetiology of congenital adrenal hyperplasia, little is known of the causes of virilising adrenal neoplasms. Occasional reports have noted apparent associations with pre-existing conditions such as untreated congenital adrenal hyperplasia (Daeschner 1965, Dluhy et al. 1971; Van Seters et al. 1981) and with nodular hyperplasia with Cushing's syndrome (Arce et al. 1978; Anderson et al. 1978). CAH, however, does not give rise to neoplasms in the vast majority of cases, and for reasons that have been detailed elsewhere (p. 126) an association with other forms of nodular change and induced hyperplasia may well be fortuitous in some cases. Virilising adrenal tumours have been recorded in the 'cancer family syndrome' (p. 116) and rare examples of sibs being similarly afflicted have been reported (p. 116). Most such tumours, cannot, however, be linked to any known predisposing condition or familial association. In utero virilisation has been reported in at least one case (Kenny et al. 1968).

Virilising tumours are more frequent in children than in adults and they are diagnosed more frequently between the second and seventh years of life (Canlorbe et al. 1971). They are particularly common, or are commonly recognised as such, in females, who outnumber males in reported series by about 3 to 1 (DeCourt and Anoussakis 1969). Virilising tumours are, in fact, the major form of functionally active adrenocortical neoplasms in children (Heinbecker et al. 1957; Kenny et al. 1968; Symington 1969; Benaily et al. 1975) with the left gland involved more frequently than the right (Tables 13.2 and 13.3). They account for the great majority of cases of adrenogenital syndrome seen by the pathologist.

In female children they almost invariably cause clitoromegaly and hirsutism and

Table 13.2. Personal series of benign adrenocortical tumours associated with virilism

Case no.	Age (yr)	Sex	Adrenal site	Weight (g)
1	5	M	Left	4
2	5	F	Right	25
3	8	M	Left	80
4	8	F	Right	400
5	8	M	Left	228
6	15	M	Left	47
7	29	F	Right	35
8	Adult	F	Not known	182

Table 13.3. Personal series of malignant adrenocortical tumours associated with virilism

Case no.	Age (yr)	Sex	Adrenal site	Weight (g)
1	47	F	Left	82
2	5	F	Left	122
3	10	F	Left	239
4	3	F	Left	265
5	12	F	Right	500
6	35	M	Not known	800
7	66	F	Left	800
8	53	F	Left	1250
9	Adult	M	Left	1500
10	25	F	Right	1500
11	52	F	Right	1847
12	52	M	Right	'Large'
13	4	F	Left	Not known

enhance growth to varying degrees. In adults oligomenorrhea followed by amenorrhea and increased musculature occur. In male children virilising tumours are associated with precocious puberty, reduced gonadotrophin levels and often spermatogenic arrest; lesions with corresponding functional properties in men usually cause no overt endocrine symptoms. Some tumours in females may be associated with simple hirsutism or minimal virilisation (Tipton et al. 1971; Hartemann et al. 1978) and in other cases signs of Cushing's syndrome may be present. Hypertension is a frequent ($<60\%$) finding in virilising tumours of the adrenal cortex (Burrington and Stephens 1969; Decourt and Anoussakis 1969; Canlorbe et al. 1971; Siegler and Rallison 1978). Problems in differential diagnosis include late-onset congenital adrenal hyperplasia, gonadal tumours and the Stein-Leventhal syndrome and CNS tumours causing precocious puberty as well as idiopathic sexual precocity, idiopathic hirsutism and 'ectopic' HCG production by, for example, hepatomas.

Functional Properties

Most adrenal tumours associated with marked abnormalities of sexual habitus seem to contain enzymatic defects reminiscent of those which channel steroidogenesis towards the production of excessive sex steroids in the congenital adrenal hyperplasia syndromes (p. 155) although unlike the latter the possibility of multiple as well as single deficiencies cannot be excluded.

In some cases active androgens such as testosterone are secreted directly by the tumour (Burr et al. 1973; Werk et al. 1973; Gabrilove et al. 1976; Larson et al. 1976; Costin et al. 1977; Smith et al. 1978; Schteingart et al. 1979; DeLange et al. 1980; Spaulding et al. 1980). Many other virilising adrenal tumours, however, secrete little or no testosterone, although a wide variety of other C_{19} steroids and their precursors emanate from such lesions (e.g. Saez et al. 1967, 1971) including androstenedione (Bardin et al. 1968) and the peripheral conversions of these steroids to testosterone may be partly responsible for virilising symptoms in these cases.

At one time the production of dehydroepiandrosterone (or its sulphate) was considered a specific feature of virilising carcinomas (Mills 1964) with correspondingly enhanced urinary 17-ketosteroids (50–400 mg/day) compared with 17-hydroxy-steroids (2–8 mg/day) (e.g. Begue et al. 1976). Further studies have, however, shown that many proved benign tumours can exhibit this steroid secretory pattern (Danowski et al. 1973; Henley 1973; Chakmakjian and Abraham 1975) and levels of precursor steroids such as pregnenolone, 17-hydroxypregnenolone, progesterone and 17-hydroxyprogesterone may also be elevated to varying degrees in both carcinomas and adenomas (Anderson et al. 1978; Granoff and Abraham 1979), as well as other adrenal C_{19} steroids such as 11β-hydroxyandrostenedione (Saez et al. 1971; Lisboa et al. 1978) and what are normally very minor products of the normal gland including androst-16-enes (Gower and Stern 1969) and 16-hydroxysteroids (Lisboa et al. 1978).

A number of adrenal tumours presenting with a predominantly virilising syndrome have also been shown, by both in vitro studies and sampling of adrenal venous effluent to synthesise glucocorticoids (Cameron et al. 1970; Saez et al. 1971; Lisboa et al. 1978; Costin et al. 1977) and steroids with mineralocorticoid activity such as deoxycortico-sterone (Schteingart et al. 1979) albeit in small amounts compared with C_{19} compounds. In general, however, Δ^5-steroids such as DHA and DHAS tend to predominate in most virilising adrenal tumours, especially in prepubertal patients, and it may be that in some cases the tumours have their origin in, or express the functions of, the fetal zone of the prenatal cortex in which these steroids predominate. 'Mixed' features of Cushing's syndrome with virilisation are not uncommon in adults particularly with malignant tumours, but are rare in children, although they do sometimes occur (e.g. Halmi and Lascari 1971).

A variety of changes in apparent steroid metabolising enzyme activities have been described in virilising tumours, and account for some of these patterns of functional activity. These include reduced 21-hydroxylase and 11β-hydroxylase activities and most commonly deficiencies in Δ^5-3β-hydroxysteroid dehydrogenase-isomerase activity (Neville et al. 1969c; Cameron et al. 1970; Huhtaniemi et al. 1978). In the latter deficiency, there may be a tendency of any residual activity to favour C_{19} rather than C_{21} steroid precursors, or vice versa (Neville et al. 1969c). Steroid sulphotransferase is normally active in these tumours, although it may be absent in some cases (Cameron et al. 1970) and, recently, increased activity of 17β-hydroxysteroid dehydrogenase has been reported (Spaulding et al. 1980).

The hormonal responsiveness of adrenal virilising tumours is variable. Responses to both ACTH (e.g. Yotsumoto et al. 1979; Table 14.1), and HCG (Blichert-Toft et al. 1975) have been noted in some predominantly DHA-secreting lesions, but many do not give overt responses in vivo. Several cases of adrenal-sited tumours responsive to gonadotrophin in vivo and in vitro and secreting testosterone without significant elevation of 17-ketosteroids have, however, now been described, notably in post-menopausal women (Pittaway et al. 1973; Werk et al. 1973; Givens et al. 1974; Larson et al. 1976; DeLange et al. 1980), where they seem to follow a benign course. This pattern of functional activity is not, as far as can be ascertained, a property of any type of normal adrenocortical cell, in which testosterone secretion is stimulated by ACTH (Cowan et al. 1977) and the clinical endocrine profile is strongly reminiscent of, and sometimes confused with, gonadal lesions. In view of the existence of what appear to be heterotopic gonadal cells in some normal adrenals, particularly in post-menopausal women (p. 285) it is a distinct possibility that some of these adrenal-sited lesions may have arisen from cells with gonadal rather than adrenocortical properties for differentiation.

However, not all testosterone-secreting tumours respond to HCG in vivo (Costin et al. 1977). In addition other C_{19} steroids may also be secreted together with small amounts of cortisol (Schteingart et al. 1979), properties that would seem to preclude an origin in ectopic gonadal cells. Most virilising adrenal-sited tumours, including typical DHA-secreting neoplasms, thus seem to express some cortical cell features and exhibit patterns of functional activity that resemble those of the various forms of congenital adrenal hyperplasia.

Differential diagnosis of virilising adrenal tumours from CAH with virilism (p. 155) can usually be achieved by dexamethasone suppression of ACTH, when the steroid output of most tumours is unaffected, although in some cases it may be paradoxically enhanced by the steroid analogue (Cameron et al. 1970; Yotsumoto et al. 1979). The distinction between adrenal and gonadal lesions can sometimes, but by no means always (vide supra) be made by ACTH and HCG stimulation tests. There are, however, no truly reliable functional criteria for distinguishing benign and malignant virilising lesions in vivo. Hypertension for example, may occur frequently with benign tumours of this type. The presence of additional stigmata of Cushing's syndrome may, however, suggest the possibility of a malignant tumour, and correspondingly excessively elevated levels of various 17-hydroxycorticosteroids and their urinary metabolites such as pregnanetriol (>50 mg/day) (e.g. Atwill et al. 1970) may also imply malignancy as opposed to benignity (Danowski et al. 1973), but no absolute distinctions can be made with this type of criterion. Changes in steroidogenic profiles during tumour progression have also been noted with virilising tumours (Halmi and Lascari 1971; Saez et al. 1971) and further complicate the assessment of such functional parameters in vivo and their prognostic significance.

Pathology

Gross appearance   Whereas in Cushing's syndrome, tumour weight and histology are moderately helpful guides to subsequent benign or malignant behaviour (p. 152), there is a considerable overlap in both features when virilising adrenocortical tumours are considered. While the larger tumours are again more likely to be malignant, tumours of up to 400 g have subsequently proved benign, and their large size at surgery compared with predominantly glucocorticoid-secreting adenomas presumably reflects the relative inactivity of their secreted steroid products (Table 13.2). We have personally seen one example of a carcinoma which weighed only 80 g (Table 13.3). Costin et al. (1977) have recorded a 17 g virilising tumour which was classified as a carcinoma on the basis of its pleomorphic histology. Nonetheless, small lesions are more likely to be benign.

Virilising tumours, like most adrenocortical tumours, are usually well encapsulated and discrete. Their cut surface usually has a uniform brown/red colour although, in smaller tumours, small yellow-coloured foci may be present (Plate B, facing p. 147). With increasing size, areas of haemorrhage, necrosis and calcification become frequent. Rarely, cyst formation may be noted.

Microscopic appearance   These tumours present a spectrum of histological features from clearly benign to malignant, but numerous 'borderline lesions' will be encountered where this distinction is undoubtedly difficult (Symington 1969; Neville and MacKay 1972).

In the small-sized adenoma, the tumour cells resemble in appearance and size the cells of the normal zona reticularis, i.e. they are compact-type cells (Fig. 13.12). They have regular, small single vesicular nuclei with eosinophilic lipid-sparse cytoplasm and are arranged in short cords or acini separated by fibrovascular trabeculae. Small foci of clear lipid-laden cells, similar to those of the zona fasciculata, may be present (Fig. 13.12) but they are infrequent compared to the benign tumours of Cushing's syndrome. Clear cells are not seen in larger-sized adenomas; individual cell necrosis (apoptosis) is frequently present (Fig. 13.12) but large areas of necrosis are usually absent. On occasion, the compact cells may contain abundant lipofuscin and thus resemble a 'black adenoma'.

In larger adenomas (100–400 g), the component cells tend to increase in size and form larger solid trabeculae or sheets punctuated by thin-walled vascular sinusoids. The cells are still compact in type with eosinophilic lipid-sparse cytoplasm, but the nuclei are enlarged, more vesicular and show prominent large nucleoli (Fig. 13.13). Cellular and nuclear pleomorphism with occasional giant or bizarre forms may be noted in tumours in this size range. These appearances are not, however, always confined to lesions of 100–400 g as they can also occur in some small tumours. All these larger lesions at the time of their initial presentation to the pathologist after surgical resection are, however, extremely difficult, if not impossible to classify prospectively as benign or malignant (Guinet et al. 1959; Kenny et al. 1968; Burrington and Stephens 1969; Symington 1969).

In proved carcinomas with virilisation, compact-type cells again comprise the lesions and form solid cords, sheets and/or trabeculae as noted previously with Cushing's syndrome (p. 144). Viable tumour cells can sometimes be found arranged in a prominent perivascular or perisinusoidal pattern with extensive areas of intervening necrosis in both types of tumour (Fig. 12.18). Commonly, the tumour cells have prominent, enlarged pleomorphic vesicular nuclei with prominent single or multiple nucleoli (Fig. 13.14). Bizarre forms and giant cells can also be found but mitotic activity is seldom prominent. Admixed with or contiguous to these enlarged or bizarre

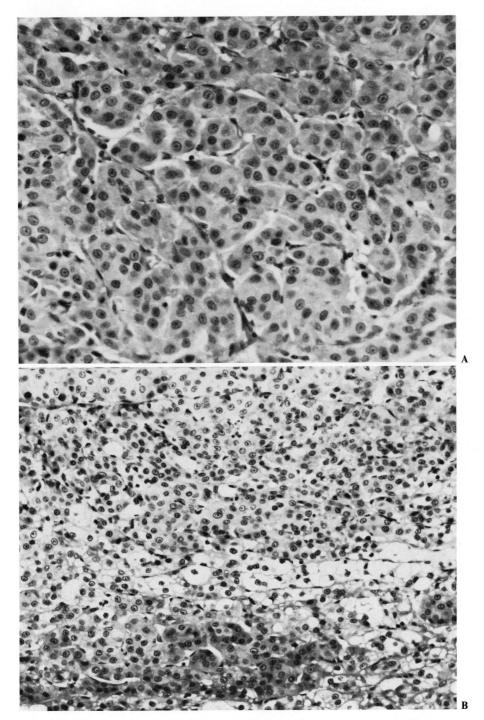

‹**Fig. 13.12.** Adrenogenital syndrome. Virilising adrenocortical adenoma (25 g). Two different aspects of a virilising tumour removed from a 5-year-old boy are shown. In **A** the cells are of normal size, are of the compact type and are arranged in short strands separated by prominent vascular spaces. In other areas of the same tumour (**B**), nests of clear lipid-laden cells may be noted. (H + E × 350 [**A**]; × 240 [**B**])

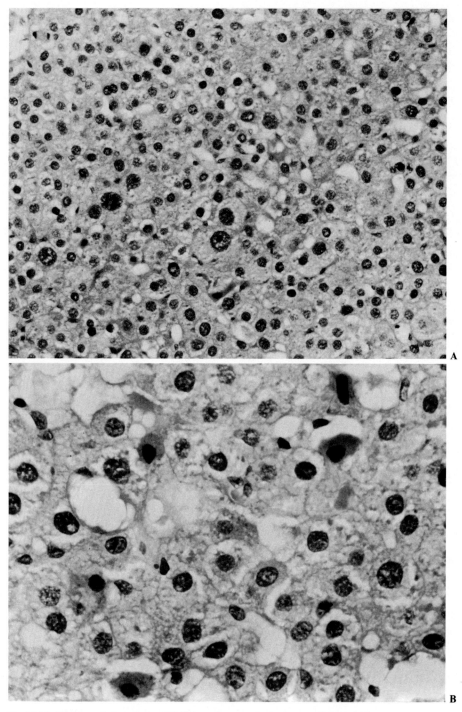

Fig. 13.13. Adrenogenital syndrome. Virilising adrenocortical adenoma (228 g). This tumour was removed from an 8-year-old boy. The constituent compact cells (**A** + **B**) are larger than normal and exhibit nuclear pleomorphism. However, prominent nucleoli are not a feature, nor are the nuclei markedly vesicular (**B**). Numerous tumour cells (**B**) also show apoptosis. (H + E × 240 [**A**]; × 500 [**B**])

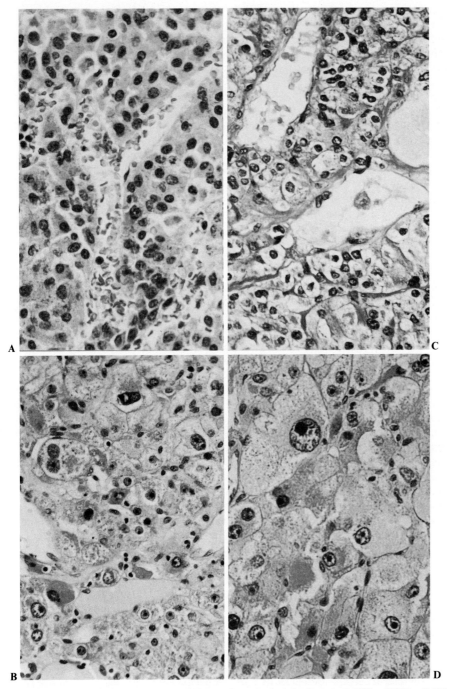

Fig. 13.14. Adrenogenital syndrome. Virilising adrenocortical carcinomas (**A** 1500 g, **B** 265 g, **C** 500 g and **D** 1500 g). The constituent cells are of the compact type, but possess different sizes, appearances, arrangements and degrees of pleomorphism in different tumours. In **A** the cells are of normal size and show little atypicality. Nuclear pleomorphism, vesicularity and prominent nucleoli are, nonetheless, the best histological guides to malignancy (**B**, **C** and **D**). Note the apparent paucity of mitotic activity. (H + E **A,B,C** and **D** × 380)

tumour cell types, one may find compact cells with regular nuclei which show little size variation from normal (Fig. 13.14). Moreover, in some of the present series of proved carcinomas, nuclear and cellular pleomorphism were not particularly conspicuous. Hence the pathological diagnosis of malignancy can be extremely difficult, and an extremely guarded prognosis must be given. Such patients should be monitored carefully.

In virilising carcinomas, foci of capsular or vascular invasion can on occasion be detected. In many, however, such features are not apparent despite a diligent search. Hence the moderately clear-cut morphological patterns found in Cushing's syndrome are not so apparent in virilising tumours at the light-microscopical level.

Ultrastructure   The ultrastructural appearances of most virilising adrenal tumours are consistent with their steroidogenic activity. These appearances obviously also reflect for example the relative predominance of clear or compact-type cells within the lesions; they are not, however, sufficiently distinctive in themselves to permit an unambiguous differentiation between androgen and corticosteroid-secreting neoplasms on solely structural criteria. Although they also reflect the pleomorphism and disorganisation apparent in the more frankly malignant lesions, ultrastructural characteristics do not, we believe, enable a reliable distinction to be made in 'borderline' cases in respect of potential malignancy.

In virilising adenomas the mitochondria tend to be circular in outline with both lamellar and sparse, generally peripherally located, vesicular cristae (Fisher and Danowski 1973; Tannenbaum 1973); mitochondrial granules may also be prominent. Membrane bound lysosomes and large lipofuscin granules are also frequently observed, and a sacculo-tubular SER and short strands and/or stacks of RER are moderately prominent. In general these are the characteristics of typical compact-type cells of the zona reticularis. Nevertheless, cells of this type are frequently observed in benign tumours causing Cushing's syndrome (p. 141) and may in some cases comprise the predominant cell type (Kovacs et al. 1976).

Larger virilising tumours frequently diagnosed as benign show most or all of the above characteristics, as do many frankly malignant lesions (Figs. 13.15, 13.16, 13.17) although marked variations may be seen in the appearance of the organelles in individual cells (Gorgas et al. 1976), which often diverge from the specific morphology of individual normal zones to present a non-specific steroidogenic appearance (Huhtaniemi et al. 1978). From published reports (Akhtar et al. 1974; Valente et al. 1978) and personal observations on larger virilising lesions of both benign and malignant varieties it seems that the SER is often exceptionally prominent, especially in the prepubertal tumours, often forming dense convoluted networks of tubules that occupy virtually the entire cytoplasm (Fig. 13.17). However, contrary to some suggestions (Tannenbaum 1973; Valente et al. 1978) organised lamellar stacks of SER can also be found in virilising tumours (Neville and O'Hare 1979) and are not confined to cases of hypercortisolism. In some cases the SER may form loose concentric laminations (Akhtar et al. 1974). In malignant lesions associated with the 'mixed' Cushing's syndrome with virilisation, however, the SER may be more limited in extent

Fig. 13.15. Adrenogenital syndrome. Virilising adrenal tumours. The ultrastructural appearance of two ▷ different tumours occurring in (**A**) 4-year-old and (**B**) 7-year-old girls causing the adrenogenital syndrome are shown. The cytoplasm in **A** is packed densely with round aberrant mitochondria of differing size showing prominent intramitochondrial inclusions (lipofuscin). A similar appearance was seen in all cells examined. The light-microscopical appearances of this lesion were consistent with the diagnosis of carcinoma and are illustrated in Fig. 14.1B. In **B** the mitochondria are small but show typical steroidogenic features, including peripherally located vesicles. The basement membrane surrounding this cell is continuous (*arrows*). Both children are well 2 and 2½ years after surgery, respectively. (**A** × 12 900; **B** × 16 500)

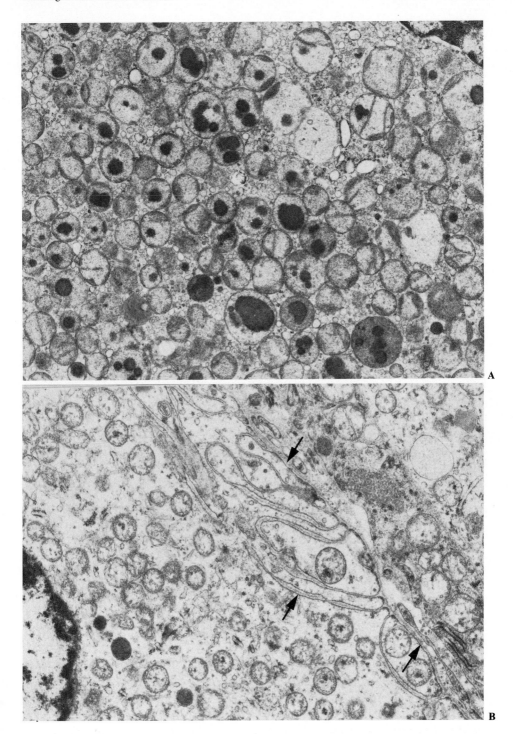

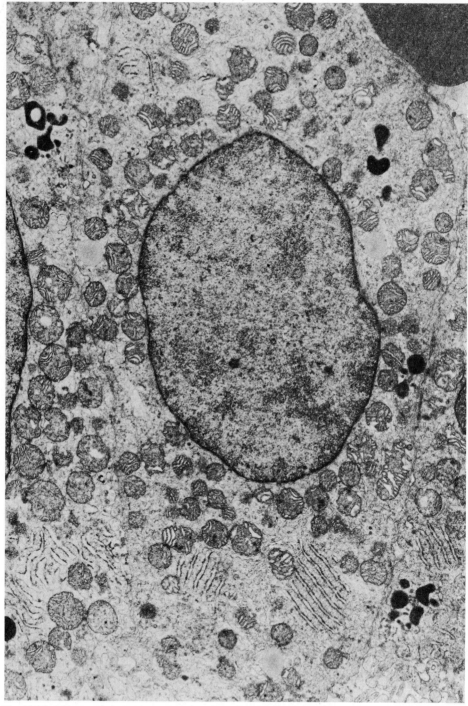

Fig. 13.16. Adrenogenital syndrome. Virilising adrenal tumour. The ultrastructural appearance of a cell from a 800 g tumour causing virilisation in a 28-year-old woman is shown. None of its features materially assist in the diagnosis of malignancy/benigness in this lesion, the light-microscopic appearance of which is illustrated in Fig. 14.1B. ($\times 12\,900$)

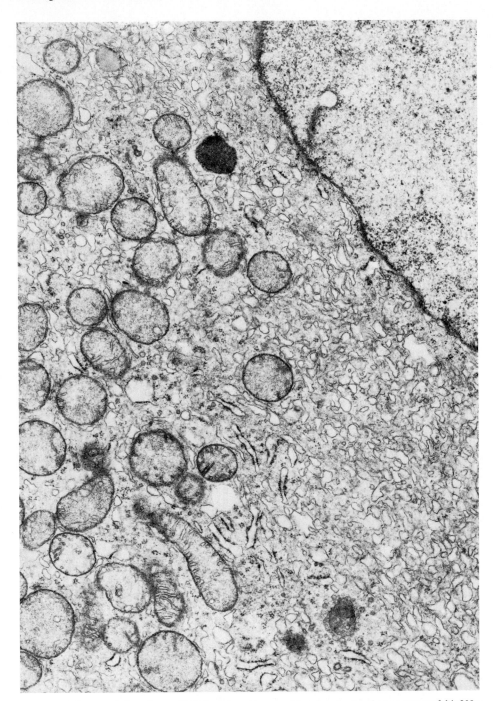

Fig. 13.17. Adrenogenital syndrome. Virilising adrenal tumour. The ultrastructural appearances of this 239 g tumour, which was removed from a 9-year-old girl with the adrenogenital syndrome, in no way indicates its malignant status. A dense mass of smooth endoplasmic reticulum was seen in almost all of the cells and the mitochondria show a variety of lamellar, tubular and vesicular internal structures demonstrating its steroidogenic nature. This tumour had metastasised at the time of surgery and its light-microscopical appearance was consistent with the diagnosis of carcinoma. (× 21 000)

and we have observed prominent elongated and ovoid mitochondria with vesicular cristae (Fig. 12.23), even when virilisation has been the predominant symptom.

The claim that partial disruption of the basement membrane of the tumour cells adjacent to vessels is a prognostic guide to malignancy has been registered with virilising lesions (Valente et al. 1978) as well as other types of tumour (p. 152). It is our experience, however, that the often convoluted microvillous membranes of the cells make this proposition very difficult to verify in many cases, or to assess quantitatively and to distinguish from fixation or sectioning artifacts.

Prognosis

Abatement of most of the signs of hyperandrogenisation will occur over several months after the removal of benign virilising adrenal tumours, although residual hirsutism may persist considerably longer. Recurrence in cases of malignancy is almost invariably fatal, although temporary remission of symptoms may be obtained with o,p'-DDD in some cases (e.g. Korth-Schutz et al. 1977). As a group, however, 'pure' virilising tumours are slow to metastasise compared with, for example, carcinomas causing Cushing's syndrome or hyperaldosteronism and such tumours often have a good prognosis. Symptoms extending over many years or even decades before the final demise of the patient have been observed in some cases (Dluhy et al. 1971; Nogeire et al. 1977).

Adrenal Tumours Causing Feminisation

Incidence and Symptoms

Adrenocortical tumours causing feminisation are the rarest type of lesion associated with hypercorticalism (Table 11.1). Bilateral gynaecomastia is the almost invariable ($>98\%$) presenting feature alerting the clinican to the presence of the tumour. Its differential diagnosis includes testicular neoplasms, Kleinfelter's syndrome, iatrogenic or idiopathic gynaecomastia, and rare forms of congenital adrenal hyperplasia (p. 159) in males, and idiopathic isosexual precocity in females. Measurement of urinary steroids, dexamethasone suppression tests and a careful history usually suffice to distinguish these conditions from the rarer feminising tumours.

The first reported case was that of Bittorf (1919) and in 1965 Gabrilove et al. reviewed a total of 52 examples. Since then, over 20 further cases have been recorded, and with the present series of five patients studied personally (Table 13.4) brings the

Table 13.4. Personal series of adrenocortical tumours associated with feminisation

Case no.	Age (yr)	Sex	Site	Weight (g)
1	59	Male	Left	1200
2	37	Male	Left	1250
3	51	Male	Left	2000
4	57	Male	Right	2400
5	72	Female	Right	3500

total to about 80 cases (Table 13.5). The vast majority (90%) have been reported in males, mostly in adults and of the female examples 75% were prepubertal and the

Table 13.5. Age incidence of 80
adrenocortical tumours causing
feminisation

Age (years)	Adenomas	Carcinomas
0–10	7	4
11–20	–	3
21–30	2	14
31–50	2	29
51–60	2	14
>60	–	3
Total	13	67

remainder postmenopausal. For obvious reasons lesions causing hyperoestrogenism are difficult to detect on the basis of endocrine signs and symptoms in adult females and the deficit of female cases is probably accounted for by categorisation of such tumours as causing Cushing's syndrome or virilisation when, as is sometimes the case, 17-hydroxysteroids and/or 17-ketosteroids are also elevated, or as 'non-functioning' tumours when the excess is confined to oestrogens. In prepubertal females isosexual precocity may occur, as described in detail in a recent case report from the Massachusetts General Hospital (Scully et al. 1979) and by Drop et al. (1981); details of another six feminising tumours in prepubertal females have been reviewed by Nottelet et al. (1976). In elderly women post-menopausal bleeding may occur (Table 13.6).

Table 13.6. Feminising tumours in females, children and post-menopausal women.

Case no.	Age[a]	Site	Size/Weight	Histological diagnosis	Reference
1	9 yr	L	6 × 4 × 2 cm	Adenoma	Walters et al. 1934[b]
2	23 mo	L	45 g	Adenoma	Kepler et al. 1938[b]
3	4 yr	R	10 g	Adenoma	Snaith 1958
4	6 yr	R	1000 g	Carcinoma	Peluffo et al. 1962[b]
5	23 mo	L	'size of mandarin'	Carcinoma	Ferrante et al. 1963[b]
6	10 yr	R	1275 g	Not stated	Benaily 1972[b]
7	6 yr	R	47 g	Adenoma	Scully et al. 1979
8	21 mo	R	200 g	Carcinoma	Wohltmann et al. 1980
9	6½ yr	L	650 g	Carcinoma	Drop et al. 1981
10	55 yr[c]	L	4 cm	Carcinoma	Mathur et al. 1973
11	65 yr[d]	R	200 g	Carcinoma	Monsaingeon et al. 1963
12	72 yr	R	3500 g	Carcinoma	Personal series

[a] At time of surgery.
[b] For details of reference see Nottelet et al. 1976.
[c] Post-menopausal bleeding.
[d] Associated with mixed Cushing's syndrome and post-menopausal bleeding.

Little or nothing is known of the aetiology of feminising adenocortical tumours. In one instance another member of the same family developed a rhabdomyosarcoma (Halmi and Lascari 1971), but, this case apart, no familial tendency has been recorded.

The majority of feminising tumours (>80%) showed malignant features (vide infra) and occurred with approximately equal frequency in either gland. One early example (Frank 1937) apparently arose from an adrenal rest in the testis.

Most benign feminising adrenal tumours have been detected in children before the age of ten years, while carcinomas affect all age groups, but seem to be diagnosed mostly between the third and sixth decades (Table 13.5).

Functional Properties

In functional terms, the differences between tumours causing virilism in females and feminisation in males are minimal. In one case an adrenal carcinoma which caused virilism in a child as its primary presenting symptom, recurred with feminisation after treatment (Halmi and Lascari 1971).

As with virilising tumours the steroid secretion patterns of feminising tumours, and some in vitro metabolic studies, suggest the presence of various enzyme defects, particularly with regard to 11β-hydroxylation (West et al. 1964; Bryson et al. 1968). All tend to channel steroidogenesis towards sex steroid formation (Axelrod et al. 1969; Rose et al. 1969; Mathur et al. 1973; Boyer et al. 1977) and oestrogen excretion rates rise to adult female levels, or above (1–4 mg/day), with oestrone/oestradiol/oestriol ratios typical of normal females in most cases. As a consequence of 11β-hydroxylase deficiencies a number of feminising tumours (like virilising tumours) show an increased output of both 11-deoxycortisol (Dempsey and Hill 1963; Gabriolove et al. 1970; Boyar et al. 1977) and deoxycorticosterone (Rose et al. 1969); consequently some patients will be hypertensive (West et al. 1964). C_{19} steroids such as DHA are also elevated in most patients, with this compound accounting for up to 50% of total urinary 17-ketosteroids (Saez et al. 1967) even in cases with a 'pure' feminising syndrome (Bhettay and Bonnici 1977). Testosterone levels, on the other hand, are often within the normal range in feminising tumours (Gabrilove et al. 1970); androgen:oestrogen interconversions are probably disturbed in many cases and their ratios rather than absolute levels are probably the most important factor in determining the degree of feminisation (Gabrilove et al. 1970). Occasional tumours also produce cortisol and may be associated with Cushing's syndrome as well as feminisation (Breustedt et al. 1977; deAsis and Samaan 1978); cases of concurrent virilisation (e.g. phallic enlargement, enhanced musculature and acne) and feminisation (gynaecomastia and increased oestrogen excretion) have also been reported in a prepubertal case (Bacon and Lowrey 1965) as well as consecutive virilisation and feminisation (Wohltmann et al. 1980).

In at least two cases (Dempsey and Hill 1963; Breustedt et al. 1977), a feminising tumour in a male has been shown to respond to HCG, but not ACTH although indirect mechanisms, such as the conversion of gonadal androgens to oestrogens by the tumour, were not excluded. In one case an in vitro response to prolactin has been claimed (Millington et al. 1976) but without proof of the purity of the hormone (p. 90). 'Ectopic' production of gonadotrophin has been suggested, but not proved in two cases (Rose et al. 1969; Boyar et al. 1977) and immunoreactive PTH, apparently causing hypercalcaemia, was noted in association with one such tumour (deAsis and Samaan 1978).

Pathology

Gross appearance   The gross features of feminising adenocortical tumours are similar to those causing virilisation, with pinkish-grey or brown cut surfaces and, in our experience substantial areas of necrosis. Occasionally calcification has been noted.

Most adenomas are small (<5 cm diameter) although larger lesions have been found which have pursued a benign course (e.g. Snaith 1958). Most proved carcinomas, on the other hand, weighed >1 kg (41/52 cases in which weights were noted) (Table 13.4). Many feminising tumours are thus large enough to be detected by palpation at the time of primary diagnosis (Migeon 1980). There were examples of carcinomas, however, which were <200 g in weight. Thus, as with the virilising

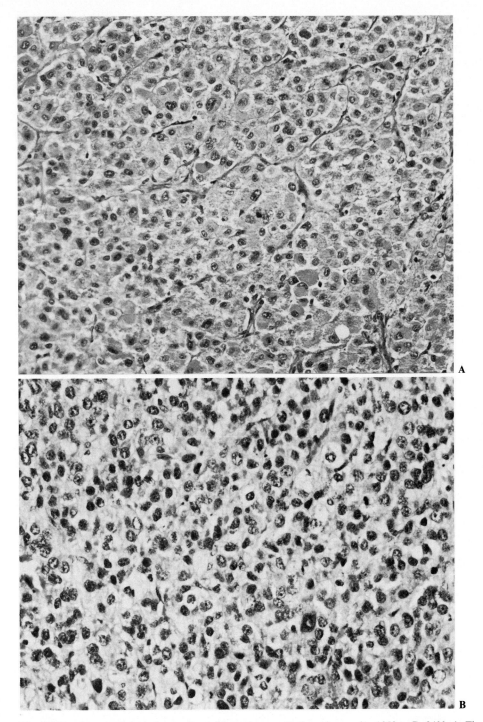

Fig. 13.18. Adrenogenital syndrome. Feminising adrenocortical carcinoma (**A**, 1250 g, **B**, 2400 g). The tumour cells are of the compact lipid-sparse type arrayed in large alveoli (**A**) or sheets (**B**). The cells are not markedly pleomorphic in either lesion, although many of the nuclei are more vesicular and have prominent nucleoli. (H + E **A** × 180, **B** × 250).

tumours there may be a marked overlap between benign and malignant feminising lesions in size and weight. It is important to stress that several smaller tumours weighing 175–244 g were originally regarded as adenomas on the basis of size and histology, only to be found to have metastasised several years after surgery (Dohan et al. 1953; Bacon and Lowrey 1965; Gabrilove et al. 1965, 1970).

Microscopic appearance   Histologically the appearances of virilising and feminising tumours are also similar and no distinction between the syndromes of hormonal excess can be made on this basis. Thus the tumour cells are usually compact in type with eosinophilic lipid-sparse cytoplasm (Fig. 13.18) arranged in solid trabeculae, sheets or large acini punctuated by fibrovascular septae. The tumour cells may be similar in size to normal compact cells and possess regular vesicular nuclei but with prominent nucleoli. Apoptosis is often present while pleomorphism and mitotic activity may be inconspicuous. Such appearances would often seem to be banal and have led on occasion to a diagnosis of adenoma. This type of tumour, in our experience, however, behaves as a carcinoma.

More commonly, feminising tumours while containing areas similar to above, tend to be composed of larger compact cells with enlarged vesicular pleomorphic nuclei with prominent nucleoli (Fig. 13.18). Giant cell and bizarre cellular forms are often present. In such lesions, the tumour cells may have a perivascular arrangement, form solid trabeculae or cords or be arranged in small acini. Thus, the appearances of such tumours are similar to the spectrum of appearances noted in virilising lesions.

In only two cases (Mitschke et al. 1978; Scully et al. 1979) has a feminising adrenal tumour been examined ultrastructurally. Both tumours contained abundant rather small mitochondria, with predominantly lamellar but some tubular cristae varying in amount from sparse to numerous in different mitochondria; the SER was rather poorly developed in one case (Mitschke et al. 1978) but was present in more typical amounts for a steroidogenic tumour in the other (Scully et al. 1979). We have seen essentially similar appearances in virilising tumours as well (Figs. 13.15, 13.16) and it seems doubtful whether the ultrastructure yields significant information of prognostic value or in respect of the specific steroidogenic nature of the lesion. Both of the above cases (a 120 g tumour in a 29-year-old male and a 50 g tumour in a female of $6\frac{1}{2}$ years) were diagnosed as adenomas, but insufficient time has elapsed to allow this prognosis to be verified (vide infra).

Prognosis

In view of the fact that metastases may be delayed for nearly a decade (e.g. Bacon and Lowrey, 1965) all feminising lesions, irrespective of their histology, are, in our opinion, best regarded as potentially malignant and treated and followed-up accordingly. The only exception may be the small prepubertal lesion, the majority of which thus far reported appear to follow a benign course at least in the short term (<5 years) (e.g. Leditschke and Arden 1974; Bhettay and Bonnici 1977; Howard et al. 1977; Wohltmann et al. 1980). Reliance on weight or steroid excretion patterns is not recommended as a prognostic guide in these cases, although the few prepubertal tumours which pursued a rapid malignant course were large (>200 g) lesions.

Testicular Changes

The appearances of the testis will vary depending on age and duration of the feminising syndrome. It may be normal with a normal seminal sperm count; more frequently however, some testicular tubules will be hyalinised and show maturation arrest. Others may consist only of Sertoli cells with interstitial fibrosis and Leydig cells few in number or apparently absent. These changes may be due to reductions in pituitary gonadotrophin levels and to direct effects of tumour oestrogens on the testis.

Attached and Contralateral Adrenal Gland in the Adrenogenital Syndrome with Tumours

It will be readily apparent from the foregoing descriptions that the functional assessment of a particular adrenocortical tumour from histological criteria is seldom possible. While the adenomas associated with Conn's syndrome (vide infra) and Cushing's syndrome (p. 139) can most often, but not always, present characteristic and diagnostic morphological patterns, compact cell carcinomas and adenomas can be associated with each clinical subdivision of hypercorticalism. Clues to their functional capacity, however, can be gauged by examining the attached and/or contralateral adrenal glands.

In the 'pure' form of the adrenogenital syndrome uncomplicated by the secretion of steroids other than androgens and/or oestrogens and caused by a tumour the cortex is normal in both weight and histological appearance (Kenny et al. 1968). However, if as is sometimes the case the adrenogenital syndrome-causing tumours are also associated with some degree of increased cortisol production (vide supra) then atrophy of the cortex to variable degrees can be expected and steroid replacement therapy may be required temporarily after surgery. In some instances, foci of metastatic cancer will occur in the contralateral adrenal gland (e.g. Nichols 1968).

Non-tumorous Adrenal Feminisation

Occasionally otherwise normal male subjects have presented with infertility due to spermatogenic maturation arrest (Gabrilove et al. 1973). There is no genital hypoplasia or pseudohermaphroditism, and gynaecomastia is often but not always present. No adrenal tumour is demonstrable in these cases but the urinary outputs of 17-ketosteroids and oestrogens are raised. The administration of dexamethasone or similar therapies results in an improved sperm count and a decrease in the steroid excretion rates. These cases have been referred to as the so-called 'male feminising adrenogenital syndrome'. The adrenal changes remain to be described in detail, although the cortex has been stated to 'reveal hypertrophy' in at least one case (Gabrilove et al. 1973). However, it is not known whether the primary site of defective steroidogenesis is the testis or adrenal in such cases, although the adrenal gland may be the more likely in view of the dexamethasone suppression data. Such cases should not be confused with CAH with typical Δ^5-3β-hydroxysteroid dehydrogenase-isomerase or 17α-hydroxylase defects, in which male pseudohermaphroditism and gynaecomastia can occur (p. 159, 165) although some may conceivably represent attenuated forms of these conditions.

Chapter 14

The Distinction Between Benign and Malignant Adrenocortical Tumours causing Cushing's and/or the Adrenogenital Syndromes: Structural and Functional Criteria

One of the principal problems facing the diagnostic histopathologist is the differentiation of benign from malignant adrenocortical neoplasms. Such a prognostic problem is not unique to the adrenal but is common to all endocrine tumours. From the foregoing account, it is clear that many of the classical histological criteria of malignancy such as capsular and vascular invasion and prominent mitotic activity are not present, or are not prominent, in adrenocortical tumours causing hypercorticalism and which were subsequently shown to be carcinomas by their ability to metastasise. In this section we will describe and discuss some alternative approaches to assist reaching a more precise distinction of benign from malignant based on in vitro functional assessments of such lesions and their relationship to tumour structure.

Morphology

The small adenomas causing 'pure' Cushing's syndrome and composed of a mixture of clear and compact cells (Fig. 12.15) should not prove a diagnostic problem. Likewise the smaller (<50 g) compact cell lesions associated with virilisation can usually be reliably distinguished (Fig. 13.12). Weight can be an important factor in the final decision. As a rule of thumb 100 g can be taken as a watershed above which most, but not all, lesions are probably malignant, and below which most, but again not all (Tables 12.7, 12.8, 13.2, 13.3), are benign. Therefore this guide is at best an approximation.

The greatest difficulty is probably encountered with compact cell tumours of 100–500 g, irrespective of whether they are associated with pure or 'mixed' Cushing's syndrome or the virilising form of the adrenogenital syndrome. In our experience prominent nuclear pleomorphism, a high nuclear:cytoplasmic ratio and enlarged vesicular nuclei with one or more prominent nucleoli are criteria of especial value, together with the presence of distinct areas of necrosis as opposed to individual cell apoptosis (Fig. 14.1).

Fig. 14.1. Adrenal tumours. Virilising adrenogenital syndrome. The lesion shown *above* (**A**) is a 800 g tumour ▷ which caused virilism. Its ultrastructure is illustrated in Fig. 13.16. Although there is nuclear enlargement and pleomorphism, they are not markedly vesicular and prominent nucleoli are not noted. No recurrence has developed in a 2½-year period. The cells of the other tumour (**B**) also caused virilism in a 4-year-old girl. Note the enlarged cells and nuclei, their pleomorphism, nuclear vesicularity and prominent nucleoli and inclusions. This tumour has not recurred over a 2-year peroid. Note the apoptotic cells (*lower right, arrows*). (H + E × 250 [**A** and **B**])

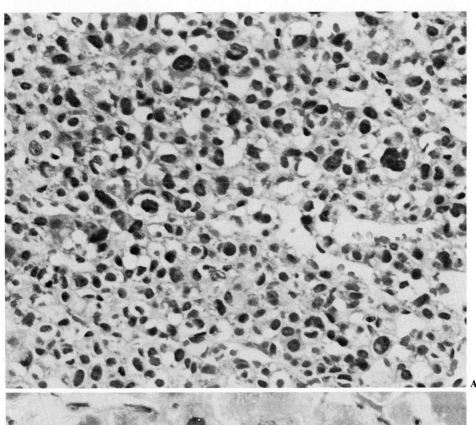

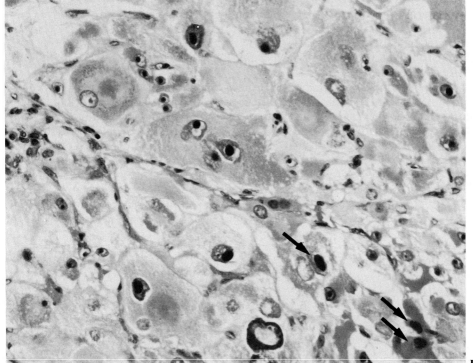

Regrettably we have not found electron microscopic studies of significant help in prognostication. Thus, while differences can undoubtedly be detected at the ultrastructural level between various benign and malignant lesions, these often reflect the different appearances seen by light microscopy (Fig. 14.2). They do not afford further help in evaluating the 'borderline' cases (such as that illustrated in Fig. 13.16). An individual tumour often shows features common to most cells within it, yet such features are not necessarily shared by other tumours causing the same syndrome (e.g. Fig. 13.15).

The regularity of organisation of cytoplasmic organelles and discontinuity of surrounding basement membrane material are two specific ultrastructural features that have been proposed as criteria of malignancy in adrenocortical tumours (MacKay 1969; Mitschke et al. 1973). On the basis of our further experience we do not believe that they are sufficiently consistent to be of diagnostic or prognostic value (Fig. 14.2). It is also important to appreciate that neither the light nor the electron microscopical appearance of these tumours can be used to assess the secretory status or type of syndrome with which they may be associated in the case of lesions causing Cushing's syndrome and/or virilisation. Conn's syndrome, is however, a different case (p. 206).

Function

As a further aid to prognosis we have, therefore, examined the functional and structural properties of nearly twenty such tumours in monolayer cell cultures, using methods we have developed for the maintainance of cells from the normal adult human cortex in vitro (Neville and O'Hare 1978). Details of some of these cases have been published elsewhere (O'Hare et al. 1979) and these, plus some additional tumours are summarised in Table 14.1. All examples referred to as carcinomas have had either histological features we consider consistent with this diagnosis (vide supra), or have subsequently been noted to metastasise. The adenomas were of the 'classical' histological pattern (Fig. 12.15) or were 'black' adenomas (Fig. 12.18) both types being associated with Cushing's syndrome. None has recurred in the 1–6 years that have elapsed since their surgical removal.

We have adopted a consistent in vitro culture and functional assessment protocol for these lesions, based on our experience of the behaviour of normal human adrenocortical cells under similar conditions (O'Hare et al. 1978). Cultures are set up from surgically-derived material and are maintained without hormonal additives for 10–14 days, following which they are exposed to $ACTH_{1-24}$ or mono- or dibutyryl cyclic AMP in maximally stimulating doses (1 $\mu g/ml$ and 0.5 mmol/l respectively) for a further seven days. Any proliferative activity of the cortical tumour cells is also assessed. In some, but not all cases, we have also treated cultures with a variety of other polypeptide hormones including LH, HCG, prolactin and TSH, at equivalent levels, to test whether the tumour cells exhibit 'ectopic' hormonal responses (vide infra). In all cases the steroid output of the cultures was assessed quantitatively and qualitatively by high performance liquid chromatography techniques (O'Hare et al. 1976; O'Hare and Nice 1981), and the pattern of both free and conjugated radiometabolites formed from

Fig. 14.2. Ultrastructure of compact cells in a 5 g adenoma causing Cushing's syndrome. This area of the ▷ tumour shows numerous macrophages (M) amongst the cortical cells (C). No basement membrane material is visible along the boundaries of the cortical cells despite the benign nature of the neoplasm. The prominent collagenous stroma (*arrows*) is suggestive of benignity but can be seen also at the light-microscopical level. (× 12 900)

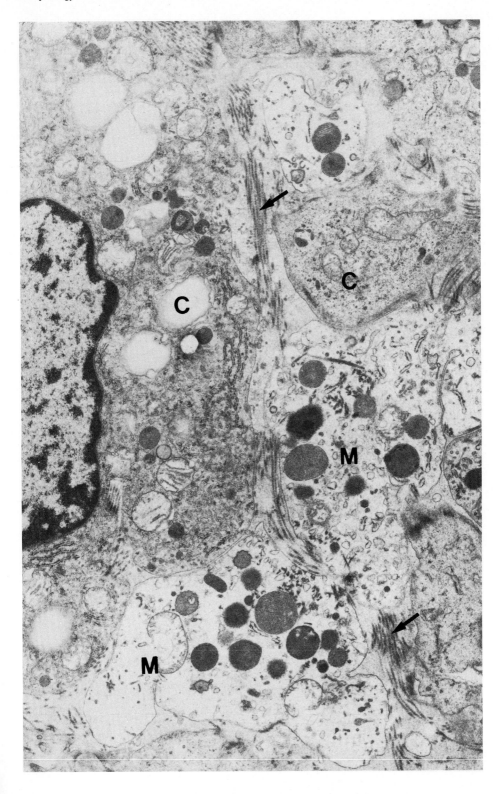

(³H)-pregnenolone and other steroid precursors was determined immediately after preparation of the cultures, and at intervals thereafter.

The results obtained with the histologically and clinically benign lesions have been exactly the same in all seven examples that caused Cushing's syndrome. All such tumours when cultured have given steroid profiles similar to normal cortical cells. The

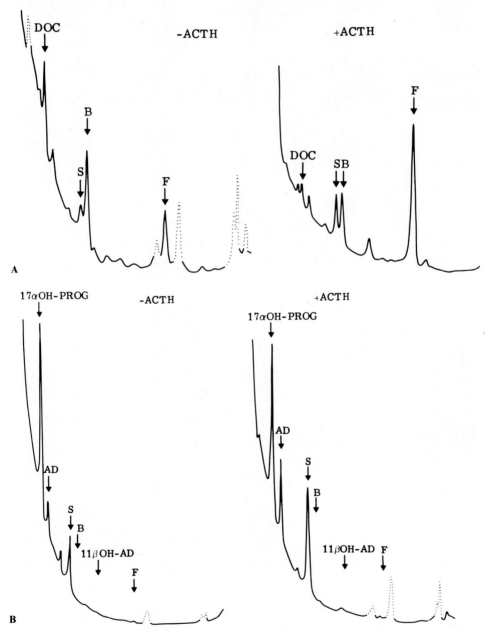

Fig. 14.3. Steroid profile (HPLC) of a benign (**A**) and a malignant (**B**) tumour associated with Cushing's syndrome in the presence and absence of ACTH in monolayer culture. See O'Hare et al. (1976) for further details of method used.

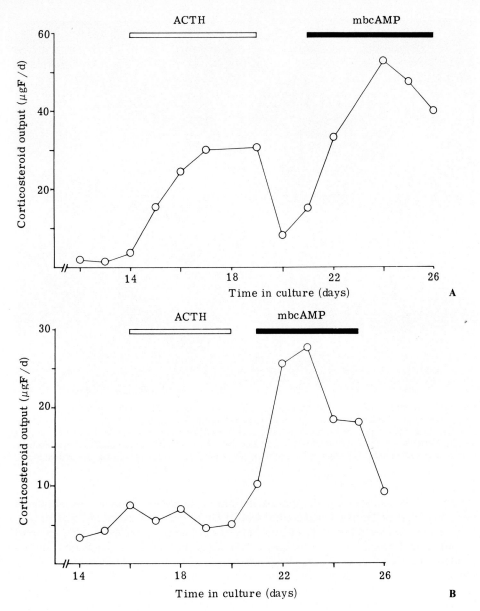

Fig. 14.4. Steroidogenic responses to ACTH and cyclic AMP by a benign (**A**) and malignant (**B**) tumour in monolayer culture.

only material difference has been the somewhat greater output of corticosterone compared with cortisol at the outset (Fig. 14.3). All benign lesions have, without exception, responded equally to ACTH and cyclic AMP with an increment in steroid output closely approximating that of normal cells (Fig. 14.4). ACTH and cyclic AMP also elicited a retraction response by almost all of the cortical tumour cells (Fig. 14.5). None of these benign tumour cells proliferated in vitro.

We have only studied one lesion causing simple virilism where there was a possibility that the tumour was benign in type. It was, however, relatively large (800 g) and some

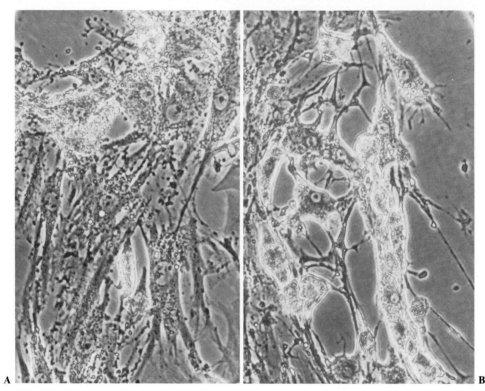

A   B

Fig. 14.5. Adrenocortical adenoma in culture. The phase-contrast photomicrographs ($\times 200$) of a monolayer culture prepared from a 15 g tumour causing Cushing's syndrome show the appearance of the cells before (**A**) and after (**B**) exposure to $ACTH_{1-24}$. The retraction response seen after 1–2 days treatment with the hormone is typical of both normal adrenocortical cells and all benign tumours causing Cushing's syndrome including 'black' adenomas. No proliferation of the cortical tumour cells has been noted in any case.

histological features of the compact-cell tumour suggested reservations about its benignity (Fig. 14.1); its ultrastructural features have been illustrated in Fig. 13.16. In culture this tumour secreted large amounts of conjugated steroids ($\sim 80\%$ of total output) and formed 11β-hydroxyandrostenedione and DHA as its major unconjugated products (Fig. 14.6). It too responded to both ACTH and cyclic AMP, albeit to a quantitatively lesser degree than the Cushing's tumours; the cells nevertheless all gave a distinct retraction response (Fig. 14.7). The behaviour of small indisputably benign compact cell lesions causing virilisation would make an interesting comparison. Nonetheless, these functional derangements may indicate an uncertain prognosis so that the further progress of this patient needs to be followed closely. At the time of writing, $2\frac{1}{2}$ years after surgery, she is alive and well.

All the histologically defined malignant lesions which we have studied in culture were responsible for a variety of 'mixed' symptoms, viz.: Cushing's syndrome with mild or severe virilisation, and marked hypertension in several cases. Table 14.1 summarises the in vitro behaviour of these lesions. All showed at least one major difference from normal cortical cells or cultured benign tumours. Some secreted only precursor steroids such as 17-hydroxyprogesterone, 11-deoxycortisol or deoxycorticosterone as their major products, while other tumours which did secrete cortisol did not respond in a normal manner to ACTH (see cases 2 and 9, Table 14.1) and/or showed a

Table 14.1. Structural and functional responses of cultured adrenocortical tumour cells

Case no.[a]	Syndrome[b]	Tumour weight (g)	Histology	Morphology	Morphologic response to ACTH	Growth	Functional response ACTH (1 μg/ml)	mbCAMP (0.5 mmol/l)	Major UV-absorbing steroids in vitro
1	C	15	Adenoma[c]	Epithelioid	++++	−	+++	++++	F+B
2	C/V	92	Carcinoma	Spherical aggregates	−	++	+	+++	F
3	C/H	125	Carcinoma	Fibroblast-like	±	+++	+	++	S+DOC[e]
4	C	420	Carcinoma	Fibroblast-like	−	+++[d]	(+)[f]	(+)[f]	17OH-PROG+S
5	C/V	880	Carcinoma	Fibroepithelioid	−	−	−	++	S
6	C/V	1850	Carcinoma	Attached spherical aggregates	−	+	−	−	S
7	V	239	Carcinoma	Fibroblast-like	−	++	++	++	11βOH-AD
8	V	800	Borderline	Epithelioid	++++	++++[d]	++	++	11βOH-AD
9	C	120	Carcinoma	Epithelioid	±	±	++	+	F+B
10	C/V	650	Carcinoma	Fibroblast-like	−	−	−	−	11βOH-AD+F
11	H	>1 kg	Carcinoma	Fibroblast-like	−	−	−	−	DOC+PROG
12	H	>1 kg	Carcinoma	Epithelioid	−	−	±	±	B+18OH-B (+ALDO)
13	C	125	Probable carcinoma	Epithelioid	+++	−	+++	+++	F+B
14	C	200	Carcinoma	Fibroblast-like	−[g]	−	−	+	F

[a]For further details of some of these cases see O'Hare et al. (1979).
[b]C: Cushing's syndrome; C/V: Cushing's syndrome with virilisation; C/H: Cushing's syndrome with hypertension; V: Virilisation or adrenogenital syndrome; H: Hypertensive syndrome.
[c]The same functional and structural responses were seen in all benign tumours causing Cushing's syndrome that were cultured (7 cases including 2 'black' adenomas).
[d]Rapid proliferation of tumour cells but for 3–4 weeks only.
[e]Reverting to 11β-hydroxysteroids (F+B) with ACTH.
[f]Qualitative but no quantitive changes.
[g]Retracted in response to dbCAMP, but not ACTH.

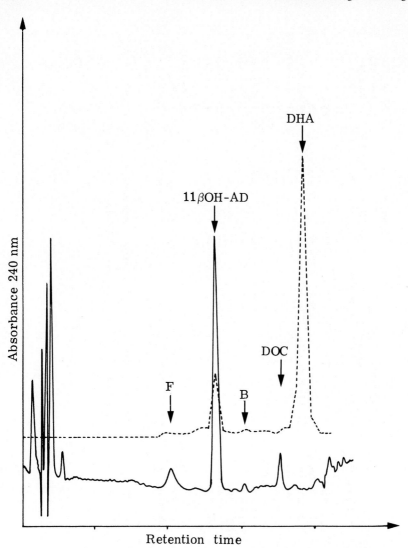

Fig. 14.6. Steroid profile (HPLC) of endogenous UV-absorbing hormones (*solid trace*) and radiometabolites formed from (^{3}H)-pregnenolone (*dotted line*) by an 800 g virilising tumour in monolayer cell culture. 11β-Hydroxyandrostenedione (11βOH-AD) and dehydroepiandrosterone (DHA) were the major products in each case (cf. Fig. 14.3). The light-microscopical and electronoptical appearances of this lesion are illustrated in Fig. 14.1 and 13.16 respectively and its appearance in culture in shown in Fig. 14.7.

marked discrepancy between the effects of the hormone and cyclic AMP (Figs. 14.3B, 14.4B). This is in marked contrast to the cultures of benign tumours (Figs. 14.3A, 14.4A). The adrenocortical carcinomas also showed a wide variety of morphological and proliferative responses. Thus, growth was marked in some instances, but not in others (Table 14.1). Some lesions formed well-spread monolayers of irregular, fibroblast-like cells, while others formed tightly packed islands of more epithelioid cells; in one case (Fig. 14.8) the tumour cells would not attach to the substrate at all but grew as free-floating aggregates. None have, however, formed continuous cell lines (Neville and O'Hare 1978); only one such line with steroid metabolising properties has been reported elsewhere (Fang 1977) and this does not, apparently, synthesise steroids

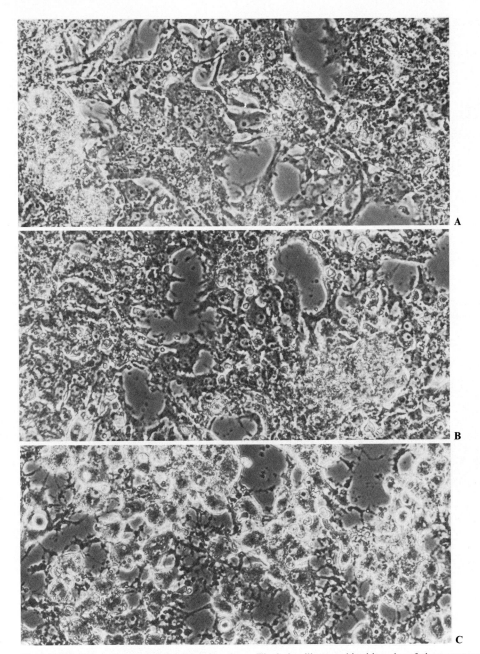

Fig. 14.7. Virilising adrenocortical tumour in culture. The lesion illustrated in this series of phase-contrast photomicrographs (× 200) caused virilism in a 28-year-old woman. Its ultrastructural appearances in vivo are shown in Fig. 13.16 and its light-microscopic features in Fig. 14.1. The tumour cells maintained without hormonal additions (**A**) show a relatively regular monolayer, although minimal nuclear pleomorphism can be seen. Addition of HCG (100 I.U/ml for 7 days) caused no visible change (**B**), but $ACTH_{1-24}$ ($1\mu g$/ml for 7 days) resulted in marked retraction of all cells (**C**). This tumour secreted 11β-hydroxyandrostenedione and DHA in vitro (Fig. 14.6) and responded to ACTH and dbcAMP (Table 14.1); unlike all benign lesions causing Cushing's syndrome, however, the cells from this tumour proliferated rapidly for 1–2 weeks when introduced into culture. Prognosis in this case must be guarded, despite the innocuous appearance of the primary lesion (Fig. 14.1).

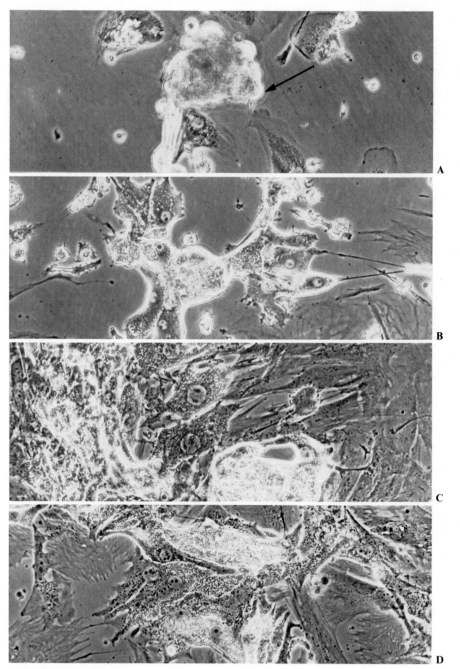

Fig. 14.8. Adrenocortical carcinomas in culture. Phase contrast photomicrographs ($\times 200$) of monolayer cultures prepared from malignant adrenocortical lesions. The tumours illustrated in **A**, **B** and **D** caused Cushing's syndrome, that illustrated in **C** the adrenogenital syndrome in a 9-year-old girl, (cf. Fig. 14.7). All cells were photographed 7–10 days after introduction into culture. The lesions shown here demonstrate the spectrum of morphological appearances seen in culture. These range from free-floating aggregates as seen in **A** (*arrow*), tightly organised groups of attached cells (**B**) as well as more extensively spread tumor cells intermingling with fibroblasts (**D**) from which they can be distinguished by their granular, lipid-laden cytoplasms.

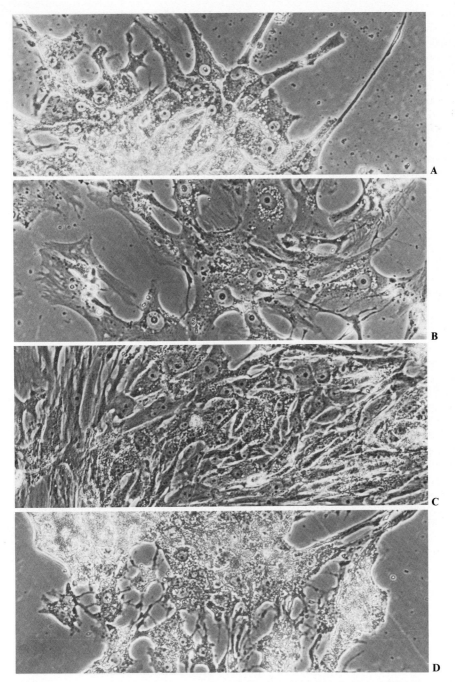

Fig. 14.9. Adrenocortical carcinomas in culture. Phase-contrast photomicrographs (× 200) of a further series of four different lesions causing Cushing's syndrome. These illustrate the pleomorphic nature of many of the cells (**A, B, C**) although the appearances of the tumour illustrated in **D** (a lesion of approximately 100 g did not differ markedly from adenomas we have cultured cf. Fig. 14.5). The cells from the tumour shown in **B** proliferated rapidly in culture for 2–3 passages but subsequently ceased dividing; those from the other lesions illustrated showed little or no propensity to divide in culture, despite their malignant nature, and were eventually overgrown by fibroblast-like cells.

de novo, although it will aromatise androgens. Many of the undoubtedly malignant lesions did not proliferate at all in vitro, an experience not, unfortunately, confined to adrenocortical tumours (O'Hare et al. 1978). The differing appearances of a number of these carcinomas in culture are shown in Figs. 14.8, 14.9.

These results suggest, therefore, that while no single feature is pathognomonic of malignancy, the presence of one or more specific morphological, functional or proliferative aberrations compared with normal cortical cells in vitro should be regarded as presumptive evidence of malignancy, in view of the uniformly normal behaviour of benign tumours studied in this manner. These functional aberrations of the malignant tumours should not, however, be seen as causing malignancy, but simply an associated phenomenon. A limited number of other culture studies (Israeli et al. 1975; Szabo et al. 1975) and short-term in vitro experiments (Oshima et al. 1969; Voigt et al. 1975) by and large substantiate our conclusions regarding the different behaviour of the benign and malignant tumours causing Cushing's syndrome and/or virilisation.

The opportunity to carry out in vitro experiments of the type outlined above is obviously limited by both access to fresh surgical material and the capability of processing it for long-term tissue culture studies. It is therefore, germane to ask whether the behaviour of such lesions in vitro is representative of their properties in vivo. We cannot verify this proposition in all cases due to a lack of relevant in vivo data, but several recent examples have confirmed our belief in the validity of these methods. Thus, a malignant tumour causing hypertension and simulating Conn's syndrome was studied by us in vitro and found to secrete no aldosterone, but synthesised instead predominately deoxycorticosterone and progesterone. Multiple hormone assays in vivo confirmed these results, and established that the hypertensive syndrome was in fact due primarily to the hypersecretion of DOC, circulating levels of which were about 40 times normal (Davies et al. 1981).

A significant proportion of the malignant tumours have shown a propensity to release enhanced levels of 11-deoxysteroids (Table 14.1). This is also a common feature of many such tumours in vivo (Lipsett and Wilson 1962; Boyar et al. 1977; Tan et al. 1977; Kelly et al. 1979). Some possible reasons why this particular aberration should be so frequently encountered are discussed below. It does, however, emphasise the need for multiple hormone assays, including precursor steroids, in the diagnosis and monitoring of subsequent disease (O'Hare et al. 1979) and this is indeed now being carried out with some degree of success by some workers (Kelly et al. 1979).

Hormonal responses to ACTH in culture afford another good discriminant, as about 80% of the malignant tumours we studied showed attenuated or absent responses, particularly when compared with cyclic AMP responses. In vitro methods seem here more valuable than studies in vivo. Thus while all benign lesions causing Cushing's syndrome that we have examined, including two 'black' adenomas, giving a total of seven cases, have shown an essentially normal response to ACTH only about half such lesions respond in vivo to an acute stimulus (Soffer et al. 1957; Saez et al. 1975; Scott et al. 1977; Nishikawa et al. 1979). The difference probably relates to the duration of stimulus. Thus compact-cell lesions seem relatively refractory to short-term ACTH treatment (1–2 h) in vitro (Hasegawa et al. 1975), a situation strongly reminiscent of the normal zona reticularis under similar conditions (Griffiths et al. 1963). In culture, however, prolonged exposure to the hormone for several days elicits a response from both normal and benign neoplastic compact cells. The discrimination of benign and malignant tumours is thus improved as only a minority of malignant lesions respond to ACTH in culture, and equally few respond in vivo (Saez et al. 1975).

The discrepancy between the responses to ACTH and cyclic AMP observed with some malignant lesions in culture is of interest in the light of various functional abnormalities of the ACTH-cyclic AMP system demonstrated using homogenate methods by Saez and his colleagues (1975). In their study of membrane-bound adenylate cyclase in ten carcinomas and three adenomas, six tumours contained enzyme which as with the normal cortical cells could be activated by both ACTH and prostaglandin E_1. In six other lesions it was insensitive to ACTH but not PGE_1, and in one neoplasm it responded to neither. Furthermore, in two cases in which the adenylate cyclase was sensitive to ACTH, glucocorticoid secretion by the intact cells was not enhanced. These results clearly demonstrate that several different defects can occur in the ACTH-cyclic AMP mechanism in tumours (Fig. 8.9). Although two 'adenomas' in Saez's study did not respond to ACTH, both were large lesions (72 and 80 g) and they were apparently virilising tumours as 17-ketosteroids but not 17-hydroxysteroids were elevated (compare case 1; Table 14.1). The Cushing's adenoma studied was, however, ACTH-responsive, a result consistent with our observations.

Further studies by this group (Riou et al. 1977; Saez et al. 1978) have shown that even when ACTH binding is normal in some tumours protein kinase activity may be altered, and conversely protein kinase may be normal while ACTH is not bound. The results we have obtained with intact cells, viz.: a few carcinomas responding to both ACTH and cyclic AMP, the majority primarily to cyclic AMP alone, and some to neither (Table 14.1), are thus probably explicable on the basis of specific lesions in each of the moeties involved in the intracellular mechanism of ACTH action (Fig. 8.9). We would suggest, furthermore, that the presence of any of these defects, particularly in tumours associated with Cushing's syndrome, is strongly suggestive of potential malignancy.

Autonomy

There is also some evidence from studies of adrenal homogenate preparations that the membrane-bound adenylate cyclase of some human adrenal tumours can be 'ectopically' activated by hormones other than ACTH (e.g. TSH and LH) (Hinshaw and Ney 1974; Matsukura et al. 1980). It has been further suggested that such effects may account for the functional 'autonomy' of the lesions (Schorr et al. 1972). We have, however, observed no such responses in the form of enhanced steroid output in cultures of four different adrenocortical carcinomas exposed to these stimuli. Recent studies have shown that adrenal tumour slices are also refractory, even in cases where membrane preparations can be activated ectopically (Matsukura et al. 1980). It seems unlikely, therefore, that this is the explanation of tumour autonomy in the vast majority of cases.

The apparent functional autonomy of these lesions is, in our opinion, most likely to be a function of residual 'baseline' levels of steroidogenesis corresponding to those seen in normal human cortical cells deprived of ACTH (Fig. 8.6). The onset of clinical hypercorticalism with such tumours is thus probably determined simply by (a) the functional normality (or otherwise) of the tumour tissue in respect of secretion of biologically active hormones, and (b) its increasing mass.

Aetiology of the Abnormal Steroidogenesis

This concept of functional abnormality versus normality as a general correlate of malignancy versus benignity entails a further prediction. Tumours causing syndromes of steroid excess due to overproduction of what are normally very minor products of the normal cortex, such as oestrogens, and those tumours which produce no active steroids at all (p. 242) are all likely to behave in a malignant fashion. This is precisely what is observed.

The secretion of high levels of sulphoconjugated steroids and C_{19} steroids such as 11β-hydroxyandrostenedione and DHA, on the other hand, appears to be part of the normal function of inner zone compact cells (O'Hare et al. 1980a; Fig. 10.2). Thus tumours with these properties may include benign lesions.

No pattern of functional activity can, however, be deemed the exclusive property of benign tumours. We have observed some lesions with apparently normal steroidogenic profiles (e.g. case 2; Table 14.1) which were small at the time of surgery, but which nevertheless pursued a rapidly malignant course. Thus, functional abnormality is, in our experience, strongly correlated with malignancy, but apparent functional normality in respect of steroidogenesis does not preclude it. Functional parameters should therefore be given equal consideration with structural histological criteria in the assessment of borderline lesions when it is possible for them to be determined in one or more of the manners we have outlined above.

The potential lesions in the ACTH-cyclic AMP-protein kinase mechanisms than can result in functional abnormalities in neoplasms have already been considered. The particular propensity of some tumours to form excessive amounts of 11-deoxysteroids does, however, warrant some further comment. This is frequently, but not exclusively, observed in tumours causing virilisation and feminisation (e.g. West et al. 1964; Bryson et al. 1968) and a possible role of the sex steroids themselves inhibiting 11β-hydroxylase activity must be considered. Nevertheless, some observations we have made on the behaviour of cultured normal adult human adrenocortical cells, and the effects of cell density on their steroidogenic profiles (Neville and O'Hare 1978) suggests another possibility.

In dense (i.e. confluent) monolayer cultures such normal cells predominantly secrete the 11-hydroxysteroids (Fig. 14.10) that might be anticipated from their attributes in

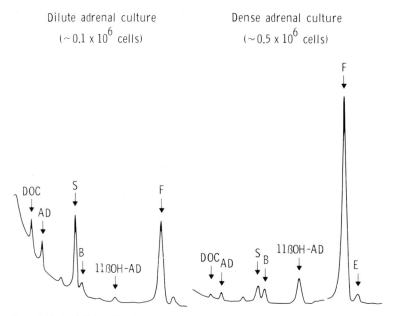

Fig. 14.10. Steroid profiles (HPLC) of dense and dilute cultures of normal adult human adrenal cells in monolayer culture.

vivo. Dilute (i.e. non-confluent) cultures of the same cells secrete, on the other hand, predominantly 11-deoxysteroids (Fig. 14.10) (Neville and O'Hare 1978; O'Hare et al. 1978). They thus resemble many of the tumour cultures prepared from malignant lesions. As this density dependence of patterns of steroidogensis is shared by benign tumours, it is mandatory that all neoplasms are studied in dense and confluent cultures to obviate such effects distorting steroid profiles. As an added precaution steroidogenesis by such lesions should be examined immediately after their introduction into culture to check that no marked changes ensue in long-term culture. However, setting these practical considerations aside the density-dependent effect observed with normal cells, and their capacity to simulate some types of malignant neoplasm when maintained in dilute cultures suggests that cell-cell contact may play a vital role in ensuring the normal patterns of steroidogenesis. As a corollary, one may speculate that any disruption of such putative interactions in tumours, notably those of the malignant variety, may specifically alter the steroidogenic capabilities of the lesions in such a way as to favour 11-deoxysteroid secretion, and cause a reduction in the output of the normal 11β-hydroxylated glucocorticoids.

Conclusions

The gross and light-microscopical features of a particular tumour provide valuable, but not necessarily invariably accurate prognostic indices. Assessment of various in vivo and particularly in vitro functional parameters should also be effected whenever possible. Abnormal responses to ACTH, cyclic AMP and/or the predominant production of precursor-type steroids are important factors in arriving at a more accurate diagnosis particularly in the case of the histologically 'borderline' tumours.

Chapter 15

Hyperaldosteronism and Related Syndromes of Mineralocorticoid Excess

The syndrome of hyperaldosteronism with low plasma renin (so-called 'primary' aldosteronism) was recognised as a specific clinicopathological entity by Conn in 1955. It is typified by hypokalaemic alkalosis, hypertension and muscle weakness, and is usually referred to as Conn's syndrome, particularly when associated with a solitary aldosterone-secreting adrenal adenoma. Similar symptoms also occur when steroids, other than aldosterone, with mineralocorticoid activity are secreted in excess, as sometimes occurs in association with malignant adrenocortical tumours (p. 231).

Pathological secondary hyperaldosteronism, with elevated plasma renin and angiotensin levels, is found in several oedematous disease states including the nephrotic syndrome, liver cirrhosis and some, but not all cases of congestive heart failure, as well as in other conditions (e.g. renin-secreting tumours; malignant hypertension).

Hyperaldosteronism With Low Plasma Renin (Primary Aldosteronism)

Symptoms and Incidence

Symptoms of excessive production of aldosterone stem from its effects on the kidney and the consequent secondary electrolyte disorders. In primary aldosteronism, this is due to its autonomous or semi-autonomous hypersecretion by the adrenal cortex.

Aldosterone excess causes, initially, enhanced renal sodium retention leading to expansion of the extracellular fluid volume and hypervolaemia. Subsequently, urinary sodium excretion comes into balance with sodium intake due to the so-called 'renal escape' phenomenon, and fluid retention ceases; oedema is, therefore, not a feature of this disease state. Hypervolaemia persists, nevertheless, and the potassium depletion, which continues unabated, results in a state of chronic hypokalaemia. Primary aldosteronism is consequently characterised by plasma sodium levels that are within the normal range or are only slightly elevated in most cases, plasma aldosterone levels that are usually only moderately elevated ($\sim$30 ng/100 ml; Davies et al. 1979) but which are not suppressed by sodium loading ($>$50 ng/100 ml on 200 mEq/d sodium; Cain et al. 1972) and a plasma potassium that is in the range 2.5–3.0 mmol/l in about 80% of cases (Weinberger et al. 1979). In some patients these 'classical' chemical features may be absent (Conn et al. 1964).

The hypokalaemic state, which often waxes and wanes during the course of the disease, is responsible for most of the symptoms which include, in approximate order of frequency, muscular weakness, nocturia, persistent frontal headaches, polydipsia, paraesthesia, visual disturbances, temporary paralysis, cramps and tetany (Conn et al. 1964). The volume-dependent hypertension while usually not malignant in intensity and not causing for example retinopathy, may on occasions be quite severe ($\sim$200/

116 mm Hg mean) (Cain et al. 1972). This causes the major threat to life with ensuing nephrosclerosis, cardiac enlargement and increased risk of cardiovascular or cerebral accidents. The physical signs and symptoms of primary hyperaldosteronism are not, however, always easily distinguished from 'essential' hypertension without laboratory studies.

No specific familial associations or predisposing conditions have been identified in the majority of cases of primary aldosteronism, although one rare form of the disease, dexamethasone-suppressible hyperaldosteronism (vide infra) is a familial disorder and appears to be transmitted by an autosomal dominant gene (New et al. 1980). It may, in fact, be a form of congenital adrenal hyperplasia (vide infra).

The incidence of primary aldosteronism as a cause of hypertension has been subject to widely varying estimates. Although many hypertensive patients present abnormalities in renin, angiotensin and aldosterone levels it now seems that despite early claims to the contrary the excessive secretion of aldosterone does not play a primary pathogenic role in the great majority of cases. The consensus is that perhaps 1%–2% of unselected hypertensives have demonstrable primary aldosteronism (Brown et al. 1972b; Kaplan 1974).

Pathology

Our association over the past 15 years with the Medical Research Council Blood Pressure Unit in Glasgow, together with an extensive referral practice, has given us the opportunity to study 153 examples of the adrenal changes in hyperaldosteronism with low plasma renin (Table 15.1). It is associated with three types of adrenal pathology viz.: tumours (both benign and malignant), nodules, and hyperplasia of the zona glomerulosa. These may occur in combination within one gland or as a single feature (Neville and Symington 1966; Ferriss et al. 1970; Neville and MacKay 1972).

Table 15.1. Classification of adrenal changes in hyperaldosteronism with low plasma renin based upon 153 personally studied cases[a]

Group	Histological subdivisions	Incidence	
1. Adrenocortical tumour	Adrenal adenoma with hyperplasia of zona glomerulosa	50	
	Adrenal adenoma with hyperplasia of zona glomerulosa and with nodules	70	82%
	Adrenal carcinoma[b]	5	
2. No adrenocortical tumour	Hyperplasia of zona glomerulosa	4	
	Hyperplasia of zona glomerulosa with micronodules	14	18%
	Hyperplasia of zona glomerulosa with micronodules and macronodules	5	
	Normal zona glomerulosa with micronodules	5	

[a]Some of the cases have been reported by Neville and Symington (1966); Ferris et al. (1970) and Neville and MacKay (1972)

[b]Attached and/or contralateral gland was not available for study in the examples personally studied.

The pathological changes can, however, be classified into two major groups, i.e. tumourous and non-tumorous hyperaldosteronism. Each group may be further sub-classified according to the precise adrenocortical morphology and their relative frequencies in our own series are shown in Table 15.1

About four-fifths of patients exhibit tumours, almost all of which are benign and solitary (Table 15.1). Although multiple tumours have been reported to occur, we have personally seen only one such example. As previous studies have not appreciated that a tumour and a large adrenocortical nodule simulating a tumour can occur in the same or contra-lateral gland (a feature we have seen on several occasions) it may well be that multiple neoplastic lesions are significantly rarer than originally recorded.

Approximately one-fifth of the patients with hyperaldosteronism and low plasma renin comprise the second group (Table 15.1) of non-tumorous changes, most of whom will show hyperplasia of the zona glomerulosa. However, such lesions are seldom seen by the pathologist because they are now detected preoperatively by various diagnostic techniques such as multidimensional computer-assisted quadric (Ferriss et al. 1970; Aitchison et al. 1971) or multiple logistic (Luetscher et al. 1974) analyses, the dexamethasone-modified adrenal scintiscan with ^{131}I-19-iodocholesterol (Seabold et al. 1976), or ^{131}I-6β-iodomethyl-19-norcholesterol, as originally introduced by Conn et al. (1971, 1972), Sakar et al. (1977) and more recently with ^{75}Se-selenomethylcholesterol (Shapiro et al. 1981) and differential venous sampling of steroid levels from each gland (Melby et al. 1972; Weinberger et al. 1979). They are perhaps somewhat less reliably distinguished by the anomalous response of plasma aldosterone to postural changes in tumour-bearing patients (Ganguly et al. 1973; Ganguly and Weinberger 1979) and adrenal venography (Horton and Finck 1972). Sodium depletion, potassium loading, cortisol, ACTH, DOCA and fludrocortisone administration do not distinguish reliably these two conditions (Padfield et al. 1975). This distinction is important because cases of bilateral zona glomerulosa hyperplasia are best treated medically as remission of their hypertensive syndrome seldom occurs after adrenalectomy ($<20\%$ of cases) (Baer et al. 1970; Ferriss et al. 1975).

In a previous retrospective survey (Ferriss et al. 1970), we distinguished a third, smaller, group of patients who presented with a unilateral adrenal lesion of 1–2 cm in diameter which defied accurate classification as an adenoma or macro-nodule despite the use of multiple histological criteria (Table 15.6). However, with the introduction of computer-assisted differential diagnosis (Aitchison et al. 1971) and in vitro studies of steroid biosynthetic potential (vide infra), these ambiguous cases should be significantly reduced in number. Such cases in our original series, therefore, have been omitted from the present revised classification.

Incidence of Pathological Adrenal Changes in Primary Aldosteronism

As mentioned above, several independent series have shown that between 65%–85% of patients with hyperaldosteronism and low plasma renin have an adrenal tumour (Neville and Symington 1966; Ferriss et al. 1975; Conn et al. 1977) (Tables 15.1, 15.2 and 15.3) almost all of which are benign. Malignant tumours causing hyper-aldosteronism are exceedingly rare. Both adenomas and carcinomas are commoner in females than in males and occur mostly between the ages of 30–50 years of age in both sexes (Table 15.2); rarely, an ectopic location has been noted (Flanagan and McDonald 1975). Benign tumours of this type can also occur in children (Table 15.2) but they are proportionately rare in contrast to the high frequency with which other forms of hypercorticalism in children are caused by tumours (see Kafrouni et al. 1975 for collective review of 'aldosteronomas' in children). Non-tumorous hyper-aldosteronism by contrast, tends to occur in slightly older persons (Davies et al. 1979)

Table 15.2. Age distribution of 266 tumours of the adrenal cortex in hyperaldosteronism with low plasma renin[a]

Adrenal changes (no. of cases)	Sex	15–20	21–30	31–40	41–50	51–60	61–70	>70	Total
				Age (years)					
Adenoma (241)	Female	6	16	59	67	17	5	1	171
	Male	2	7	20	28	9	3	1	70
Carcinomas (25)	Female	–	2	5	3	5	1	–	16
	Male	–	1	4	1	2	1	–	9

[a]Data from the present series together with those previous reviewed (Neville and Symington 1966). See Table 15.6 for the details of the carcinomas reported in the literature to date.

Table 15.3. Primary aldosteronism: analysis of 240 patients with benign tumours of the adrenal cortex

	Male	Female
Sex incidence	30%	70%
Modal age incidence (years)	30–50	30–50
Site of tumours (left:right)		
Single	1:1	7:4
Multiple	1:4	4:1
Weight of tumours (g)		
<2	34%	
<4	58%	

and with an approximately equal frequency in either sex (Ferriss et al. 1970; Neville and MacKay 1972; Table 15.1), although again children are not entirely exempt (Grim et al. 1967).

Adrenocortical Tumours

(1) Adenomas

Gross appearance   Over 90% of adenomas causing Conn's syndrome are single. In females, they are found more often in the left than the right gland. In males they occur with an approximately equal frequency in either gland (Table 15.4). The typical adenoma of Conn's syndrome is a circumscribed encapsulated lesion with a distinctive, golden-yellow cut surface (Plate A, facing p. 146). This appearance often contrasts with the paler yellow colour of the non-functioning nodule particularly the larger macronodules, and can be readily distinguished from the yellow/brown mottled appearance of the adenoma associated with Cushing's syndrome (Plate A). Rarely, foci of calcification may be seen in such small tumours (Kelch et al. 1973). Most aldosterone-producing adenomas are small when removed at surgery. In our own series 34% weighed <2 g and 58% were <4 g (Table 15.5). Nonetheless, occasional adenomas can weigh >70 g and we have seen one recent adenoma which weighed 200 g.

In view of their small size, many adenomas are wholly intraglandular and only detected on sectioning the gland after operation. At one end of the spectrum, we have seen examples measuring only 2–3 mm in diameter and weighing <100 mg. Larger tumours, on the other hand, project from one or other pole of the adrenal gland and

Table 15.4. Hyperaldosteronism with low plasma renin. Site distribution of adrenal adenomas in 218 patients[a]

Site	No. of patients		Total
	Males	Females	
Single			
Right adrenal	22	37	59
Left adrenal	25	70	95
Bilateral	2	1	3
Unknown	14	40	54
Subtotal	63 (91%)	148 (93%)	201 (92%)
Multiple			
Right adrenal	4	2	6
Left adrenal	1	8	9
Bilateral	1	1	2
Unknown	–	–	–
Subtotal	6 (9%)	11 (7%)	17 (8%)
Total	69 (30%)	159 (70%)	218 (100%)

[a]Data culled from present series and from the cases reviewed by Neville and Symington (1966).

Table 15.5 Hyperaldosteronism with low plasma renin (Conn's syndrome). Weights of 151 adrenal adenomas

Weight (g)	No.	(%)
<2	51	(34%)
2–4	36	(24%)
4–5	16	(11%)
5–10[a]	26	(17%)
10–20	11	(7%)
20–30	3	(7%)
>30	8	
Total	151	(100%)

[a]Data culled from present series and from the cases reviewed by Neville and Symington (1966).

with increasing size, foci of necrosis, and cystic change may be found. We have seen one adenoma which was almost entirely cystic with only a thin rim of viable neoplastic tissue around its periphery.

Microscopic appearance   Adenomas have a characteristic and somewhat unexpected histological appearance typified by a protean cellular morphology (Neville and Symington 1966; Symington 1969; Neville and MacKay 1972; Maltini et al. 1973). Four

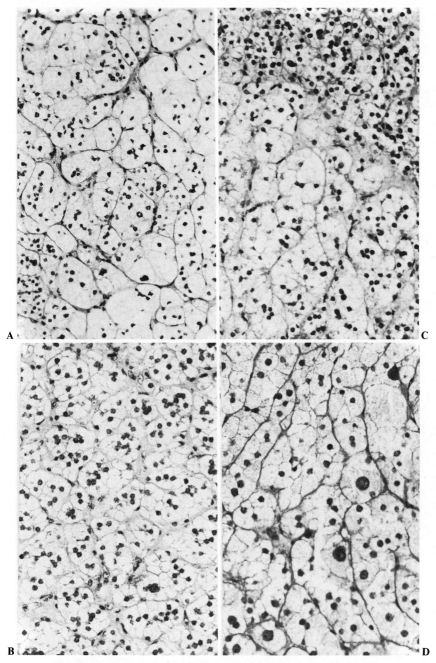

Fig. 15.1. Hyperaldosteronism with low plasma renin. Adrenocortical adenomas (**A**, 1.5 g; **C**, 2.4 g; **D**, 2.09 g; **B**, a 1-cm macronodule) The commonest cellular patterns are illustrated in Fig. **A, C,** and **D** and may be compared with that of a macronodule (**B**). The cells (**A**) are normal in size, and are of the large clear lipid-laden zona fasciculata type arranged in cords and nests. There is little pleomorphism. In **C**, the intermediate-type cells may be seen at the *top right*, while in **D**, nuclear pleomorphism is present. By comparison, the cells of the nodule (**B**) are normal in size and only of the zona fasciculata type. The fibrovascular trabeculae may be more prominent but the appearances can be difficult to distinguish from **A** unless different cell types or pleomorphism is present. (H + E × 150 [**A, B,** and **C**]; × 240 [**D**])

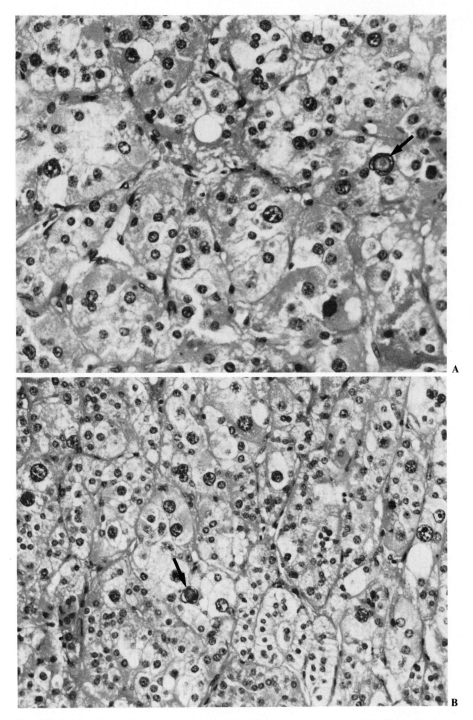

Fig. 15.2. Hyperaldosteronism with low plasma renin. Adrenocortical adenomas. The illustrations are taken from two tumours, one (**A**) weighing 2.9 g and the other (**B**), 3.5 g. The cells are of the larger clear lipid-laden type and have giant, pleomorphic nuclei, some of which also show inclusions (*arrows*). (H + E × 375 [**A** and **B**])

distinct cell types can be distinguished in such lesions – large and small clear lipid-laden cells, zona glomerulosa-type and zona reticularis-type (compact) cells. The small clear cells were formerly referred to as 'hybrid' cells (Neville and Symington 1966); we now prefer to call them 'intermediate' cells, in view of other current connotations of the former term. Very few adenomas ($<10\%$) consist of a single cell type and all four cell types can be found in a single tumour in most instances, if carefully sought.

The commonest cell type encountered in these lesions consists of large lipid-laden clear cells similar to those of the zona fasciculata in appearance, size and nuclear:cytoplasmic ratio (Fig. 15.1). The tumour cells are arranged in short cords or nests, separated by a fine fibrovascular connective tissue stroma. However, the nuclei are more vesicular than normal and often contain vacuolated inclusions (Fig. 15.2). Pleomorphism is usually present but is seldom marked, although occasional giant or bizarre nucleated forms can be detected (Fig. 15.2).

While large lipid-laden clear cells may occur alone, when the distinction of tumour from non-functioning nodule may be difficult (Fig. 15.1), they are found more commonly in association with smaller lipid-rich cells also arranged in nests and cords. Such cells also have vesicular nuclei but their nuclear:cytoplasmic ratio is similar to that of normal zona glomerulosa cells although they contain more visible lipid. Thus, this cell type seems to have the cytological characteristics of both zona glomerulosa and zona fasciculata cells; these are the 'intermediate' cells (Fig. 15.1).

In these adenomas, groups of typical zona reticularis-type compact cells are also occasionally noted in association with the other cell types (Fig. 15.3). In rare instances

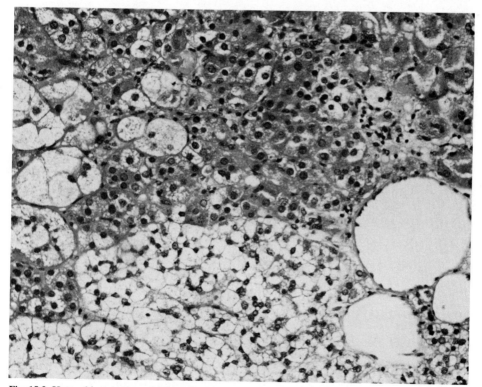

Fig. 15.3. Hyperaldosteronism with low plasma renin. Adrenocortical adenoma (3.1 g). All four cell types which can occur in benign tumours causing hyperaldosteronism with low plasma renin are shown. Clear zona fasciculata-type cells are present (*left*), with intermediate cells (*below*), compact zona reticularis-type cells (*top right*) and between them zona glomerulosa-type cells. (H + E × 200)

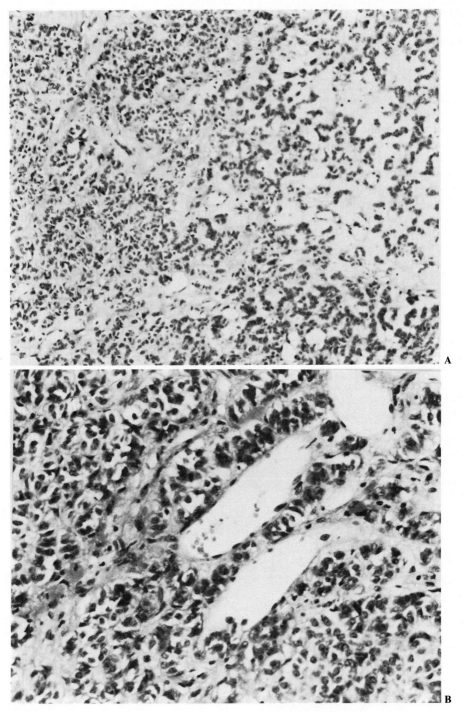

Fig. 15.4. Hyperaldosteronism with low plasma renin. Adrenocortical adenoma (7.4 g). This benign tumour contained, almost exclusively, cells of the zona glomerulosa type arranged in cords, strands and nests. Areas of stromal myxomatous change were also present (**A**) together with prominent vascular sinusoids (**B**). (H + E **A** × 150; **B** × 300)

they may be the predominant cell type and when filled with abundant lipofuscin granules they may give the appearance of a so-called 'black adenoma', as in the case reported by Caplan and Virata (1974). Such lesions (which we have not seen) are apparently indistinguishable microscopically from the 'black adenomas' associated with other hypercortical states (p. 139).

In many adenomas recognisable zona glomerulosa-type cells are also present (Figs. 15.4 and 15.5). In rare instances they, or cells of similar appearance (Fig. 15.4) may be the sole component (Symington 1969). While such cells may appear on cursory

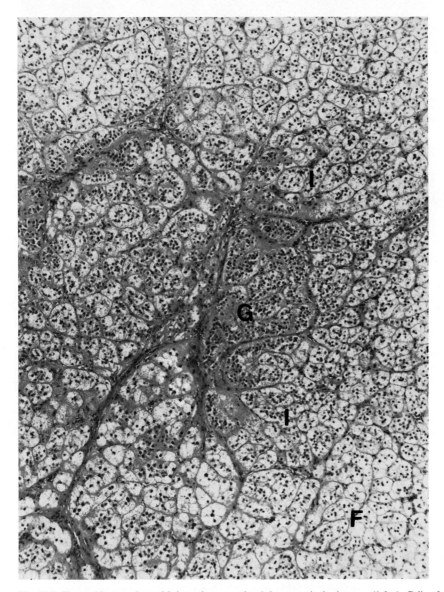

Fig. 15.5. Hyperaldosteronism with low plasma renin. Adrenocortical adenoma (1.0 g). Cells of the large clear type (F) are the main constituents of this tumour. Toward the periphery of the lesion, numerous fibrovascular trabeculae dip into the tumour and appear to carry with them zona glomerulosa-type cells (G). Intermediate cells (I) are present between the zona glomerulosa type and large clear cells. (H + E × 100)

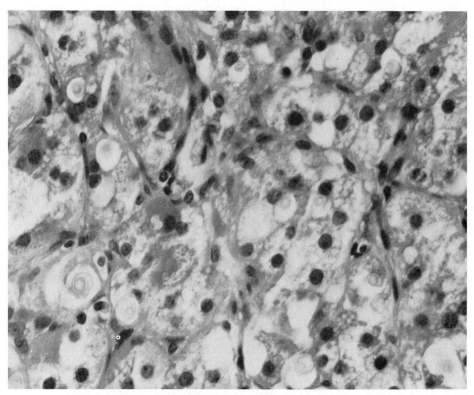

Fig. 15.6. Hyperaldosteronism with low plasma renin. Spironolactone bodies. Numerous spironolactone bodies are present in the tumour, occuring in cells of the clear lipid-laden zona fasciculata type. In other lesions, we have noted them also in zona glomerulosa-type cells. ($H + E \times 600$)

examination to occur more or less at random in the substance of such tumours, our observations indicate that they are often found in nests, short cords or trabeculae predominantly around the periphery of the lesion, dipping into the substance of the tumour in a tongue-like manner accompanied by fibrovascular trabeculae derived from the capsule (Fig. 15.5).

Table 15.6. Pathological features of most value in differentiating between adrenocortical adenomas and nodules in hyperaldosteronism with low plasma renin[a]

Feature	Adenoma	Nodule
Gross colour	Golden-yellow	Lighter yellow
Cell type	Mixed; rarely (6%) clear cells only	Clear cells only
Nuclear and cellular pleomorphism	Generally present	Absent, although may be present in focal areas
Nuclear character	Vesicular	Hyperchromatic
Nuclear inclusions	Present	Absent
Ultrastructure	Features of zona glomerulosa cells	Features of zona fasciculata cells
Spironolactone bodies	May be present	Absent

[a]From the data of Ferriss et al. 1970.

In patients with adenomas given the drug spironolactone for several weeks or months prior to surgery to control their hypertensive symptoms, so-called 'spironolactone bodies' (p. 64) can be detected in some cells in the adenoma (Fig. 15.6) as well as in the attached and contralateral adrenal glands in most cases. Our experience to date suggests that such bodies are not detected in lesions that have the microscopical characteristics of nodules associated with this syndrome and we believe therefore, that this feature can be of help in distinguishing nodules from adenomas (Ferriss et al. 1970). A complete list of the criteria we have found important in discriminating between adenomas in Conn's syndrome and non-functioning nodules is summarised in Table 15.6.

Ultrastructure   Several electron microscopic studies of Conn's syndrome adenomas have now been reported (MacKay 1969; Reidbord and Fisher 1969; Sommers and Terzakis 1970; Tannenbaum 1973; Kovacs et al. 1974; Beskid et al. 1978; Kano et al. 1979). They have tended to concentrate upon the ultrastructural features of both the most commonly occurring clear and intermediate cell types. These studies have shown that, in general, these cells have ultrastructural features such as mitochondria with tubulo-lamellar cristae, interdigitating cell membranes and moderately developed smooth endoplasmic reticulum and sparse rough ER that are in part akin to normal zona glomerulosa cells or are intermediate between this cell type and typical zona fasciculata cells (Fig. 15.7). Individual cells within such adenomas may, however, show wide differences in ultrastructural features that mirror the cellular heterogeneity found at the light microscopic level.

The aetiological significance of these intermediate cells and the other structural features of typical adenomas found in Conn's syndrome, notably the relative paucity of cells with a typical zona glomerulosa appearance in most tumours is discussed later (p. 233).

(2) Carcinomas

Nearly 30 adrenal carcinomas associated with the clinical signs and symptoms of Conn's syndrome and with evidence of aldosterone secretion have now been reported (Table 15.7). The first case of tumorous hyperaldosteronism recorded in the literature was, in fact, due to a malignant tumour (Foye and Feichtmeir 1955). Estimates of their general incidence indicate that perhaps $<5\%$ of tumorous hyperaldosteronism is caused by a malignant adrenal tumour (Table 15.1; Salassa et al. 1974; Conn et al. 1977).

Although the symptoms in these cases are generally similar to those found with benign lesions, the classic triad of hypertension, hypokalaemic alkalosis and muscle weakness may be accompanied by abdominal pain and sometimes fever. Unlike the adenomas, there may also be an excess secretion of a variety of steroids in addition to aldosterone, so that elevated urinary 17-keto and/or 17-hydroxysteroids occur in many but not all cases (see Alterman et al. 1969 for a review of clinical features of some early cases). One example we have recently studied in vitro secreted large amounts of 18-hydroxycorticosterone and corticosterone as well as aldosterone (p. 238). However, symptoms of concurrent hypercortisolism, virilism or feminisation are seldom seen in cases in which hyperaldosteronism is chemically proved. It should be remembered that other malignant tumours may also cause clinical signs and symtpoms of hyper-mineralocorticoidism without, however, secreting aldosterone (p. 231).

Benign and malignant 'aldosteronomas' may be detected and be distinguishable clinically from one another in some cases by venography, angiography, CAT scanning and scintiscans (Conn et al. 1977; Britton 1979; Dunnick et al. 1979; Linde et al. 1979).

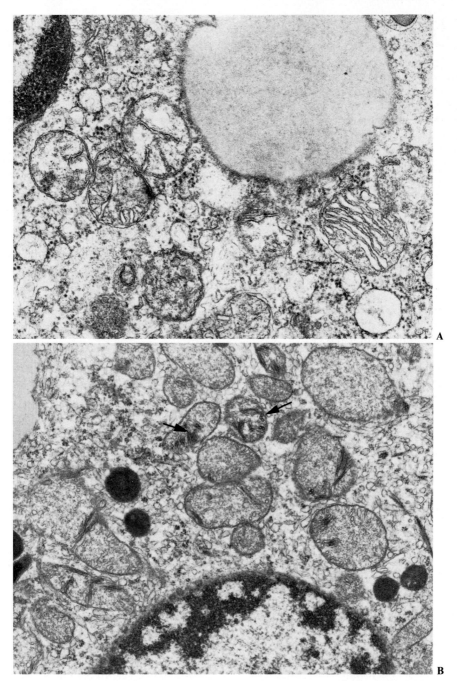

Fig. 15.7. Hyperaldosteronism with low plasma renin. The ultrastructure of a zona glomerulosa cell from the attached gland (**A**) and of an 'intermediate' cell from the adenoma itself (**B**). The glomerulosa cell in the attached gland still shows typical lamellar cristae in the mitochondria while the adenoma cell contains mitochondria with tubulo-vesicular cristae more akin to those of fasciculata cells. Tubular arrays (*arrows*) are also seen in these tumour cells but not, apparently, in the normal cortex. Both cells possess a more extensive smooth endoplasmic reticulum than the normal zona glomerulosa cells, particularly in the adenoma. This patient had been treated with spironolactone prior to surgery. ([**A**] × 45 000; [**B**] × 21 000)

Table 15.7. Malignant adrenocortical tumours associated with the clinical features of Conn's syndrome and suspected or proved hyperaldosteronism

Case no.	Age (yr)	Sex[a]	Adrenal site[a]	Weight (g) or (size)	Reference
1	60	M	R	(4 cm)	Foye and Feichtmeir 1955
2	40	M	L	1400	Brooks et al. 1957[d]
3	44	F	L	NS	Kandrac et al. 1957[d]
4	38	F	R	583	Zimmerman et al. 1959[d]
5	32	F	L	40; 65[b]	Conn et al. 1964
6	46	F	NK	NS	Brorson 1964
7	50	F	R	90	Santander et al. 1965
8	64	F	L	1010	Crane et al. 1965[d]
9	24	M	R	(12 × 15 cm)	Andrade et al. 1965[d]
10	26	F	R	2032	Neville and Symington 1966
11	68	M	L	30	Alterman et al. 1969
12	52	M	L	900	Salassa et al. 1974
13	NS	NS	NS	1050	Salassa et al. 1974
14	NS	NS	NS	250	Salassa et al. 1974
15	NS	NS	NS	260	Salassa et al. 1974
16	54	F	NS	650	Six et al. 1972
17	35	M	L	1000	Brooks et al. 1972
18	34	F	R	320	Filipecki et al. 1972
19	31	M	L	450	Miyazaki et al. 1973
20	37	M	L	600	Huguenin et al. 1975
21	NS	NS	NS	NS	Cathelineau and Poizat 1976
22	32	F	NS	246	Schambelan et al. 1976
23	55	F	L	(8 cm)	Schambelan et al. 1976
24	24	F	R	(2 cm)[c]	Conn et al. 1977
25	31	F	R	(6 × 3.5 × 3 cm)	Revach et al. 1977
26	48	M	L	(12 cm)	Present series
27	60	F	L	(7 cm)	Present series
28	51	F	L	1000	Present series
29	56	F	L	NS	Present series

[a]NS, not stated; F, female; M, male; L/R, left/right; NK, not known.
[b]Two tumours removed from the gland 1 year apart.
[c]Malignancy not proved.
[d]For details of references see Alterman et al. 1969.

Table 15.8. Hyperaldosteronism with low plasma renin. Weights of 25 adrenal carcinomas[a]

Weight (g)	Number
<30	1[b]
30–100	5
100–200	3
200–500	4
500–1000	6
1000–2000	5
>2000	1

[a]For details see Table 15.7 (in cases in which weights have not been given these have been estimated from the reported dimensions of the tumour).
[b]Malignancy not proved; case 24 in Table 15.7.

Gross appearance   Many carcinomas causing hyperaldosteronism are relatively large lesions when they are detected, frequently weighing >500 g at surgery (Table 15.8). However, a significant number of smaller tumours which have subsequently been shown to be carcinomas by their ability to metastasise have been found with weights (30–100 g) which overlap those of the benign tumours (e.g. Santander et al. 1965; Alterman et al. 1969; Salassa et al. 1974; Conn et al. 1977). The gross features of all such lesions, large or small, are broadly similar to other malignant adrenal tumours associated with hypercorticalism. Their cut surface is reddish-brown or grey-pink in many cases and as such may be readily distinguished from the characteristic golden-

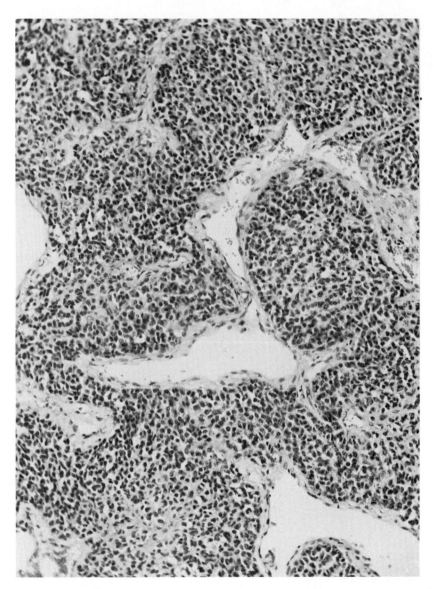

Fig. 15.8. Hyperaldosteronism with low plasma renin. Adrenocortical carcinoma (2 000 g). The tumour cells are of the zona glomerulosa type and are arranged in characteristic large trabeculae separated by prominent fibrovascular trabeculae. (H + E × 160)

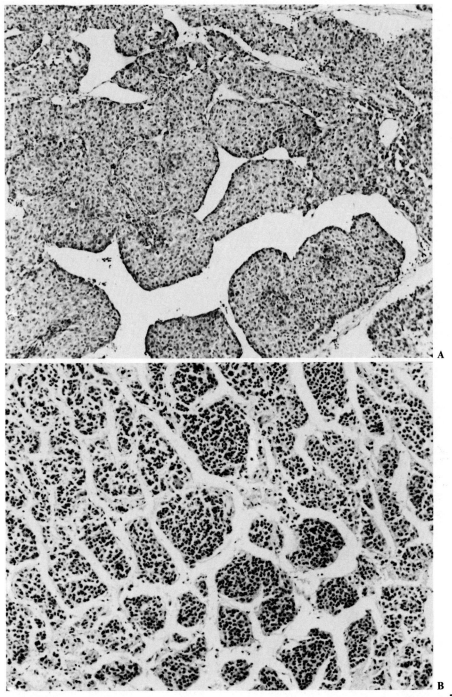

Fig. 15.9. Hyperaldosteronism with low plasma renin. Adrenocortical carcinomas (**A**, 7 cm diameter). Two further different cellular patterns associated with hyperaldosteronism are shown. In **A**, the cells are of the intermediate type and arranged as in Fig. 15.8 in large trabeculae with intervening dilated vascular spaces but without prominent stromal connective tissue. In **B**, the tumour cells are of the compact type and form large cords and trabeculae separated by fibrovascular septae. (H+E **A** ×100; **B** ×140)

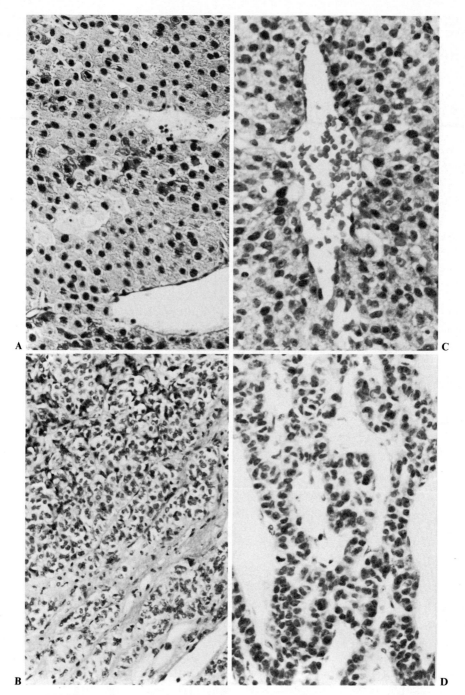

Fig. 15.10. Hyperaldosteronism with low plasma renin. Adrenocortical carcinoma. Four different cell types and patterns of arrangement are seen in the same carcinoma. In **A**, the cells are of the compact type arranged in sheets with interposing sinusoids. In **C**, the cells are intermediate and assume a pattern which radiates away from the sinusoids. In **B** and **D**, the cells are of the glomerulosa type and form cords and strands interspersed by sinusoids (**D**) or fibrovascular septae (**B**). Compare with the benign tumour shown in Fig. 15.4. (H + E [**A**] × 375; [**B**] × 180; [**C** and **D**] × 375)

yellow of typical adenomas (Plate A, facing p. 146). Malignant tumours causing hyperaldosteronism are very vascular in many reported cases, and with increasing size areas of haemorrhage, necrosis, cystic change and calcification are more frequently encountered.

Microscopic appearance   In our experience carcinomas associated with a biochemically proved syndrome of aldosterone excess often present a characteristic microscopic appearance if the five cases that we have seen are representative (Table 15.7). The tumour cells are arranged in large trabeculae, punctuated and separated by prominent vascular sinusoids, surrounded by broad collagenous bands (Fig. 15.8); many tumour cells are of recognisable zona glomerulosa-type with a finely granular but not overtly vacuolated cytoplasm and a high nuclear:cytoplasmic ratio. These cells may form single columns, strands, or double layers arranged in a cord-like fashion reminiscent of the definitive cortex of the neonatal gland (Fig. 15.9, 15.10). They are not entirely dissimilar to the cells in those rare adenomas composed of zona glomerulosa-type cells (Fig. 15.4). With increasing size in the cases we have examined, necrotic areas are a prominent feature of these tumours and may come to form wide areas separating trabeculae of viable tumour cells; numerous intravascular thrombi may also be present. This trabecular appearance, while characteristic of many malignant 'aldosteronomas' is not exclusively confined to them and we have seen similar patterns in a malignant tumour causing Cushing's syndrome (Fig. 15.11).

The trabecular cellular arrangement described and illustrated above and the highly vascular nature of the lesions have been observed in a number of other cases (Santander et al. 1965; Filipecki et al. 1972; Miyazaki et al. 1973; Revach et al. 1977) although more lipid-rich cells similar to 'intermediate' cells in adenomas have been described in some of these lesions (e.g. Santander et al. 1965; Huguenin et al. 1975) as well as compact-type eosinophilic cells (Miyazaki et al. 1973). One of the tumours we have examined has also contained a variety of clear, compact and intermediate cell types arranged in large trabeculae separated by dilated vascular sinusoids (Fig. 15.9, 15.10), with zona gomerulosa-type cells tending to occur at the periphery of the tumour, in a manner reminiscent of that which occurs in benign tumours (p. 211).

Other workers (e.g. Filipecki et al. 1972) have reported tumour cell invasion of the trabeculae or capsule, together with increased mitotic activity (Brooks et al. 1972) as characteristic of these malignant lesions. However, these features have not been prominent in most of the tumours that we have studied although significant mitotic activity was seen in one lesion (Fig. 15.10). Despite this fact all underwent a rapid malignant course. Moreover, cellular and nuclear pleomorphism, as reported by some authors (Alterman et al. 1969; Brooks et al. 1972) have not, in our experience, been as marked as in many other types of malignant adrenocortical tumours associated with hypercorticalism, with the possible exception of those causing feminisation (p. 184). Undue reliance on these criteria (Salassa et al. 1974) may result in erroneous histopathological identification of malignant lesions with hyperaldosteronism as being benign (e.g. Huguenin et al. 1975; Revach et al. 1977). Indeed nuclear pleomorphism is often more marked in the benign tumours causing this syndrome (Fig. 15.2).

Ultrastructure   No reports have been published of the ultrastructure of a malignant 'aldosteronoma'. We therefore present here findings on one such case in our series (no. 29; Table 15.7). This tumour was also cultured in vitro and various functional studies were carried out (p. 238).

This lesion, the histological appearance of different areas of which is shown in Fig. 15.10, consisted ultrastructurally of cells similar in size and general appearance. Pleomorphism was notable only in so far as mitochondrial size was concerned

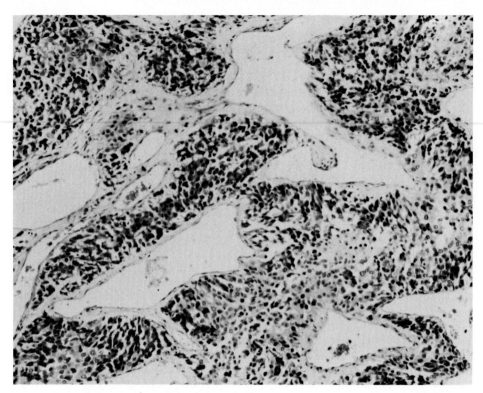

Fig. 15.11. Cushing's syndrome. Adrenocortical carcinoma (650 g). This carcinoma was associated with a 'mixed' pattern of Cushing's syndrome with virilisation but not with aldosterone excess. The cells are compact in type and are arranged in large trabeculae separated by thick-walled vascular sinusoids. The ultrastructural appearance of the tumour is illustrated in Fig. 12.24. (H + E × 120)

(Fig. 15.12). These organelles, generally round but markedly variable in size had a sparse internal structure with mostly lamellar or tubulo-lamellar cristae. The SER was moderately well developed. The RER was more extensive than we have noted in many carcinomas, although organised as long strands rather than stacks, and polyribosomal complexes were particularly numerous. Few lysosomes were visible in the cells and liposomes were rare. The free edges of the cortical tumour cells were smooth with occasional interrupted patches of basement membrane material, and were without notable microvilli or interdigitations, but junctional complexes between adjacent tumour cells seemed fairly frequent, compared with other carcinomas. In some areas (Fig. 15.13) the component cells were ultrastructurally very similar to normal zona glomerulosa cells.

Prognosis

The behaviour of malignant lesions with hyperaldosteronism is extremely aggressive although there are exceptions (Miyazaki et al. 1973). In some cases survival following removal of the primary tumour is a matter of months rather than years. Although responses to o,p'-DDD have been noted (e.g. Six et al. 1972) experience with this category of tumour is not yet sufficiently extensive to state whether this form of chemotherapy is more or less effective than with other forms of tumorous hypercorticalism. Symptomatic relief may be obtained with spironolactone in some cases (Salassa et al. 1974).

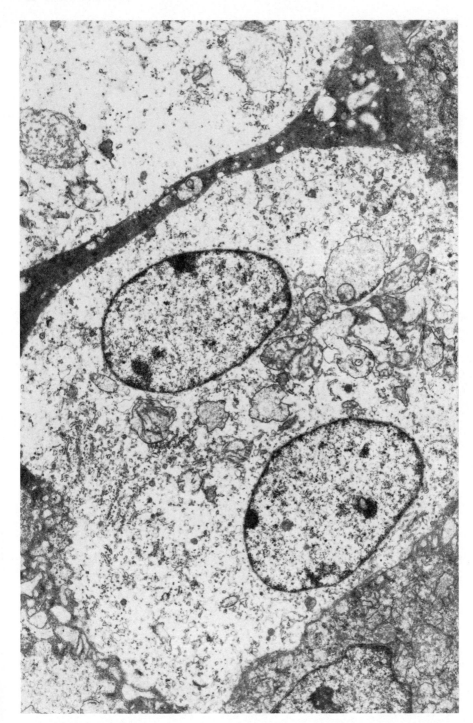

Fig. 15.12. Hyperaldosteronism with low plasma renin. Ultrastructure of a malignant tumour causing hyperaldosteronism. The light-microscopical appearances of this lesion are illustrated in Fig. 15.10. Mitochondrial pleomorphism is notable in this region of the tumour, which corresponds to the compact cell type seen in areas of the tumour. (× 9900)

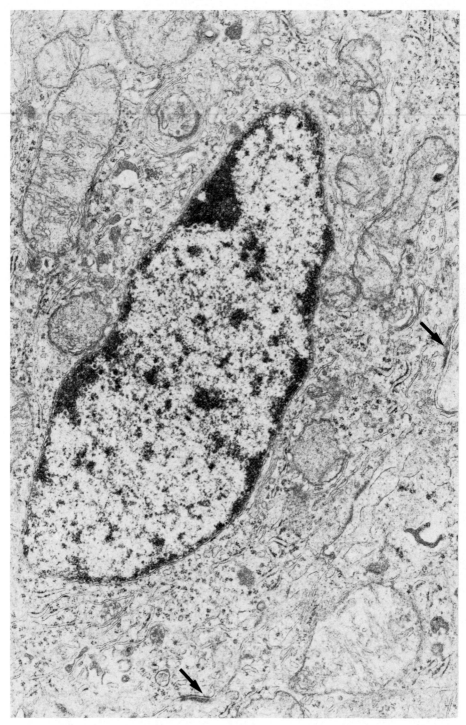

Fig. 15.13. Hyperaldosteronism with low plasma renin. Ultrastructure of another region of the tumour illustrated in Fig. 15.12, corresponding to the glomerulosa-type cells therein. Junctional specialisations (*arrows*) were prominent between these cells. (× 21 000)

By contrast, the typical adenoma causing Conn's syndrome is an entirely benign lesion whose surgical removal is associated with recovery and an almost complete restoration of normal physiological parameters in the majority of cases (Ferriss et al. 1975). We have seen recurrence of another adenoma in the contralateral gland in only one case, an experience comparable with that of other groups (Hunt et al. 1975).

The Attached and Contralateral Adrenal Gland in Tumorous Primary Aldosteronism

The adrenal gland attached or contralateral to benign aldosterone-producing tumours often contains clear-cell nodules of varying sizes. These nodules are similar in histological and gross appearance to those which occur in Cushing's syndrome and which are also a frequent autopsy finding in normal subjects (p. 53). They vary from microscopic dimensions, so-called *micronodules*, to approximately 2–3 cm in diameter, so-called *macronodules*. Most are multiple and generally bilateral, although some macronodules may be single and unilateral, simulating a 'tumour'. In these cases very careful examination of its histology (Figs. 6.16A, 15.1) should resolve the question, failing which an investigation of its steroidogenic potential in vitro should clinch the matter. Studies in tissue culture have recently shown that nodules cannot form aldosterone and do not contain significant quantities of aldosterone when analysed by HPLC (p. 57). They also lack the ultrastructural features associated with aldosterone formation. We believe, therefore, that they probably stem from, rather than cause, the hypertension.

The attached gland in most cases shows hyperplasia of the zona glomerulosa, such increased prominence being a feature noted in the original case reported by Conn (1955). Most frequently it is present around the entire periphery of the cortex and is increased in width (Fig. 15.14). In focal areas tongue-like projections may extend into the cortex when they are often associated with a prominent capillary supply. Spironolactone bodies (p. 64) will also be found in the cytoplasm of cells of the zona glomerulosa and the cells of the outer part of the zona fasciculata in patients treated preoperatively with this drug (Kovacs et al. 1974). In some cases of glands with an adenoma removed at surgery an appearance reminiscent of the stress-related reversion pattern (p. 39) may be seen (Fig. 15.14).

In most instances the adrenal cortex of the attached and contralateral gland appears thinner than normal (Fig. 15.14). This tendency to cortical atrophy is probably related to the fact that such adenomas also contain and are capable of producing cortisol and corticosterone (p. 234) and may be in part under ACTH control (see below).

Certainly, there is no evidence that the attached and contralateral glands with such benign adenomas are themselves hyperactive in respect of aldosterone secretion, despite their histological appearance. Removal of the unilateral adenomas causes a temporary hypoaldosteronism unless patients receive prior spironolactone therapy (Morimoto et al. 1971) and the aldosterone content of attached glands is much lower than in the adenomas when measured by HPLC (O'Hare and Nice 1981), a result consistent with studies by other workers (Bailey et al. 1960; Biglieri et al. 1963; Vecsei et al 1969; Lucis and Lucis 1971; Dahl et al. 1976).

We have not had the opportunity to make a detailed examination of the attached and contralateral glands in cases of malignant 'aldosteronomas'.

Non-Tumorous Hyperaldosteronism with Low Plasma Renin

There are now many well-documented examples of patients with hyperaldosteronism and low plasma renin in whom no adrenal tumour is found at operation (Ferriss et al.

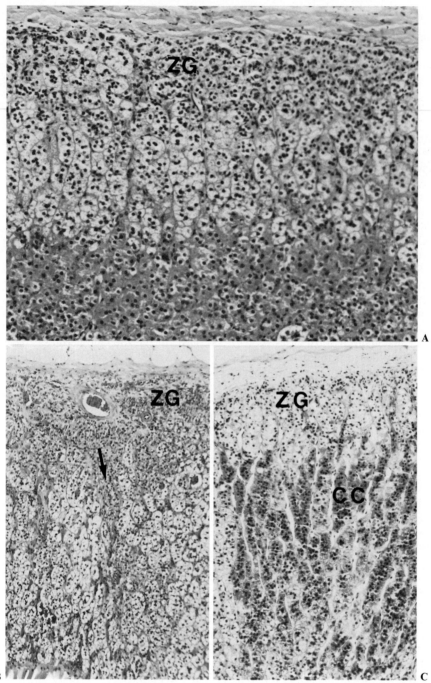

Fig. 15.14. Attached adrenal gland. Hyperaldosteronism with low plasma renin with adrenocortical adenomas. Various different patterns are shown. The cortex may be seen to be narrower than normal, particularly in (**A**) and in each there is hyperplasia of the zona glomerulosa. Tongues of zona glomerulosa (ZG) cells can extend down into the substance of the cortex (*arrow*) (**B**). Not infrequently, below the zona glomerulosa, short columns of compact cells (CC) may extend into the cortex, reminiscent of the so-called 'reversion pattern'. (H + E × 150 [**A**]; × 120 [**B**]; × 120 [**C**])

1970, 1975) a condition originally described by Laragh et al. (1967) and Davis et al. (1967). Various terms have been applied to this condition, including idiopathic hyperaldosteronism and pseudo-primary hyperaldosteronism (Baer et al. 1970); we prefer the term 'non-tumorous hyperaldosteronism' as there is now increasing doubt as to whether this condition is truly 'primary' in nature (Padfield et al. 1981).

There are a variety of adrenal changes associated with the disorder and it is possible that the syndrome has multiple aetiologies. Plasma aldosterone levels in these cases tend to be lower, on average, than in tumorous hyperaldosteronism and hypokalaemia may not be as profound (Davies et al. 1979). As mentioned previously, it is important to detect this entity prior to operation as surgical intervention is generally without benefit, patients just exchanging their aldosteronism for Addison's disease while the hypertension remains unabated in almost all cases (Ferriss et al. 1975). The crucial test is the demonstration of bilaterally elevated aldosterone levels in the adrenal venous effluent, but non-invasive methods such as a computerised quadric analysis of plasma electrolyte and hormone levels as developed by the MRC Blood Pressure Unit in Glasgow (Aitchison et al. 1971) have proved extremely reliable in distinguishing this condition from tumorous hyperaldosteronism. Treatment of these patients should be medical (Ferriss et al. 1975).

As mentioned above, in our series obtained prior to the advent of these methods approximately 15%–35% of cases with hyperaldosteronism and low plasma renin presented with a non-tumorous adrenal pathology (Table 15.1). However, in only 23 were the full clinical and biochemical studies carried out to substantiate the diagnosis (Table 15.9). Their age and sex incidences are noted in Table 15.10.

Table 15.9. Personal series of 23 cases of non-tumorous hyperaldosteronism[a]

Case no.	Sex	Age (yr)	Adrenal gland weights (g) Left	Right
1	F	41	2.8	NR[b]
2	M	50	NR	NR[b]
3	F	40	3.4	NR
4	M	48	–	9·8
5	F	47	7.7	NR
6	M	57	3.5	3.2
7	F	54	3.4	2.2
8	F	62	6.1	2.6
9	M	38	5.4	NR
10	M	48	NR	NR
11	M	57	4.9	NR
12	F	–	6.5	4.0
13	M	58	6.7	6.4
14	F	–	6.4	6.6
15	F	59	–	7.0
16	F	–	4.3	3.8
17	M	–	1.3	8.0
18	M	48	7.5	5.5[c]
19	M	59	NR	NR[c]
20	M	13	–	6.3[b]
21	F	17	5.0	3.7[b]
22	F	9	11.5	9.0
23	F	19	4.0	1.5

NR Not recorded.
[a]Some previously recorded by Ferriss et al. 1970.
[b]Bilateral hyperplasia of zona glomerulosa only.
[c]Deoxycorticosterone secretion and not aldosterone responsible for the clinical syndrome.

Table 15.10. Non-tumorous hyperaldosteronism with low plasma renin: age and sex incidence of 23 cases

Sex	Age incidence							
	<20	21–30	31–40	41–50	51–60	61–70	Not known	Total
Male	1	–	1	3	5	–	1	11
Female	3	–	1	2	2	1	3	12

Gross appearance   The appearances of such adrenal glands at operation are extremely variable. Many are of normal size, weight and gross appearance (Table 15.11). Occasionally glands of less than normal weight are found (cases 1, 2, 5, 6 and 7: Table 15.9). In other patients, they are of increased size and weight. This is generally caused by the presence of nodules, in particular macronodules, which usually measure between 0.25 and 1 cm in diameter, but can be up to 2–3 cm in size.

Table 15.11. Non-tumorous hyperaldosteronism with low plasma renin: adrenal gland weights in the present series of 23 cases

Site	Adrenal gland weights (g)						
	<3	3–4	4–6	6–8	8–10	>10	Not recorded
Left	1	4	4	7	–	1	5
Right	2	4	1	5	2	–	6

On sectioning the gland may appear superficially normal, with a narrow inner brown zone corresponding to the zona reticularis and a prominent outer yellow zone corresponding to the zona fasciculata. More often small, yellow-coloured nodules are found often only intra-glandularly and even intra-cortically and frequently sited near the central vein. In addition larger nodules may be found towards one pole or, again within the gland. Such nodules are generally multiple, but macronodules may occasionally be single and unilateral, simulating an adenoma (Fig. 15.15). This distribution of nodules often accounts for the marked disparity in size and weight which can occur in such glands (Table 15.9).

Microscopic appearance   In general, the appearance of the glands is identical to those already described in association with the neoplasms which cause hyperaldosteronism with low plasma renin, i.e. hyperplasia of the zona glomerulosa with or without nodules both of macroscopic and microscopic size.

The commonest findings are in our experience hyperplasia of the zona glomerulosa and micronodules. However, in some instances when we have examined single sections of the adrenal gland, we have found that the zona glomerulosa is focal and apparently normal in its distribution, or it may be difficult to see in the areas where it has been compressed by nodules. Other sections of the adrenal gland, however, have shown marked hyperplasia of the zona glomerulosa (Fig. 15.16). In this context, therefore, many sections of the gland are usually required to reach an appropriate anatomical diagnosis.

In spironolactone-treated patients spironolactone bodies are usually found in the cells of the zona glomerulosa and also undoubtedly occasionally in clear cells of the outer zona fasciculata. In some adrenal glands a distinct zone of 'intermediate'-type cells with a high nuclear-cytoplasmic ratio and a lipid-containing but moderately

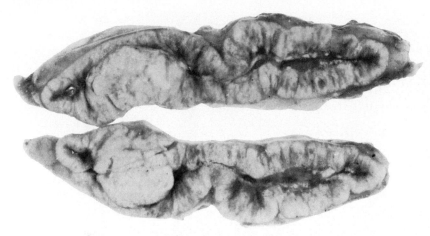

Fig. 15.15. Hyperaldosteronism with low plasma renin. Bilateral nodular hyperplasia. Of the two glands received from this 57-year-old man, only the left gland was weighed (4.89 g). It has been opened to show a 0.6-cm yellow intraglandular nodule. Numerous micronodules are just discernable in the remainder of the gland. (× 4)

eosinophilic cytoplasm may be present immediately below the hyperplastic zona glomerulosa (Fig. 15.16). These form columns of cells that extend downwards and merge with the underlying clear-cells of the zona fasciculata and may even reach the more strongly eosinophilic zona reticularis compact-cells. The significance of these cells is obscure. Although this pattern is reminiscent of a stress-related reversion pattern (p. 39) there is no reason to suppose that these patients are especially stressed. It is conceivable that they represent a form of functionally intermediate cell (p. 237).

The possible aetiologies of 'primary' hyperaldosteronism with non-tumorous zona glomerulosa hyperplasia and its relationship with 'essential' hypertension is discussed later (p. 240). However, one rare form of the disease in which the cause appears to be distinct is the so-called dexamethasone (glucocorticoid)-remediable hyper-aldosteronism (Sutherland et al. 1966; Salti et al. 1969). This familial condition appears to be a non-HLA-linked disorder (New et al. 1980) that may be a form of congenital adrenal hyperplasia with a partial 17α-hydroxylase defect (New and Petersen 1967; Miura et al. 1968; New et al. 1973). It appears to be an autosomal dominant inheritance (Giebink et al. 1973). We have not had the opportunity of seeing this disease at the pathological level, but reported changes included hyperplasia and nodules. Further studies (New et al. 1976) have indicated that as well as hypersecretion of aldosterone, other unidentified mineralocorticoids (p. 230) may be secreted in some of these cases.

Hyperaldosteronism with High Plasma Renin (Secondary Aldosteronism)

Elevated aldosterone, in response to increased levels of circulating renin and angiotensin, is a concomitant of a variety of extra-adrenal diseases, and, unlike primary aldosteronism, is usually associated with oedema, commonly of renal, cardiac or hepatic origin as the renal 'escape' mechanism is inoperative (Brown et al. 1972b). Non-oedematous diseases associated with secondary hyperaldosteronism include hyperthyroidism, some cases of essential hypertension (15%–20%), renal artery stenosis and malignant hypertension.

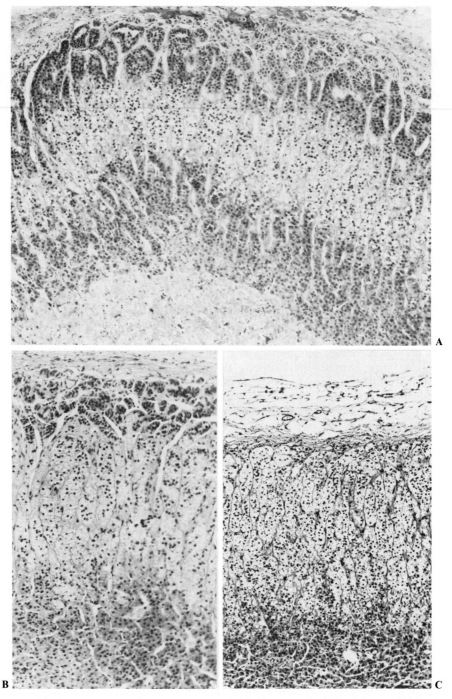

Fig. 15.16. Hyperaldosteronism with low plasma renin. Bilateral hyperplasia of the zona glomerulosa. The zona glomerulosa is more prominent than normal exhibiting focal (to the *right* in **A**) and diffuse hyperplasia (**B**). The related vascular sinusoids are also more prominent than usual. In **A**, short compact cell columns reminiscent of the reversion pattern are seen in this operatively removed gland. A normal cortex (**C**) is shown for comparison. (H + E × 100 [**A**]; × 100 [**B**]; × 60 [**C**])

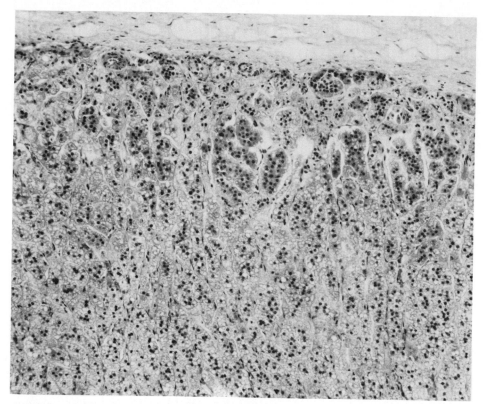

Fig. 15.17. Secondary Aldosteronism. Bilateral hyperplasia of the zona glomerulosa. This male patient had essential hypertension with raised plasma renin and aldosterone levels. The glands weighed 18.0 g and 20.0 g and show diffuse hyperplasia of the zona glomerulosa together with a broadened cortex in which 'reversion changes' may be seen beneath the zona glomerulosa. ($H + E \times 120$)

Pitcock and Hartroft (1958) originally reported that in these cases in which plasma sodium was low and the juxtaglomerular apparatus was hypergranular, indicating hypersecretion of renin, the width of the zona glomerulosa was correspondingly enhanced. The cases that we have seen have followed this pattern with focal or diffuse zona glomerulosa hyperplasia (Fig. 15.17). In addition, all the glands have exhibited compact cells columns extending from the zona glomerulosa down into the substance of the cortex. As these glands were obtained at autopsy, it is not possible to state whether they are identical in a functional nature to the similar changes noted in operation glands removed from non-tumorous aldosteronism (Fig. 15.16) or whether they represent the so-called reversion pattern in response to stress (Fig. 5.5).

Bartter's Syndrome (Tertiary Aldosteronism)

In 1962, Bartter et al, described a new syndrome of hypokalaemic, hypochloraemic alkalosis with elevated plasma renin, angiotensin II and aldosterone levels, presenting in infancy and during adult life, and, in at least some cases, inherited as an autosomal recessive condition. Unlike other forms of secondary hyperaldosteronism, such as that caused, for example, by renin-secreting tumours of the juxtaglomerular apparatus, this condition is not associated with hypertension.

Further studies have revealed a significant resistance to the pressor effects of angiotensin II. It is now clear that its aetiology involves the overproduction of prostaglandins, notably PGE_2, but also possibly the more potent, albeit labile, prostacyclin (Zipser et al. 1979). The syndrome's symptoms are alleviated by administration of prostaglandin synthetase inhibitors such as indomethacin. The inappropriate PG secretion appears to arise from the hyperplastic renal medullary interstitial cells in this disorder (Verberckmoes et al. 1976) with the PGs causing renin hypersecretion and juxtaglomerular (JGA) hyperplasia which is pathognomonic of this syndrome (Bartter et al. 1962). Increased PG synthesis is reflected by an increased urinary prostaglandin level (Gill et al. 1976) and this, together with JGA hyperplasia, distinguishes it from salt-losing chronic glomerulonephritis.

Adrenal changes in Bartter's syndrome have not been adequately documented. Early cases in which bilateral adrenalectomy was carried out in an unsuccessful attempt to ameliorate hypokalaemia showed 'grossly normal glands' (Trygstad et al. 1969), and biopsy specimens have reportedly shown glomerulosa hyperplasia (Bartter 1977); the extent and ubiquity of these changes together with alterations, if any, in the remainder of the cortex have not been recorded.

Syndromes of Mineralocorticoid Excess Without Hyperaldosteronism

It has long been known that adrenal steroids such as deoxycorticosterone, and corticosterone by virtue of their intrinsic, albeit low, mineralocorticoid activity will cause hypertension and hypokalaemic alkalosis when secreted in excess (Table 8.4). Hence their secretion by tumours or other conditions (Biglieri et al. 1968; Brown and Strott 1971) may simulate Conn's syndrome with hyperaldosteronism.

Thus, isolated hypersecretion of deoxycorticosterone, and also to some extent corticosterone, can result in the symptoms of Conn's syndrome without concomitant hypercortisolism. This is due to the very limited glucocorticoid activity of DOC ($<0.5\%$ of cortisol) and in the case of corticosterone, which is a much more potent glucocorticoid (30% of cortisol activity), notably its very rapid hepatic metabolism to reduced compounds inactive as glucocorticoids.

Mineralocorticoid and hypertensogenic activity has also been claimed on behalf of a variety of minor adrenal products including 18-hydroxydeoxycorticosterone (Melby et al. 1972), 16β-hydroxydehydroepiandrosterone (Liddle and Sennett 1975) $16\alpha,18$-dihydroxy DOC (Dale and Melby 1973), 5α-dihydrocortisol (Marver and Edelman 1978), 17α-hydroxy-20α-dihydroprogesterone (Coghlan et al. 1976) and most recently 19-nor-DOC (Hall et al. 1979). However, neither 16β-OH-DHA (Gomez-Sanchez et al. 1976) nor 5α-dihydrocortisol possess significant intrinsic mineralocorticoid activity in vivo (Adam et al. 1978), although they may, like the hydroxyprogesterones and 16α, 18-dihydroxy DOC, amplify the effects of aldosterone by an as yet unknown mechanism. The mineralocorticoid activities and circulating levels of 18OH-DOC and 16α, 18-dihydroxy DOC are also probably too low to cause hypertension (Ulick 1976a) and 18-hydroxycorticosterone (Fraser and Lantos 1978) is also devoid of significant activity. 19-Nor-DOC, however, has 2–3 times the mineralocorticoid activity of DOC (Gomez-Sanchez et al. 1979).

Potentially, therefore, at least some of these steroids and corticosterone and deoxycorticosterone may cause syndromes of mineralocorticoid excess when pathologically elevated due to congenital, acquired or neoplastic adrenocortical lesions.

Congenital

The classical form of hypertensive congenital adrenal hyperplasia with an 11β-hydroxylase defect and elevated DOC and/or 11-deoxycortisol has already been discussed and the adrenal changes described (p. 160).

Juvenile hypertension with enhanced 5α-dihydrocortisol excretion (Ulick et al. 1977) and a deficiency of cortisol 11β-ketoreductase has been described in a patient with hyporeninism and hyposecretion of all known corticosteroids (New et al. 1977); a similar case has recently been reported by Shackleton et al. (1980) where deficient hepatic metabolism of adrenal steroids seemed to underly the defect. The aetiological role of this reduced steroid metabolite remains debatable however (vide supra). The adrenal structural changes in this congenital disorder, if any, have not been recorded.

Acquired

Non-Tumorous

In studies of non-tumorous hypertension with low renin, the MRC Blood Pressure Unit have identified a number of cases in which there was an apparently isolated hypersecretion of deoxycorticosterone (Brown et al. 1972b). These cases were distinguishable from classical cases of 11β-hydroxylase and 17α-hydroxylase deficiency by the absence of abnormalities of sex differentiation, normal levels of plasma cortisol and corticosterone and normal responses to ACTH. Aldosterone levels were normal. Two such cases were examined histologically (18 and 19; Table 15.9). Both showed bilateral hyperplasia of the zona glomerulosa, an appearance indistinguishable from proved cases of non-tumorous hyperaldosteronism (Fig. 15.16).

The aetiology of this disorder is obscure but it is responsive to spironolactone therapy and the DOC levels are not suppressed by dexamethasone. It is conceivable that it might represent an attenuated late-onset form of 11β-hydroxylase defect occurring only in zona glomerulosa cells and sparing the inner zones. Aldosterone levels would be in the normal range because of zona glomerulosa hypertrophy.

In cases of Cushing's syndrome due to the 'ectopic ACTH' syndrome, plasma DOC may be elevated to levels (>100 ng/100 ml) where a significant mineralocorticoid effect may be obtained (Brown and Strott 1971; Schambelan et al. 1971); this does not occur in pituitary-dependent Cushing's disease, and should be distinguished from its secretion by an adrenocortical tumour.

Adrenocortical Tumours

Reference has already been made to the frequency with which 11-deoxysteroids, including DOC, are elevated in cases of adrenocortical carcinomas causing Cushing's syndrome. When plasma DOC levels rise one or two orders of magnitude above normal (~ 200 ng/ml), hypokalaemic alkalosis and hypertension may dominate the clinical picture even when there is concurrent hypercortisolism (e.g. Biglieri et al. 1968; Tan et al. 1977). Cases of mixed virilism and Conn's syndrome (Marquezy et al. 1965; Herbeuval et al. 1968) have been reported in association with malignant tumours with predominant DOC secretion, as well as pure hypermineralocorticism (Powell-Jackson et al. 1974; Davies et al. 1981). One case of hypermineralocorticism with isolated DOC secretion has been recorded in association with a purportedly benign adrenal tumour

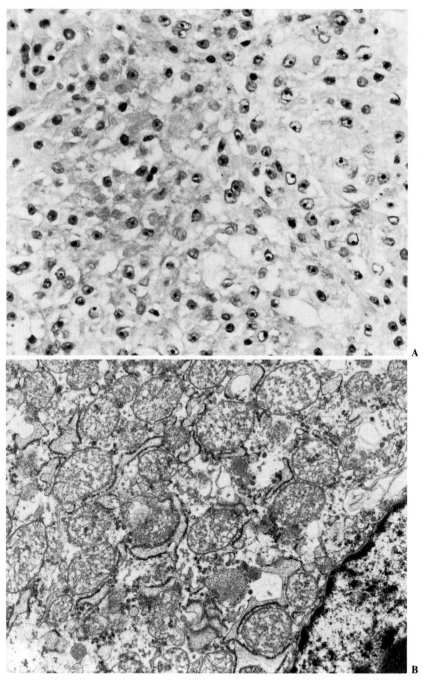

Fig. 15.18. DOC-secreting adrenocortical carcinoma from a hypertensive hypokalaemic female patient aged 51 years. The primary tumour was unresectable (>1 kg) and hepatic metastases were seen at surgery. Circulating DOC levels were about 40 times the normal mean (12 nmol/l) (Appendix A). The tumour cells form sheets interspersed by small sinusoids. The cells are of the compact type with lipid sparse eosinophilic cytoplasm. Marked nuclear vesicularity with prominent nucleoli may also be seen at the light microscopical level (**A**). (**B**) Ultrastructurally this lesion showed typical steroidogenic-type mitochondria with an unusual pattern of surrounding dilated saccules of rough endoplasmic reticulum seen in most of the cells examined. (H + E × 300 [**A**]; × 21 000 [**B**])

weighing 240 g (Kondo et al. 1976). In the light of our experience with the functional assessment of benign and malignant tumours in vitro (p. 193), however, we would view with suspicion in respect of potential malignancy, all tumours with such a functional abnormality.

Hypersecretion of corticosterone by tumours simulating the signs and symptoms of hyperaldosteronism has also been noted in several instances (Fraser et al 1968; Mills et al. 1980), although other cases in which cortisol has also been elevated presented with Cushing's syndrome with severe hypokalaemic alkalosis (Krølner et al. 1979). Corticosterone-secreting tumours with minimal endocrine abnormalities have, however, also been found (Weinstein et al. 1970). Oedema has been a feature in some of these cases.

The adrenocortical tumours causing hypermineralocorticism without excessive aldosterone that we have seen have had histological features indistinguishable from carcinomas causing Cushing's syndrome (Fig. 15.18); most have not resembled the characteristic picture of the malignant 'aldosteronoma' (Fig. 15.8). The ultrastructural features of one such tumour with corticosterone secretion have been illustrated by MacKay (1969). The mitochondria contained well-marked tubulo-vesicular cristae, a feature that we have also seen in a case associated with DOC hypersecretion (Davies et al. 1981) (Fig. 15.18). Such tumours seem to be aggressive rather than indolent in their behaviour.

Aetiology and Correlation of Structure and Function in Conn's Syndrome

The histological changes in the adrenal in Conn's syndrome have been both puzzling and apparently paradoxical. First, benign tumours in this disorder do not, in the great majority of cases, contain zona glomerulosa cells, while malignant tumours may so do. Second, the gland attached to an adrenal tumour shows apparent hyperplasia of the zona glomerulosa, despite the fact that both angiotensin and potassium levels are reduced. Third, the precise aetiological relationship of the hyperplastic glomerulosa in non-tumorous primary aldosteronism with the hypertensive syndrome, and the relationship of the adrenal cortex to other 'low-renin' forms of 'essential' hypertension remains obscure.

Tumour Structure and Function

Based on our studies of the behaviour of rodent and human aldosterone-secreting cells in monolayer culture, and our revised concepts of adrenocortical functional zonation (p. 108), we can now explain the apparent paradoxical nature of the cells comprising the benign lesions in Conn's syndrome.

The adrenal adenomas are the major source of aldosterone excess in this syndrome as determined by their HPLC steroid profiles (Fig. 15.19). When these cells are introduced into culture they form monolayers with an appearance identical to those of benign adenomas causing Cushing's syndrome, and normal zona fasciculata cells (Fig. 15.20A). In all 16 tumours that we have cultured we have noted this morphological appearance and the presence of a typical ACTH-induced retraction response (Fig. 15.20B). Furthermore, examination of their steroid secretion profiles after several days culture revealed, in all cases, little or no aldosterone secretion. Such cultures did, however, secrete more corticosterone than cortisol (Fig. 15.21) in a

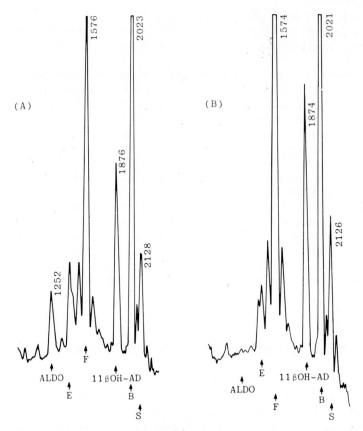

Fig. 15.19. Hyperaldosteronism with low plasma renin. Steroid profiles (HPLC) of hormones extracted from an adenoma causing Conn's syndrom (**A**) and the gland attached to the tumour (**B**). Note the presence of a distinct, albeit small, peak of aldosterone in the former but not the latter. The numbers appended to major peaks indicate their retention times in seconds; several peaks (e.g. F and B) are off-scale at the attenuation used to demonstrate the aldosterone peak.

manner reminiscent of benign tumours associated with Cushing's syndrome. When the tumour cultures were exposed to ACTH, the 17-hydroxysteroids rose in almost all cases to become the predominant class of steroid, typically represented by cortisol (but also including some 11-deoxycortisol in dilute cultures of tumour cells). Almost all aldosterone-producing adenomas are also responsive to ACTH in vivo (Slaton et al. 1969).

An examination of steroid secretion by a typical tumour during the first few days revealed the reason for the discrepancy between the steroid content of the intact tissues (Fig. 15.19) and the steroid secretion by the cultures (Fig. 15.21). Within four days of dispersion and introduction into monolayer culture, aldosterone secretion by the tumour had fallen to the levels of the attached gland (Fig. 15.22). Their complete steroid profile as revealed by HPLC (Fig. 15.23) showed, furthermore, that the loss of aldosterone was accompanied by a corresponding decline in 18-hydroxycortico-sterone, but that their immediate precursors and other glucocorticoids, including cortisol rose. A similar phenomenon has been observed in cultures of rat glomerulosa cells (Hornsby et al. 1974; Hornsby and O'Hare 1977); here, the glucocorticoids

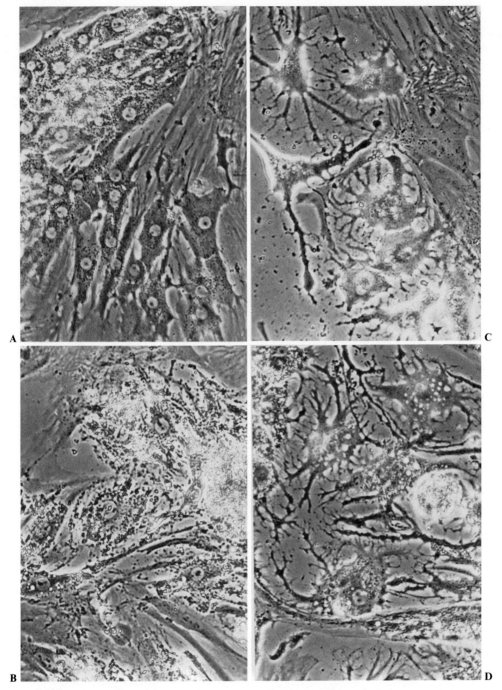

Fig. 15.20. Benign aldosterone-secreting tumours in culture. Phase-contrast photomicrographs (× 180) of two such tumours in monolayer culture show (**A**) the more rarely encountered pattern of rather small regular epithelioid cells and (**B**) the common appearance of such lesions with well-spread lipid-laden cells, indistinguishable from normal zona fasciculata cells in culture. Both types of cell show a marked retraction response (*right*) when exposed to $ACTH_{1-24}$ (1 μg/ml); neither type of cell continued to secrete aldosterone in vitro in significant quantities in long-term culture despite the presence of this steroid in the solid tumour tissue and during the first few days of culture.

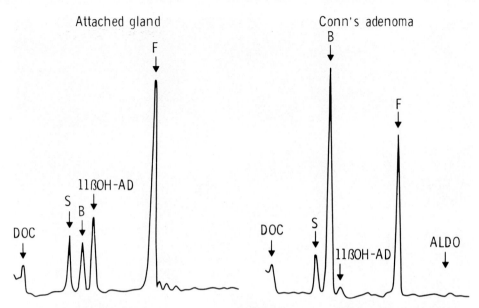

Fig. 15.21. Hyperaldosteronism with low plasma renin. Steroid profiles (HPLC) from a two-week-old monolayer culture of a Conn's adenoma compared with that of the attached gland. Note the relative preponderance of corticosterone (**B**) in the former, but the absence of detectable aldosterone (ALDO). See O'Hare *et al* (1980b) for methods.

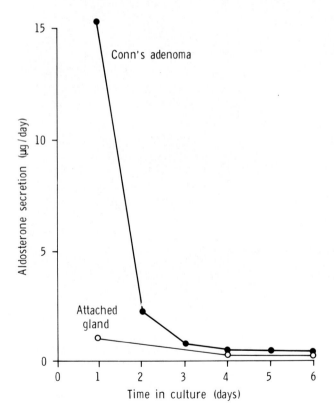

Fig. 15.22. Hyperaldosteronism with low plasma renin. Aldosterone secretion by an adenoma (*closed rings*) compared with the attached gland (*open rings*) during the first week of monolayer cell culture.

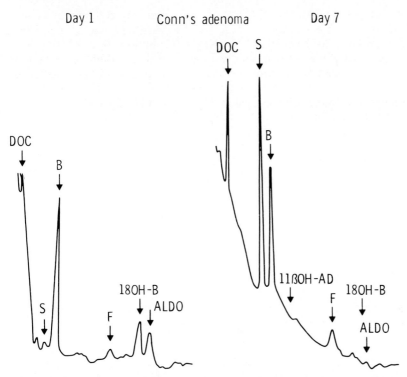

Fig. 15.23. Hyperaldosteronism with low plasma renin. Steroid profiles (HPLC) of hormones secreted by an adenoma causing Conn's syndrome after 1 day and 7 days in monolayer culture. This lesion was relatively small (0.5 cm diameter); many larger tumours secreted less aldosterone and more cortisol at the outset (cf. Fig. 15.19).

themselves suppress aldosterone directly. While we cannot definitively exclude the possibility that the aldosterone-secreting cells simply failed to survive in culture, it seems far more likely that the tumour cells show the same sort of functional shift from a glomerulosa to fasciculata phenotype that we have noted in cultured rat cells.

If we conclude from these observations that the glomerulosa-type cells in these benign lesions are subject to the same steroid suppressive effects in vivo, then the histological heterogeneity of the tumours becomes explicable. Thus, disruption of the normal patterns and pathways of vascularisation in the tumours as they enlarge could result in a change in the local cellular microenvironment, such that they can no longer sustain the glomerulosa phenotype and come to assume a zona fasciculata-like appearance and produce cortisol. It is noteworthy that such zona glomerulosa cells as are apparent in these lesions appear to be confined to the vicinity of vascularised connective tissue trabeculae peripherally placed or dipping down into the tumour from the overlying cortex (Fig. 15.5).

In the rare zona glomerulosa-type benign lesions it may be that this switch has not occurred because of a 'normal' cell:vascular relationship. Certainly this type of lesion appears well supplied with blood and contains numerous vascular sinusoids. The 'intermediate'-type cells in the typical adenoma in Conn's syndrome may well also represent an intermediate form between zona glomerulosa and zona fasciculata from a functional point of view. Possibly they secrete corticosterone rather than cortisol, but lack aldosterone-synthesising capabilities. Such properties, while essentially specu-lative, would account for the propensity of these lesions to contain high levels of corticosterone, compared with cortisol (Kaplan 1967), and they certainly agree well with the ultrastructural appearance of these lesions (Reidbord and Fisher 1969; Sommers and Terzakis 1970; Neville and MacKay 1972; Kovacs et al. 1974).

In the one malignant aldosteronoma that we have cultured, a different pattern of behaviour was noted. This tumour contained substantial amounts of corticosterone and 18-hydroxycorticosterone as well as aldosterone (Fig. 15.24). 18-Hydroxycorticosterone is, of course, also found in benign lesions (Marusic and Mulrow 1969) but not in such disproportionately large amounts as were detected in this malignant tumour

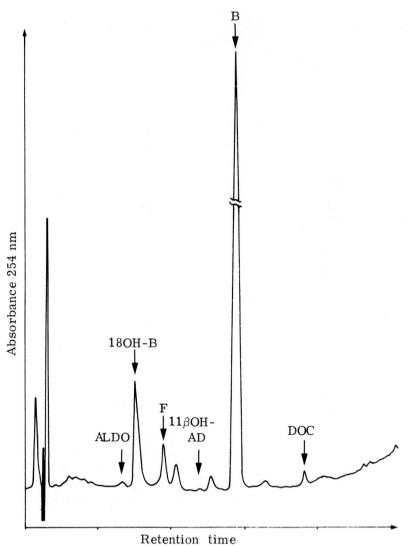

Retention time

Fig. 15.24. Hyperaldosteronism with low plasma renin. Steroid profile (HPLC) of a freshly disaggregated malignant adrenocortical tumour associated with a hypertensive syndrome (Case 29 Table 15.7). In contrast to most benign tumours associated with Conn's syndrome (Fig. 15.19) this lesion secreted little cortisol (F); large amounts of corticosterone (B) and 18-hydroxycorticosterone (18OH-B) were formed, together with small but detectable quantities of aldosterone (see O'Hare et al. 1980 for further details of separation of 18-hydroxysteroids by HPLC). Its responses to ACTH and dbcAMP in vitro were small (<50%) and transient (24–48 h only).

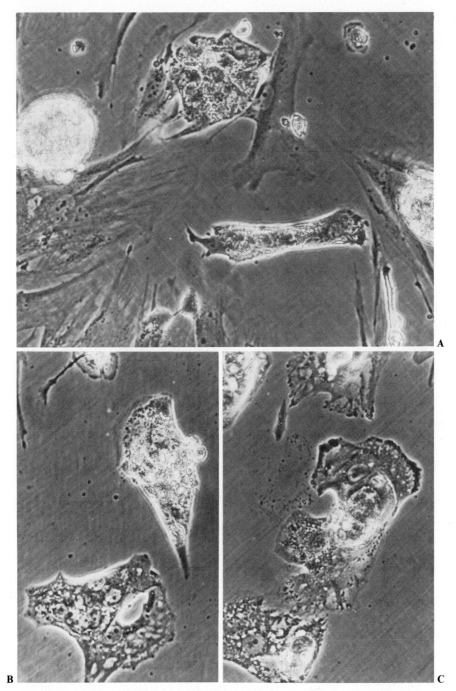

Fig. 15.25. Malignant aldosterone-secreting adrenocortical tumour in culture. Phase-contrast photo-micrographs (× 200) show the pleomorphic irregular nature of these carcinoma cells (cf. Fig. 15.20) when maintained without hormonal or other additions (**A**). Neither dbcAMP (0.5 mmol/l (**B**) nor ACTH$_{1-24}$ (lμg/ml (**C**) caused any perceptible alteration in cell morphology, in marked contrast to the behaviour of benign tumours causing Conn's syndrome. The light-microscopical and electronoptical appearances of this lesion in vivo have been shown in Figs 15.10 and 15.12/13 respectively.

(compare Figs. 15.9A and 15.25). In culture, the carcinoma cells continued to secrete both 18-hydroxysteroids and aldosterone and, while a small amount of cortisol was formed, it never became the major product. The tightly associated islands of small lipid-sparse cells seen in these cultures (Fig. 15.25) were in marked contrast to the benign lesions (Fig. 15.20). This lesion also showed functional abnormalities in hormonal responsiveness, failing to give a sustained response to either ACTH or cyclic AMP comparable with the (5–8-fold) increment seen in all benign lesions.

Structure and Function of the Attached Gland

The apparent hyperplasia of the zona glomerulosa of the attached gland in cases of tumorous primary aldosteronism is more difficult to explain satisfactorily, particularly as the constituent cells do not appear functionally hyperactive, on the basis of the steroid content of the attached gland (Fig. 15.19B) and the hypoaldosteronism that ensues when the tumour is removed (contralateral glands also show glomerulosa 'hyperplasia'). The most plausible explanation that we can offer at the present time is that possibly the hypertensive syndrome caused by aldosterone secreted by the tumour itself results, via changes in adrenal blood flow (p. 109) in a shift in the zonal boundaries within the gland, thus extending the morphological dimensions of the zona glomerulosa. In the absence of effective angiotensin stimulation of the gland in this low renin condition the cells of this extended zone may well fail to secrete significant quantities of mineralocorticoids and thus suffer what amounts to functional atrophy.

The possibility that this represents a pre-existing hyperplasia of unknown aetiology with as yet unidentified glomerulotrophins being the primary cause (Nicholls et al. 1975b; Bravo et al. 1980) on the base of which a true tumour evolves seems to us inherently less likely. Under the circumstances one would anticipate (a) that hypertension would not resolve when the tumour was removed, and (b) that further tumours would ultimately arise in the contralateral gland. Neither of these two consequences actually seems to take place.

Finally, it should be borne in mind that the zona glomerulosa hyperplasia in the attached gland may well be more prominent because of a tendency to slight cortical atrophy in some but not all such attached glands and the presence of underlying compact cells simulating a hyperplastic glomerulosa (Fig. 15.14). We believe that these latter cells have not received sufficient attention in published studies, and that while their structural and functional significance remain unknown, care should be taken in interpreting the patterns of adrenal change in Conn's syndrome.

The Relationship of Nodules and Adenomas in Conn's Syndrome: A Possible Functional Continuity?

There is an increasing body of evidence to suggest that low renin hypertension, primary aldosteronism without adrenal tumour and essential hypertension may be different aspects of a single disease spectrum rather than different conditions (Ferriss et al. 1978; Davies et al. 1979). If this is true then it is important to examine the possibility that tumorous hyperaldosteronism may also be a closely related disorder. When a tumour is composed only of zona glomerulosa cells it tends to be large or more often malignant (p. 216). When it consists of clear cells apparently alone or with intermediate cells and/or zona glomerulosa cells, then the lesion is small and frequently of lesser size than a nodule. The zona glomerulosa cells when seen are arranged peripherally in the tumour, probably in relation to the afferent vascular supply.

Is it possible that some nodules evolve from aldosterone-secreting lesions by a process of functional modulation such as we have observed in culture? Initially a small 'adenomatous' lesion composed of zona glomerulosa cells would produce aldosterone, lower the plasma renin and result in hypertension. However, with further growth, a change in the vascular relationship and microenvironment of the cells could occur which no longer permits them to produce aldosterone. Thus they would change structurally and functionally through the intermediate type cell to acquire zona fasciculata and zona reticularis properties. If this process proceeds to completion, the lesion would be indistinguishable morphologically and functionally from the typical nodule. Naturally there would be a gradual decrease in aldosterone production but hypertension could continue unabated if there are established renovascular changes.

While this sequence remains an intriguing possibility, if it were to apply universally, we would expect to have observed a high incidence of recurrent hyperaldosteronism due to the development of a further tumour in the contralateral adrenal gland. We have not personally seen this sequence in our study of 153 adrenal tumours. Moreover, adrenal nodules can be found without hypertension, and hypertension can occur without nodules being present. A test of the polyclonal or monoclonal origin of these lesions by, for example, glucose-6-phosphate dehydrogenase isozyme patterns might prove interesting in this context.

Chapter 16
'Non-Functioning' (Non-Hormonal) Adrenocortical Tumours

Incidence and Symptoms

A variety of tumours, or tumour-like lesions, not associated with signs and symptoms of overt clinical hormonal excess, may involve the adrenal cortex. These include myelolipomas (p. 290), cysts (p. 294) and tumours derived from the stroma. However by far the commonest example is the so-called 'non-functioning' nodule, often wrongly referred to as an adenoma. These have been previously discussed in detail (p. 53).

Another lesion of importance is the so-called 'non-functioning' or 'non-hormonal' adrenocortical tumour, which tends to be large and almost invariably malignant. The term 'non-hormonal' is preferred as, although there is no clinical evidence of hormonal imbalance, such tumours are not necessarily steroidogenically inert and may in some

Table 16.1. Non-hormonal adrenocortical carcinomas

Case no.	Sex	Age (yr)	Adrenal	Size (cm)	Reference
1	M	2.5	R	10 × 7.5	Lewinski et al. 1974
2	M	38	R	NK	Lewinski et al. 1974
3	F	35	L	16 cm diam	Lewinski et al. 1974
4	M	38	R	25 × 20	Lewinski et al. 1974
5	F	61	R	Fetal skull	Lewinski et al. 1974
6	F	56	L	'Large'	Lewinski et al. 1974
7	M	64	R	25 × 19 × 15	Lewinski et al. 1974
8	F	53	L	NK	Lewinski et al. 1974
9	F	48	L	11 cm diam	Lewinski et al. 1974
10	F	42	NK	20 × 20 × 20	Lewinski et al. 1974
11	F	65	R	40 × 33 × 25	Lewinski et al. 1974
12	M	66	R	NK	Lewinski et al. 1974
13	M	–	NK	36 cm diam (4500 g)	Lewinski et al. 1974
14	M	59	L	28 × 22 × 12	Lewinski et al. 1974
15	M	39	L	15 × 15 × 9	Lewinski et al. 1974
16	F	45	L	23 × 20 × 15	Lewinski et al. 1974
17	F	57	R	(1100 g)	Lewinski et al. 1974
18	M	50	L	19 × 17 × 9	Lewinski et al. 1974
19	M	14	R	18 × 15 × 13 (1520 g)	Lewinski et al. 1974
20	M	61	L	12 cm diam (700 g)	Lewinski et al. 1974
21	F	41	R	9 × 4.5 cm	Tang et al. 1979
22	M	37	R	12 cm diam	Mooppan et al. 1977
23	F	51	R	7 cm diam	Cassan et al. 1978
24	F	40	L	10 cm diam	Cassan et al. 1978
25	F	53	L	8 cm (250 g)	Cassan et al. 1978
26	M	48	L	6 cm	Smith et al. 1979
27	F	32	L	5 cm	Smith et al. 1979
28	M	31	R	17 × 15 cm	Smith et al. 1979

NK—Not known.

cases produce significant quantities of inactive steroid hormone precursors (vide infra); they are included, therefore, as examples of 'hypercorticalism' albeit of a covert type.

In 1974, Lewinski and his colleagues reviewed the world literature on non-hormonal carcinomas and, by adding 20 cases of their own, were able to present the salient features from 178 examples. Since then only sporadic cases have been reported (Hajjar et al. 1975; Bulger and Correa 1977; Mooppan et al. 1977; Cassan et al. 1978; Smith et al. 1979; Tang et al. 1979) bringing the total to about 190 (Table 16.1).

Non-hormonal adrenocortical carcinomas, therefore, are rare but not as rare as, for example, feminising tumours (Table 13.5). They occur more frequently in males than in females (2:1), usually presenting with vague complaints such as a palpable mass, abdominal pain, weakness, anorexia and, notably in some but not all cases, fever (Lewinski et al. 1974). Angiography and urography are useful diagnostic techniques. They are usually detected in the fifth to seventh decades of life (i.e. later than most adrenal tumours) although children are by no means totally exempt (Table 16.1). The left adrenal gland is somewhat more often the site of the tumour than the right (Lewinski et al. 1974). Although examples of bilateral tumours have also been recorded it is not known whether such bilateral lesions represent separate primary tumours or if one is a metastasis of the other. No significant familial associations or other predisposing conditions have been reported.

Functional Activity

Many non-hormonal adrenocortical carcinomas are not without steroidogenic activity, although they are unable to form excessive amounts of active hormones, such as cortisol, aldosterone, or various sex steroids (Fig. 8.4). Many such tumours, however, seem to be able to effect the first step in steroid biosynthesis from cholesterol producing pregnenolone (Fig. 8.4). Metabolites of pregnenolone such as pregn-5-ene-3β,20α-diol and 5-pregnane-3α,20α-diol occur in increased amounts in the urine (Fukushima and Gallagher 1963) and 16α-hydroxylated metabolites of pregnenolone may also be found (Fantl et al. 1973).

The basis of this failure of pregnenolone utilisation to form progesterone and other Δ^4-3-ketosteroids such as cortisol is not known in most cases but it could be due to enzyme defects involving the Δ^5-3β-hydroxysteroid dehydrogenase and possibly C_{17-20} desmolase systems. Other hydroxylating systems may, however, be intact in some lesions. In a recent example studied personally, cultured tumour cells from a metastasis failed to metabolise pregnenolone to active hormones and secreted no detectable Δ^4-3-ketosteroids such as cortisol is not known in most cases but it could be due to sterone, on the other hand, were converted to a variety of steroids including predominantly corticosterone (Fig. 16.1).

If in some lesions the enzymes responsible for cleaving cholesterol to pregnenolone are deficient, cholesterol together with its esters, will tend to accumulate in the cells and give them a lipid-laden clear appearance. This is also the basis of the morphology of the adrenal cortex in congenital 'lipoid' hyperplasia and may also account for the 'clear' cell morphology of a minority of these tumours (vide infra).

Therefore, in the follow-up of patients with non-hormonal carcinomas it is essential to characterise the nature of the precursor steroids being released by such tumours, if any, and to measure them in the blood and/or urine as index substances in the monitoring of the clinical status of such patients, rather than to try and make use of any of the typical adrenal products.

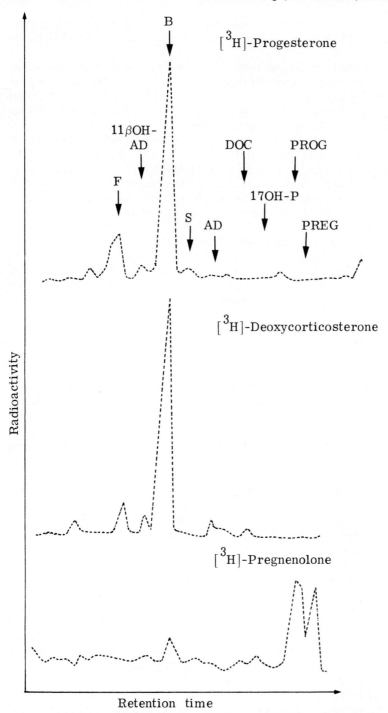

Fig. 16.1. Non-hormonal adrenocortical carcinoma. Steroid profiles (HPLC) of radiometabolites formed from a series of tritiated steroid precursors by a lung metastasis of a 'non-functioning' tumour in monolayer culture. Despite a failure to metabolise pregnenolone to active hormones both exogenous progesterone and deoxycorticosterone were converted to 11β-hydroxysteroids including cortisol (F) and corticosterone (B), respectively. The appearance of the cultured cells and the metastasis itself are illustrated in Fig. 16.3.

Pathology

Gross appearance Non-hormonal adrenocortical carcinomas have similar gross features to those of functioning adrenocortical carcinomas, although they tend to be larger than the latter, often showing more extensive areas of necrosis and haemorrhage. This increase in size is probably related to the fact that they fail to produce clinical signs and symptoms at an early stage. Weights >1 kg and sizes >20 cm are, therefore, not uncommon (Table 16.1) although non-functioning tumours as small as 5 cm have been detected (Smith et al. 1979) (Table 16.1).

Microscopic appearance Microscopically, it is our experience that the predominant cell type which comprises these lesions is an eosinophilic lipid-sparse compact cell. Some tumours, however, contain more clear cells than compact cells, and most tumours described in the literature have been stated to contain more clear than compact cells. This is at variance with our own experience, and the predominance of the lipid-sparse cells is a feature not emphasised by previous workers.

The general arrangement of the tumour cells is similar to functioning adrenal tumours associated with Cushing's and the adrenogenital syndromes (Fig. 16.2). Not infrequently non-hormonal compact cell tumours show marked nuclear and cellular pleomorphism in some areas, while in others their size and appearance does not deviate significantly from the normal compact cell. However, even these more normal-sized cells tend to have enlarged vesicular nuclei with prominent nucleoli.

As with other adrenal tumours, the usual histological criteria of malignancy are not applicable. The presence of tumour cell invasion of the capsule or the vascular spaces is, for example, not obviously related to the subsequent behaviour of the lesions. Mitotic activity is also variable and, as in many adrenocortical tumours, its absence cannot be deemed evidence of benignity. Although nuclear pleomorphism and vesicularity are guides to malignancy it is preferable at this time to regard all non-hormonal tumours as malignant, irrespective of their histology, as few authenticated long-term survivals have been reported. Patients found to have such non-hormonal lesions should be followed-up accordingly at frequent intervals when suitable steroid assays should be conducted (vide supra).

The only 'non-functioning' adrenal carcinoma to have received a detailed ultrastructural examination was a gelatinous 'myxoid' lesion (Tang et al. 1979). It showed conspicuous parallel arrays of RER, relatively sparse SER compared with most functioning tumours, and sparse mitochondria with infrequent peripherally located tubulo-vesicular cristae of a nonetheless recognisable steroidogenic type; in short, features common to a wide variety of adrenal carcinomas, and probably reflecting the persistence of at least some steroidogenic properties (vide supra).

Prognosis

The prognosis of non-hormonal adrenocortical carcinomas is poor being similar to that of the hormonally active lesions. Thus most patients with 'non-functioning' carcinomas die with metastases within one year of diagnosis (Lewinski et al. 1974), and chemotherapy is relatively ineffective in retarding the disease in many cases.

Metastases when they develop are most frequently detected in the local lymph nodes, liver, lungs and bones with characteristics similar to primary lesions (Fig. 16.3). More recently brain metastases have been recorded as frequent findings (Lewinski et al. 1974). Such lesions were formerly considered to be rare (Huvos et al. 1970; Lipsett et al. 1963). Extended survival with chemotherapy may be allowing such metastases to become overt in some cases.

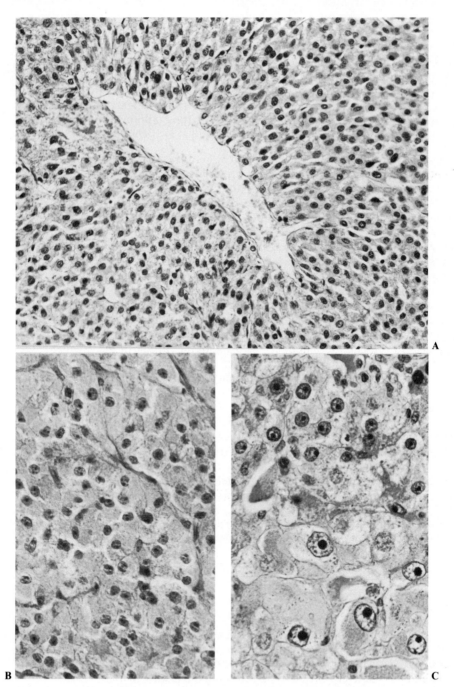

Fig. 16.2. Non-hormonal adrenocortical carcinomas. Three cellular patterns are shown. In each lesion the tumour cells are of the compact type. The example shown in **A** measured 31.6 cm in diameter. The cells are organised in broad sheets with a marked perivascular arrangement between which there is extensive necrosis. There is little pleomorphism, although the nuclei are enlarged, a feature also noted in **B** taken from a 10 × 7.5 cm tumour. In contrast, (**C**), the tumour weighed 1100 g and showed marked cellular and nuclear hypertrophy and pleomorphism. Prominent nucleoli are seen in the vesicular nuclei. (H + E [**A**] × 180; [**B**] × 240; [**C**] × 300)

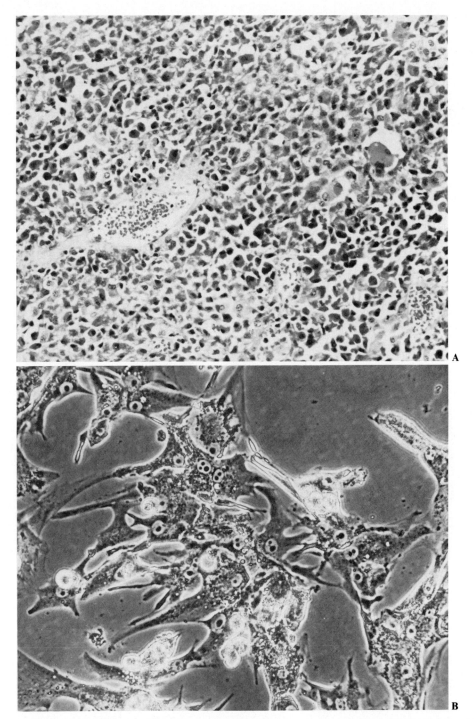

Fig. 16.3. Non-hormonal adrenocortical carcinoma. Pulmonary metastasis. A highly pleomorphic metastatic lesion is illustrated (**A**) with numerous mitoses and giant cellular forms. The constituent cells are again of the compact type. In culture (**B**) the pleomorphic multinuleate nature of many of the cells from this metastasis is further apparent. (H + E × 180 [**A**]; PC × 200 [**B**])

The Attached and Contralateral Gland in Non-Hormonal Adrenocortical Tumours

The remainder of the cortex, when available for study, shows a normal size and zonal appearance in cases of 'non-hormonal' carcinomas, in accordance with the absence of active hormones being secreted by the tumours and the failure of these patients to show any evidence of adrenal insufficiency.

Part C
HYPOCORTICALISM

Chapter 17
Acute Acquired Adrenoprivic Hypocorticalism

The commonest cause of acute acquired adrenocortical insufficiency of primary adrenal origin was formerly regarded as bilateral adrenal haemorrhage (so-called adrenal apoplexy), such as occurs in the Waterhouse-Friderichsen syndrome (p. 277) with meningococcal septicaemia. Further studies, however, have quite clearly demonstrated that bilateral adrenal haemorrhage is rarely associated with overt biochemical evidence of acute adrenal insufficiency. It is worth noting, for example, that surgical extirpation of both adrenal glands and without substitution therapy is not followed by the overt manifestation of adrenocortical insufficiency within a period of 24–48 h, such as is said to occur following adrenal haemorrhage in fulminating septicaemia. Furthermore, plasma cortisol levels have been measured in the Waterhouse-Friderichsen syndrome and found to be elevated (Migeon et al. 1967) as one would anticipate of the adrenal in response to stress. In addition, most cases of neonatal adrenal haemorrhage (p. 277), even when the haemorrhage is bilateral and massive, are still capable of a spontaneous and full recovery without the need for steroid replacement therapy (Black and Williams 1973). Hence, most cases of adrenocortical haemorrhage and necrosis can no longer be regarded as a primary cause of life-threatening adrenal insufficiency. Rather, in adults and children, it would appear to be relegated to a possible contributory factor to the demise of the patient but not a primary cause due to acute adrenocortical steroid insufficiency.

The commonest cause of acute adrenocortical insufficiency is therefore probably that which can occur in patients who are receiving substitution steroid therapy following bilateral adrenalectomy, or in patients with chronic acquired adrenoprivic hypocorticalism (Addison's disease). When such treatment is withdrawn or these patients are further stressed as, for example, by an operation or infection, then minor or even major degrees of insufficiency may rapidly evolve, if replacement therapy is not augmented. Very rarely, massive bilateral adrenal haemorrhage and hypotensive crises may follow anti-coagulant therapy (O'Connell and Aston 1974).

Chapter 18
Chronic Acquired Adrenoprivic Hypocorticalism (Addison's Disease)

All patients with chronic acquired adrenoprivic hypocorticalism present clinically with Addison's disease, the symptoms of which include weakness and fatigue, weight loss, hyperpigmentation, hypotension, hyponatraemia and gastrointestinal symptoms. Of the many causes (Table 18.1) idiopathic organ-specific autoimmune adrenalitis (idiopathic Addison's disease) (IAD) and tuberculosis of the adrenal are the commonest. Idiopathic Addison's disease now accounts for approximately 70% of all cases which occur in Europe (Mason et al. 1968), with 10%–15% of cases due to tuberculosis. A recent analysis of the aetiology in Japan, however, has shown that there tuberculosis still is the commoner cause (Ofuji et al. 1977).

Table 18.1. Causes of chronic acquired adreno-privic hypocorticalism (Addison's disease)

IDIOPATHIC
    Organ-specific autoimmune adrenalitis
INFLAMMATORY
    Granulomata
        Tuberculosis
        Sarcoidosis
    Protozoal and Fungal
        Histoplasmosis
        Blastomycosis
        Coccidiomycosis
        Candidiasis (moniliasis)
        Torulosis (cryptococcosis)
    Viral
        Cytomegalic virus
        Herpes simplex
METABOLIC
    Amyloidosis
NEOPLASTIC DISORDERS
    Metastatic carcinoma

Addison's disease is a rare disorder which occurs at most in about 60 persons/million of the population in Europe (Nerup 1974a,b). It is most commonly detected in the third to fifth decades although no age is exempt. It affects the sexes equally during the first three decades of life and thereafter is about three times as common in women (Irvine et al. 1979). When it is associated with other autoimmune disorders e.g. hypoparathyroidism, autoimmune atrophic gastritis, or autoimmune thyroiditis it is commoner in females irrespective of age.

Its differential diagnosis includes all conditions causing hyperpigmentation, chronic fatigue and chronic nausea and vomiting. Circulating ACTH levels are increased in this form of primary adrenal insufficiency, typically levels of 300–500 pg/l being noted (Besser et al. 1971), and patients fail to respond to long-term ACTH stimulation (e.g.

1 mg Synacthen depot intramuscularly daily for three consecutive days) (Irvine and Barnes 1972). In one or two cases, an ACTH-secreting adenoma has been observed to develop secondary to long-standing Addison's disease (Jara-Albarran et al. 1979).

Organ-specific Autoimmune Adrenalitis (Idiopathic Addison's Disease)

Pathology

Gross appearance   The adrenal glands are smaller than normal and are often misshapen (the 'contracted' gland of the early literature). On occasion they may not be detectable macroscopically at autopsy and can only be identified when the adrenal area is subsequently examined in minute detail microscopically.

The adrenal weight has been recorded in very few instances. Values for single autopsy glands have varied between 1.9 and 4.6 g (Sloper 1955) although in some other cases, subsequently reported, gland weights of or around 0.2 g have been noted.

Microscopic appearance   Microscopically the atrophy of the adrenal gland is seen to be diffuse and to involve the entire cortex (Guttman 1930; Symington 1969). The capsule appears thickened, probably due to the overall reduction in gland size rather than increased fibrosis. In extreme cases little or no cortical tissue remains, and only a few adrenocortical cells are detected occurring singly, in small clusters or as strands enmeshed in a condensed reticulin framework (Fig. 18.1). The cells are compact in type with eosinophilic lipid-sparse cytoplasm and, occasionally, lipofuscin pigment. In many cases these compact cells are of normal size similar to those of the normal zona reticularis. Occasionally, however, hypertrophy of the cells with large nuclei and prominent nucleoli, possibly induced by the raised plasma ACTH levels (vide supra) can be observed. In some glands, small nodules of adrenocortical cells may be present, or may occur apparently outside the capsule. Such nodules show similar changes to those found in the remainder of the cortex. The medulla appears intact and may reach the inner aspect of the capsule due to destruction of the overlying cortex.

Evidence of an immune component in this disease is provided by what is usually an extensive diffuse lymphocytic infiltrate in relation to the adrenocortical cells, together with some plasma cells and macrophages (Fig. 18.1). In severe cases germinal centres may exist. This lymphocytic infiltrate can extend into the medulla but this probably represents the residuum of a reaction with the adrenocortical cells which surround the adrenal vein. If accessory adrenocortical tissue is present, it often shows similar features (Wells 1930). The ultrastructure of adrenal cells in IAD has not been reported.

While occasional lymphocytes can be found in ~20% of autopsy adrenals, significant focal lymphocytic infiltration is uncommon in non-Addisonian cases (Petri and Nerup 1971).

The appearances of autoimmune adrenalitis require to be differentiated from the diffuse steroid-induced atrophy associated with low levels of ACTH when the cortex consists of clear lipid-laden cells only (p. 61) and also from other causes of inflammatory infiltration (pp. 261, 265).

Aetiology

This form of adrenal atrophy is now generally regarded as an organ-specific autoimmune disease in essentially the same category as Hashimoto's thyroiditis and autoimmune gastritis. It is not infrequently associated with other autoimmune diseases

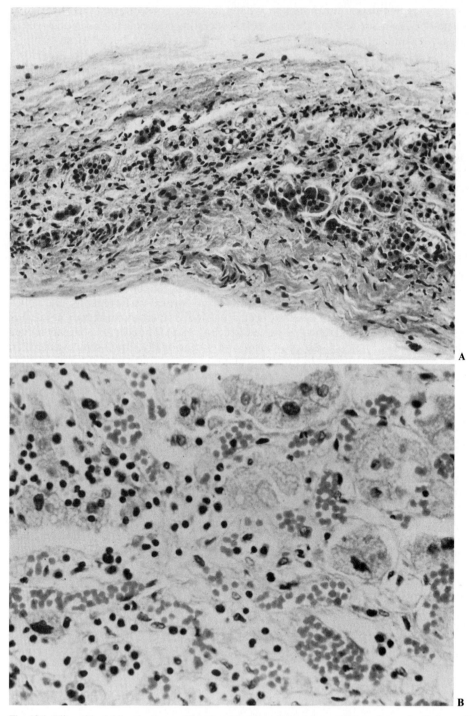

Fig. 18.1. Idiopathic Addison's disease. The atrophic adrenal gland has a thickened capsule. Only small islands of surviving compact cells (**A**) are present, although the medulla (not shown) was intact. A chronic inflammatory infiltrate is present in both glands illustrated but is seen better in **B**.
Fig. 18.1B courtesy of Professor John Anderson (Glasgow). (H + E × 180 [**A**]; × 500 [**B**])

such as those of the thyroid, with, for example, up to half the cases of IAD having concurrent thyroid autoantibodies, although not necessarily overt thyroid disease in the form of detectable hypothyroidism. The conjunction of Addison's disease with overt hypothyroidism is sometimes referred to as Schmidt's syndrome (1926) (for review see Carpenter et al. 1964). Other associations of varying frequency include pernicious anaemia, idiopathic hypoparathyroidism (with or without moniliasis), type I diabetes mellitus and premature ovarian failure (Table 18.2).

Table 18.2. Principal clinical disorders associated with Addison's disease in 383 patients[a]

	Idiopathic	Tuberculous	Other
Amenorrhea/oligomenorrhea	59	1	
Thyroid disease			
Thyrotoxicosis	16	1	
Hypothyroidism	28		
Hashimoto thyroiditis	7		
Goitre	9		
Pernicious anaemia	12		
Diabetes mellitus			
Type I	31		
Type II	6	2	
Hypoparathyroidism	18		
Vitiligo	22	1	
Asthma	9		
Coeliac disease	2		
Renal tubular acidosis	2		
Primary biliary cirrhosis	1		
Myasthenia gravis	1		
No. of Addison's patients affected	153	4	0
Total no. of Addison's patients	321	58	4

[a]Data from Irvine et al 1979.

Autoantibodies can be detected by immunofluorescence (Fig. 18.2) and complement fixation in approximately 50%–70% of patients with idiopathic Addison's disease (Anderson et al. 1957; Blizzard et al. 1967; Nerup 1974b), particularly when it is associated with the other organ-specific autoimmune diseases (Wuepper et al. 1969) noted above. Most of these autoantibodies appear to be organ-specific, but are not species-specific cross-reacting with the adrenal cortex from other mammals. The antibodies are associated with both cell-mediated (Nerup and Bendixen 1969a) and humoral immune mechanisms (Irvine et al. 1969) and many appear to be directed at cytoplasmic antigens in the mitochondria (Nerup and Bendixen 1969b) and microsomes respectively (Goudie et al. 1968). No absolute correlation has, however, been found between the occurrence of circulating anti-adrenal antibody and anti-adrenal cellular hypersensitivity. The circulating antibodies occur with a higher frequency in younger patients with idiopathic Addison's disease and tend to persist often, but not always, after diagnosis and institution of replacement steroid therapy.

In about 17%–25% of patients with idiopathic Addison's disease antibodies have been detected which react with not only the adrenal gland but also with other steroid-producing cells (Anderson et al. 1968). These so-called 'steroid cell' antibodies appear to be one of the principal causes of the onset of premature menopause and ovarian atrophy in such patients (Irvine et al. 1968; Irvine and Barnes 1974).

The relationship of the anti-adrenal autoantibodies to the genesis of adrenal atrophy is, however, far from clear, particularly since most are directed at intracellular

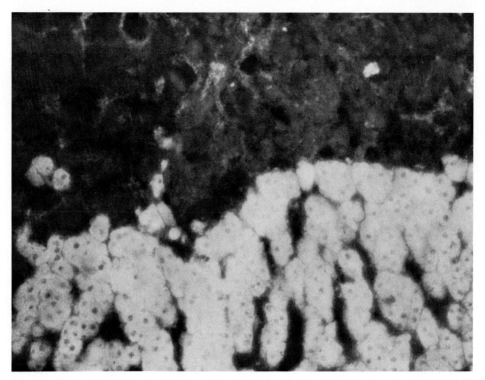

Fig. 18.2. Idiopathic Addison's disease. An immunofluorescent illustration of autoantibodies to the adrenocortical cells in a patient with hypocorticalism.
Courtesy of Professor John Anderson (Glasgow). (× 360)

components presumably inaccessible in intact cells to the antibodies. It is apparent from clinical data that such circulating autoantibodies can occur in subjects with normal adrenocortical reserve, and neither the cellular nor humoral immune parameters correlate directly with clinical parameters (Irvine et al. 1967). Moreover, they can pass from the maternal to the fetal circulation during pregnancy when no adrenal insufficiency appears to be present in the resulting offspring (Irvine et al. 1979). Delayed hypersensitivity or antibody-dependent or cell-mediated cytotoxicity seem the most likely causative mechanisms operating in IAD, with perhaps the majority of anti-adrenal antibodies detected in patients with established disease being the result rather than the cause of the autoimmune-mediated destruction of the cortex.

More recent studies have revealed the presence of a population of precipitating antibodies in some patients with idiopathic Addison's disease (Andrada et al. 1968), usually in those with the moniliasis-polyendocrinopathy syndrome (Heinonen et al. 1976). Such precipitating antibodies seem to differ from those demonstrable by complement fixation and immunofluorescence, and although some cross-react with components of animal adrenals, they do not react with other steroid-producing tissues (Heinonen and Krohn 1977). This particular group of patients, therefore, may represent a subset of those with idiopathic Addison's disease. More recently (Khoury et al. 1981) autoantibodies to cell surface antigens of the adrenal cortex have been detected in IAD. It may be that these are the antibodies which are more relevant to the genesis of hypofunction, cell death and atrophy.

Idiopathic Addison's disease may in some instances be familial, and it has been suggested that it may be inherited as an autosomal recessive trait (Irvine et al. 1979).

This seems particularly the case. but not exclusively so, when it is associated with other autoimmune syndromes (e.g. Schmidt's syndrome, or idiopathic hypoparathyroidism) (Spinner et al. 1968); many cases however, show no Mendelian pattern. Patients with IAD have an increased prevalence of HLA-B8 (risk factor x7), and of Dw3 (Thomsen et al. 1975; Irvine et al. 1979), particularly in the case of Dw3 subjects with idiopathic Addison's disease who have circulating antibodies.

Adrenoleukodystrophy (Addison-Schilder's Disease)

Incidence and Symptoms

This is a rare form of Addison's disease associated with diffuse demyelination of the central and peripheral nervous systems, originally described by Siemerling and Creutzfeld (1923). Long thought to be a coincidental association it is now known to be due to an inborn error of metabolism and is generally referred to as adrenoleukodystrophy (ALD) after Blaw (1970). It is a fatal X-linked hereditary disorder occurring only in males; females with Schilder's disease (diffuse demyelinating cerebral sclerosis) show no adrenal changes. Over 50 cases have now been described. It is not, however, the only neurological disorder reported in association with Addison's disease as cases of spastic paraplegia, idiopathic epilepsy, suspected disseminated sclerosis and mental retardation have been recorded (Irvine et al. 1979); their relation with adrenoleukodystrophy has not been positively established in all cases but some seem to represent a neurological adult-onset variant of ALD that has been termed adrenomyeloneuropathy (Schaumburg et al. 1977) and which is characterised by adrenal insufficiency since childhood and progressive spastic paraparesis developing in the third decade (Griffin et al. 1977).

Adrenoleukodystrophy generally becomes manifest in boys 5–15 years of age, although cases with a neonatal or adult onset have been recorded (Powers et al. 1980). Most affected family members show the neurological symptoms (ataxia and paresis) first and to a greater degree, although in some cases only the adrenal symptoms occur (hyperpigmentation and asthenia), others express both to varying degrees and at varying intervals (Schaumburg et al. 1975). Steroid replacement therapy does not modify the inexorable neurological changes which lead to death within 2–4 years in most cases. Adrenal biopsy is reportedly the most reliable diagnostic test.

Pathology

Adrenal Cortex

The appearances of the adrenal gland at autopsy vary, depending on the duration of the disease process. They have been described and reviewed in detail recently by Powers et al. (1980).

Gross appearance The glands although retaining their characteristic shape are smaller than normal and each weighs <2 g, often <1.0 g (normal pubertal autopsy weight 3–6 g). In some instances no adrenal tissue is detectable macroscopically.

Microscopic appearance Microscopically, the appearances vary depending upon the longevity of the disease course with progressive atrophy occurring with time (Powers et al. 1980).

The capsule appears thickened due to the atrophy of the cortex (Fig. 18.3). In the less severe cases, the zona glomerulosa appears spared, but admixed with normal inner clear zona fasciculata and compact zona reticularis cells, there appear foci of 'ballooned' cells with granular or hyaline eosinophilic cytoplasm and vesicular nuclei (Schaumburg et al. 1972) (Fig. 18.4). Some ballooned cells with vesicular or hyperchromatic eccentric nuclei also exhibit a unique striated appearance of the cytoplasm (Fig. 18.4). These cells are considered to be pathognomonic of the disease and are not seen in any other adrenal pathologies (Powers and Schaumburg 1973). Occasional binucleate forms also exist. Such groups of ballooned cells are multifocal

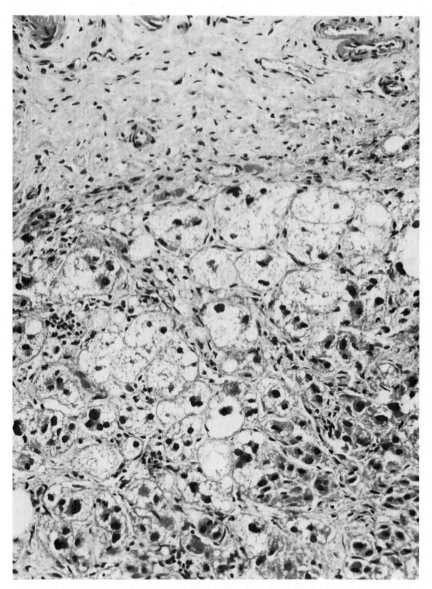

Fig. 18.3. Adrenoleukodystrophy. An early example is shown in which the adrenal gland has a broadened capsule and contains both clear and compact cells. Cellular hypertrophy ('ballooning') is most evident in the former although some cells also show striation (H + E × 160)

and often form small nodules and may undergo subsequent lysis to form macrovacuoles. Ultrastructural studies have shown that cytoplasmic ballooning and striations result from proliferation of the smooth endoplasmic reticulum and the accumulation of lamellar-lipid profiles (Powers et al. 1980) (Fig. 18.5).

With increasing severity, the number of normal cortical cells declines further and macrovacuoles and ballooned granular cells become even more prominent. In extreme cases only the medulla appears to remain although some scattered compact-type adrenal cells forming small foci may be seen internal to or within the capsule (Fig. 18.6). In these cases without 'ballooned' cells the appearance of the cortex may be indistinguishable from idiopathic Addison's disease. With further progressive change all the adrenal cells may disappear. There is thus a spectrum of change due to progressive adrenal cytolysis, and the elevated plasma ACTH levels of this disorder (Rees et al. 1975b) possibly potentiate the process of ballooning and macrovacuole formation (Powers et al. 1980). Lymphocytic infiltration is uncommon and found only in the most extensively atrophied glands, in contrast to autoimmune idiopathic Addison's disease.

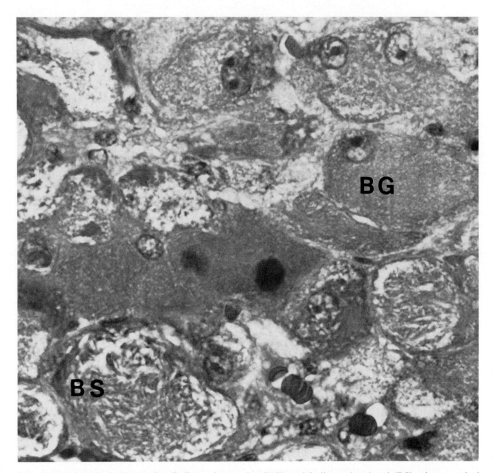

Fig. 18.4. Adrenoleukodystrophy. Ballooned granular (BG) and ballooned striated (BS) adrenocortical cells.
Courtesy of Dr. J. Powers. (H + E × 750)

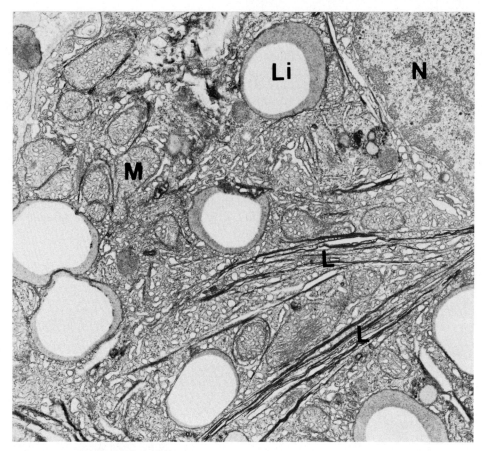

Fig. 18.5. Adrenoleukodystrophy. A striated cell is illustrated to show, in particular, the lamellar-lipid (L) profiles (Li – lipid droplet; M – mitochondria; N – nucleus).
Courtesy of Dr. J. Powers. (× 16 900)

Other Tissues

The cerebral white matter displays inflammatory and demyelinating changes (Hoefnagel et al. 1962) together with gliosis and macrophages with cytoplasmic lamellae (Schaumburg et al. 1974). The Schwann cells of the peripheral nerves and the Leydig cells of the testis are also abnormal in some cases with lipidic lamellae in their cytoplasm (Powers and Schaumburg (1974a, b). In adult onset cases (adreno-myeloneuropathy) there may be spermatogenic arrest (Powers and Schaumburg 1981). These changes closely resemble some of the changes in the adrenocortical cells and presumably stem from the same cause.

Aetiology of Adrenal Changes in Adrenoleukodystrophy

Recent studies have shown that the process of adrenal cytolysis and atrophy described above is caused by an inborn defect in fatty acid metabolism, whereby mono-unsaturated fatty acids of increasing chain length (C_{22}–C_{26}) accumulate in a variety of

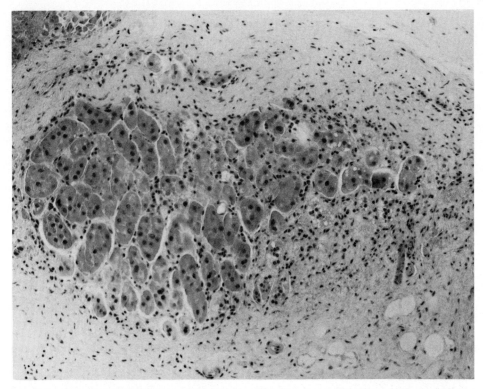

Fig. 18.6. Adrenoleukodystrophy. A small focus or nodule of compact cells remains within the thickened capsule. There is a moderate inflammatory infiltrate. No marked changes typical of adrenoleukodystrophy, i.e. 'ballooned' or striated cells, were present in this section although they were seen in other areas of the gland. ($H + E \times 200$)

tissues and are esterified with cholesterol (Igarashi et al. 1976; Menkes and Corbo 1977). The precise enzymatic defect that results in this long-chain fatty acid accumulation is not yet known with certainty but is probably due to a failure of such compounds to be degraded in a normal manner. ALD is, therefore, apparently a form of lipid storage disease.

It is known from a variety of other systems that such long-chain fatty acids are toxic and interfere with mitochondrial and microsomal enzyme activities. This probably leads to the proliferation of smooth endoplasmic reticulum noted in ALD (Powers et al. 1980). As the long-chain fatty acids esterified to cholesterol accumulate further in the cytoplasm, they solidify as crystalloids and give rise to the characteristic cytoplasmic lamellae of naked lipid or lipid-protein aggregates that are found in the adrenal and other tissues, and which are responsible for the 'striated' cytoplasm seen at the light microscopical level. The adrenal cortex is probably particularly susceptible to these effects because of its high lipid content and active metabolism of sterols and sterol esters.

Tuberculosis of the Adrenal Gland

As mentioned above, this is now a rare cause of chronic acquired hypocorticalism in Europe (10%–15% of cases). To result in Addison's disease tuberculous involvement of the adrenals must be bilateral and have caused almost complete destruction of the cortical tissue (Baker 1928; Guttman 1930). Active extra-adrenal tuberculosis is found in only a minority ($<20\%$) of such cases (Sloper 1955) and although earlier series (e.g. Coneybeare and Millis 1924) reported pulmonary foci in almost all cases, these were healed in every case and most lesions detected elsewhere were clinically latent.

Pathology

Gross appearance   The adrenal glands in tuberculous Addison's disease are usually moderately or sometimes greatly enlarged, and combined weights of up to nearly 50 g have been recorded at autopsy, with mean combined weights of about 25 g (Guttman 1930) compared with a normal combined weight of approximately 12 g. The glands have a yellowish-grey uniform appearance or a nodular mottled grey/red colour depending on the activity of the lesions. Often the capsule is adherent to surrounding structures. On sectioning, the gland is seen to be replaced by a confluent, sometimes semi-fluid, caseous mass with usually only a thin rim of surviving cortical and fibrovascular tissue. Small flecks of calcification are often present but extensive calcification is uncommon.

Microscopic appearance   Microscopically the gland is replaced by large confluent foci of caseation necrosis surrounded by a thin rim of small round cells, principally lymphocytes, with, in addition, occasional Langerhan's-type giant cells (Fig. 18.7). Lymphocytic infiltration is however, much more limited than in autoimmune adrenalitis, both in frequency and extent. Tubercle bacilli can be demonstrated in approximately 50% of these cases by the use of the Ziehl-Neilsen stain. Fibrosis in relation to such foci is minimal, possibly due to the local influence of high levels of glucocorticoids. Occasional isolated compact-type adrenocortical cells are found among the small round-cell infiltrate, some showing evidence of cell death or degenerative change. The surviving adrenocortical tissue often forms a small peripheral rim and consists of clear cells which show the effect of stress of dying in autopsy specimens. On occasion the foci of tuberculosis appear to be more prominent in nodules of the adrenal cortex, although sparing of extra-adrenal nodules has been reported.

In most instances no medulla can be identified and this is in keeping with the morphological and experimental studies which tend to indicate that it is more susceptible to tuberculosis than the cortex and that in many instances the destructive process seems to commence in the medulla and spread centrifugally (Barker 1928; Guttman 1930; Blacklock and Williams 1961). The adrenal vasculature may also be important in determining the site of onset of infection (Symington 1969).

It would appear that once tuberculosis of the adrenal gland commences it is irreversible; healing does not occur (Barker 1928; Guttman 1930) and it proceeds to progressive destruction of the gland. Where there has been complete destruction of the gland, periadrenal fibrosis with granulation tissue may be noted. Small venous thrombi may also be seen in those areas.

Extensive immunopathological studies of patients with tuberculous adrenalitis have now been carried out (e.g. Irvine et al. 1968; Wuepper et al. 1969; Nerup 1974b) and it would appear that autoantibodies are not involved in either the pathogenesis or progression of this disorder. Neither is the destruction of the cortex per se sufficient stimulus for the production of most anti-adrenal antibodies. Thus, no adrenal-specific autoantibodies have been detected in proved cases of tuberculous adrenalitis, although occasional cases have shown 'steroid-cell' antibodies (Kamp et al. 1974).

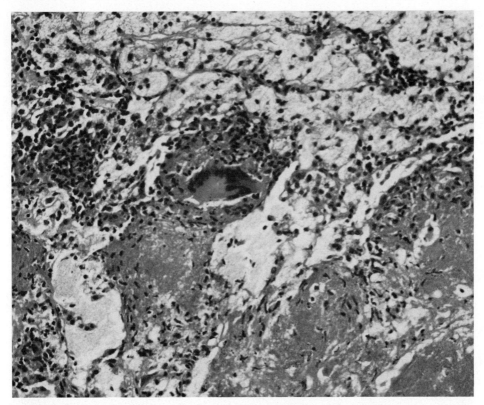

Fig. 18.7. Tuberculosis of the adrenal gland. The peripheral part of a large area of caseation necrosis is seen with a Langerhan's-type giant cell and a dense rim of small round cells. A surviving portion of the cortex is shown at the *top*. (H + E × 240)

Amyloidosis

While amyloid deposits in the adrenal gland used once to be a frequent autopsy finding, it is rare to notice this nowadays as cases of chronic sepsis become rarer and it is even rarer to find amyloidosis (β-fibrillosis) as a cause of hypocorticalism. As with tuberculosis, it requires to be bilateral and extensive to cause adrenal insufficiency and is usually found as part of a general reaction to secondary chronic infection, i.e. it is a secondary form of amyloidosis associated with the involvement of other viscera.

Pathology

Gross appearance   The adrenal gland may be normal in size or slightly enlarged in some cases, but greatly enlarged glands weighing 30–34 g per pair have been reported. On sectioning the cut surface appears greyish-yellow.

Microscopic appearance   Amyloid deposits usually occur in the zona fasciculata and the zona reticularis and are found between the adrenal cells and the capillary endothelium. Small perivascular foci of amyloid may also be found in the medulla. Gradually, with increasing deposition of amyloid the inner zone is converted to a

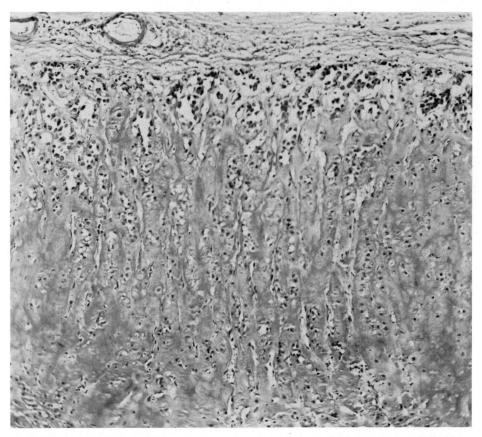

Fig. 18.8. Adrenal amyloidosis. The cortex, with the exception of the outermost zona glomerulosa, has been replaced by hyaline masses, particularly deposited between the adrenal cells and the capillaries. (H + E × 120)

hyaline acellular mass which extends peripherally to leave only a small cap or cluster of adrenocortical cells around the periphery. This is the kind of appearance found when the changes are associated with hypocorticalism (Fig. 18.8).

Smaller and lesser degrees of involvement may occur as a secondary phenomenon in association with many other diseases, when they are not associated with overt hypocorticalism.

Metastatic Carcinoma

Metastatic carcinoma in the adrenal gland is a frequent finding at autopsy in tumour-bearing patients (e.g. Lumb and MacKenzie 1959). Its reported frequency depends on the extent and care with which adrenal examination is carried out, as many deposits are only of microscopic size, although they are often multiple (Fig. 18.9).

While Addison in his first description of the disease listed metastatic carcinoma amongst its causes, it is in fact undoubtedly an extremely rare cause of hypocorticalism (Sahagian-Edwards and Holland 1954; Modhi 1981), and quite massive adrenal metastases do not neccessarily compromise cortical function (Cedermark and Sjöberg 1981).

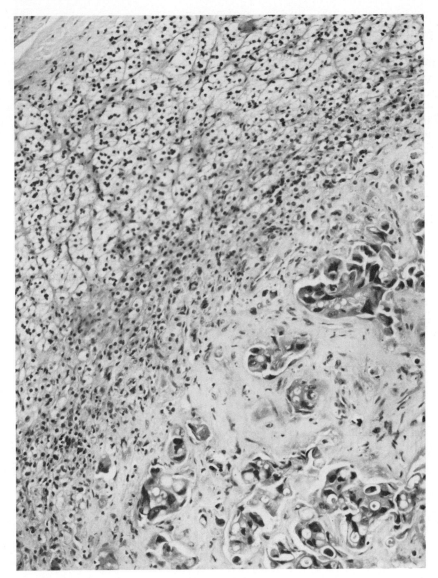

Fig. 18.9. Metastatic carcinoma of the adrenal gland. A focus of metastatic mammary carcinoma with a prominent desmoplastic response is seen in the central part of the gland related to the central vein. The surrounding cortex (*left*) is normal in appearance. (H + E × 150)

Miscellaneous Causes Including Non-Tuberculous Infections

Table 18.1 lists a variety of other potential causes of hypocorticalism, some represented only by isolated reports. Cases associated with protozoal and fungal infections have been described and illustrated by Frenkel (1960) and by Nichols (1968). Although rare in non-tropical zones they may account for a significant fraction of patients with Addison's disease in tropical areas (Del Negro et al. 1980). The high local levels of glucocorticoids in the gland may well predispose it to infections of this type, as suggested by Frenkel (1960).

Histoplasmosis (Sarosi et al. 1971) and cryptococcosis (Salyer et al. 1973) are the most frequently encountered infections of this type in sub-tropical zones, and some evidence of adrenal insufficiency may be encountered in up to half the cases of disseminated disease. Cryptococcosis is common in certain areas (e.g. Ohio and Tennessee Valley in the U.S.A.) as is paracoccidioidomycosis in Venezuela. The latter infection also commonly involves the adrenal glands causing caseation necrosis resembling tuberculous glands and results in adrenal hypofunction in a significant number of cases of systemic infection (Marsiglia and Pinto 1966). As with tuberculous lesions, inflammatory, granulomatous and fibrotic reactions are not remarkable in such fungal lesions. Even in cases without overt hypocorticalism these infections may diminish adrenal reserve (Del Negro et al. 1980).

Amongst the viral infections that can cause adrenal necrosis are those induced by the cytomegalovirus and the herpes simplex virus (Joseph and Vogt 1974; Ruiz-Palacios et al. 1977); as a cause of recognisable adrenal insufficiency both are, however, extremely rare.

Chapter 19
Congenital Adrenoprivic Hypocorticalism

Idiopathic Congenital Adrenocortical Hypoplasia and the Syndrome of ACTH Unresponsiveness

Incidence and Symptoms

Idiopathic congenital adrenocortical hypoplasia, first described by Sikl (1948), occurs in approximately 1:12500 births (Laverty et al. 1973). Most cases present in the immediate perinatal period with Addisonian crises, although the symptoms may be delayed until infancy (1–2 years), or even later (Baker et al. 1967). In the absence of prompt diagnosis and replacement steroid therapy, most affected infants die. It needs to be distinguished from commoner causes of adrenal failure such as congenital adrenal hyperplasia with enzyme deficiencies, secondary hypoplasia with CNS defects and/or pituitary hypoplasia (p. 271), and from acquired forms of perinatal insufficiency including prenatal exposure to glucocorticoids (maternal Cushing's syndrome or steroid therapy), and perinatal adrenal trauma with haemorrhage and calcification which in rare cases may cause adrenal insufficiency. A definitive diagnosis of congenital adrenal hypoplasia can, however, often be made only at autopsy, and should be accompanied by clear-cut clinical and/or chemical evidence of adrenal insufficiency.

Clinically, three variants of congenital hypoplasia are recognised, two of which are unresponsive to ACTH, indicating a primary adrenal abnormality. In the majority of instances there is a deficiency of all secreted adrenal steroids, including mineralocorticoids (Sperling et al. 1973; Pakravan et al. 1974). Less commonly the condition may present without a salt-losing syndrome indicative of aldosterone deficiency, i.e glucocorticoid deficiency only, as reported both in males (Migeon et al. 1968) and females (Franks and Nance 1970). In two brothers with true ACTH unresponsiveness, plasma DOC levels were ten times the normal value, while cortisol was in the low-normal range (Thisthlethwaite et al. 1975) suggesting a defect in steroid 17α-hydroxylation. These non-salt losing cases tend to live longer, but those that do come to autopsy show significant hypoplasia (Kelch et al. 1972). Thus, although they are sometimes distinguished clinically from the pansteroidoprivic cases, they clearly merit inclusion from a pathological point of view.

Rare cases of isolated hypoaldosteronism but without symptoms of glucocorticoid deficiency have also been noted in association with congenital adrenal hypoplasia (Ehrlich et al. 1969; Peterson et al. 1977). Their relationship to the other forms of hypoplasia and the nature of the defect remain obscure.

Although sporadic cases of congenital adrenal hypoplasia have been noted, its familial incidence (Uttley 1968; O'Donohoe and Holland 1968) indicates a strong hereditary tendency. Males outnumber females by about 6:1 (Wuchner and Meiler 1977) and an X-linked recessive mode of inheritance seems likely in many instances (Weiss and Mellinger 1970). However, the presence of both affected males and females in some sibships (O'Donohoe and Holland 1968) indicates a possible autosomal recessive mechanism of transmission in these cases. The familial ACTH-unresponsiveness syndrome (without hypoaldosteronism) also shows genetic heterogeneity. No abnormalities of the pituitary gland, gonads or external genitalia are noted at autopsy.

The possibility has been raised that some cases of congenital 'idiopathic' adrenal hypoplasia may stem from overt pituitary disturbances. Prader et al. (1975), Golden et al. (1977), Kelly et al. (1977) and Grumbach et al. (1978) have described individual cases of X-linked adrenal insufficiency with concurrent hypogonadotrophic hypopituitarism in adolescents. The precise relationship between these two conditions is not obvious; it would not appear to be a direct causal one as ACTH levels were not reduced in these cases. It may be, however, that the reduced gonadotrophins are a consequence of the absence of adrenal steroids at some early stage in development, as all cases of supposed primary congenital adrenal hypoplasia (vide infra) who have survived, have failed to undergo normal pubertal development, even those who have had normal prepubertal gonadotrophin levels (Hay 1977). By contrast, patients with classical Addison's disease usually have, when treated, no problems of sexual maturation or fertility.

Pathology

Gross appearance   Adrenal weights are markedly reduced in all clinically verified cases studied at autopsy, irrespective of the precise symptomology. Although combined gland weights of up to 2 g (i.e. 25% normal birth weight) have been noted with clinical evidence of insufficiency, most weigh considerably less (<1 g combined weights in perinatal cases). In 10%–15% of cases no adrenocortical tissue at all has been detected (Wuchner and Meiler 1977), even on microscopic examination (Pakravan et al. 1974), although in some instances careful search in the perirenal fat has revealed microscopic islands of adrenal-type tissue (Petersen et al. 1977).

Care should be taken to ensure that there is evidence of adrenal insufficiency before older infants with combined adrenal weights in the 1–2 g range are included as cases of idiopathic hypoplasia (e.g. Favara et al. 1972; Russell et al. 1977), as these may fall within the range of normal gland weights for the age (Fig. 3.2).

Microscopic appearance   The original histological descriptions of idiopathic adrenal hypoplasia (Sikl 1948; Kerenyi 1961) indicated that the glands were of a distinctly different appearance to the hypoplastic adrenals in cases of pituitary insufficiency (e.g. anencephalia) (p. 272). The cortex consisted of large irregularly arranged eosinophilic cells resembling those of the fetal zone extending out to the capsule with no clear-cut outer zone of definitive or adult cortex (Fig. 19.1). This so-called 'cytomegalic' cortex has since been seen in some infants afflicted with the presumed X-linked form of the disorder (Uttley 1968). However, both male and female sibs in families with the presumed autosomal recessive form of the disorder (O'Donohoe and Holland 1968) showed a 'miniature' type of gland with well-formed definitive cortex and little or no fetal zone (Fig. 19.2), an appearance histologically indistinguishable from that found in cases of hypoplasia secondary to pituitary insufficiency (Kerenyi 1961) (Fig. 20.1).

Such cases of the ACTH-unresponsiveness syndrome as have been studied at autopsy or by biopsy (including males with presumed X-linked inheritance) also show the 'miniature' type of hypoplastic gland (Migeon et al. 1968; Kelch et al. 1972). In the absence of functional studies, however, it is difficult to evaluate the suggestion that it is the zona glomerulosa that is preserved in these cases and that the zona fasciculata and zona reticularis are degenerate (Migeon et al. 1968), particularly as the latter zone is

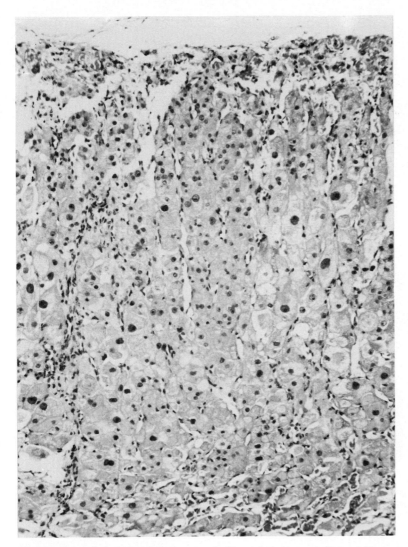

Fig. 19.1. Congenital adrenoprivic adrenocortical hypoplasia (cytomegalic type). The cortex consists of large eosinophilic cells arrayed in irregular columns reminiscent of the fetal zone and extending from the capsule to the inner vascular sinusoids. (H + E × 140)

seldom prominent in infancy (p. 49). A case of isolated hypoaldosteronism with adrenal hypoplasia in an adult (Ehrlich et al. 1969), however, showed the cytomegalic pattern, and a case of infant hypoaldosteronism revealed only 'fetal-type' cells but without overt cytomegaly (Petersen et al. 1977).

Contrary to older assertions, therefore, it is now clear that primary and secondary adrenal hypoplasia do not always present with a distinct and different histological appearance. The nature of the biochemical lesion in the primary cases is also obscure. A defect in the ACTH-receptor mechanism (p. 80) would seem a plausible hypothesis in familial glucocorticoid deficiency (Spark and Etzkorn 1977) although the pansteroidoprivic cases may well show a more fundamental aberration. Cases with isolated hypoaldosteronism may conceivably lack functional angiotensin receptors, but no in vitro studies have yet been carried out to examine these hypotheses.

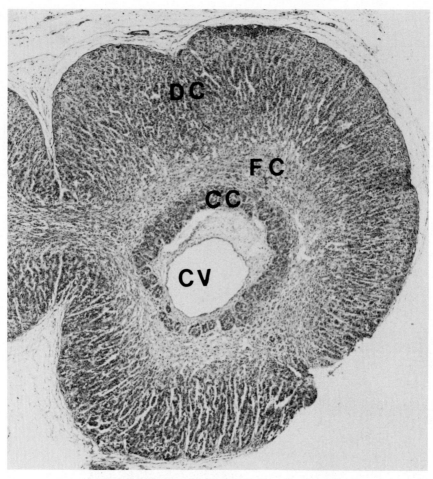

Fig. 19.2. Congenital adrenoprivic adrenocortical hypoplasia (miniature type). The section shows a miniature-type gland with a prominent definitive cortex (DC) and a small zone of fetal cortex (FC). Note the cortical cuff (CC) around the central vein (CV). (H + E × 50)

Congenital Adrenal Hyperplasia

This hereditary condition is, in several of its forms, a cause of adrenoprivic hypocorticalism. It has been described in detail and its histological features illustrated previously (p. 160).

Chapter 20
Tropoprivic Hypocorticalism

This form of hypocorticalism is characterised by low or absent plasma ACTH levels thereby resulting in adrenal atrophy and reduced steroidogenesis.

Acquired

The commonest examples of the acquired disorder usually occur as a result of exogenous steroid administration, or in association with cortisol or other glucocorticoid-producing endocrine tumours. More rarely, ACTH deficiency is acquired in later life as the result of pituitary disease.

Iatrogenic

This is the commonest example of acquired tropoprivic hypocorticalism and has both exogenous and endogenous causes. The exogenous causes result from the administration of pharmacological amounts of glucocorticoids to patients, for example those with skin disorders or endocrine-responsive neoplasms. The endogenous aetiology is typically associated with a cortisol-producing endocrine tumour, almost always of the adrenal cortex, although tumours of ectopic adrenal rests (p. 283) will have similar effects. In both instances the raised glucocorticoid levels result in decreased ACTH secretion by the pituitary and low or absent plasma ACTH levels, with the result that adrenal atrophy occurs with reduced endogenous adrenal steroidogenesis. The gross and microscopic appearances of the gland in these conditions have been described previously (p. 61).

Pituitary-Derived

In this aspect of hypocorticalism there is also a reduction in ACTH production. There are two principle causes in adults, namely Sheehan's syndrome (1939), i.e. post-partum infarction of the pituitary which results in loss of function, and Simmond's disease, or panhypopituitarism. In addition examples of the isolated deficiency of some individual pituitary hormones have recently been reported (p. 268) but this condition has only been described in relation to ACTH in a very small number of cases (Limjuco et al. 1976; Corrall et al. 1979).

If death due to Sheehan's syndrome occurs shortly after delivery this acute phenomenon will not necessarily result in any apparent morphological abnormality of the adrenal cortex. However, with extended survival and a reduction in ACTH secretion in both Sheehan's syndrome and Simmond's disease, varying degrees of adrenocortical atrophy can be anticipated, resulting in appearances which have already been described (p. 69). Adrenal atrophy will be further exaggerated by steroid replacement therapy suppressing what little, if any, ACTH secretion remains.

Congenital

Incidence

Hypoplasia of the adrenal cortex may be met with at birth secondary to a deficiency of factors concerned with adrenal growth and function.

The commonest cause of secondary adrenal hypoplasia at birth is anencephalia, which occurs in 1:450 pregnancies with females outnumbering males by 4:1 (Rimoin

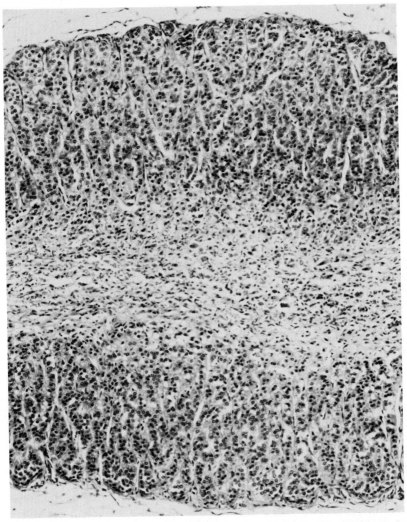

Fig. 20.1. Congenital tropoprivic hypocorticalism. The adrenal gland from an anencephalic consists of an outer definitive zone and a much reduced centrally located fetal cortex. (H + E × 150)

and Schimke 1971). In most anencephalics the neurohypophysis is usually absent or, if present, small, while the adenohypophysis is consistently present but may lack acidophils (Kerenyi 1961). The resultant hypoadrenocorticism in such monsters due to the absence of an intact hypothalamo-pituitary axis obviously presents no clinical problems, but has afforded some insight into the regulation of fetal adrenal growth (p. 99).

Other CNS defects such as microcephalia with occipital cephalomeningocoele and some cases of hydrocephalus with occipital defects have also been associated with congenital adrenal hypoplasia. Isolated cases of congenital absence or hypoplasia of the entire pituitary (Moncrieff et al. 1972) and neurohypophyseal aplasia without other CNS defects (Aimone and Campignoli 1970; Böhm et al. 1972) likewise cause adrenal hypoplasia and may be responsible for perinatal adrenal failure on very rare occasions. These infants are otherwise normal at birth, except for small external genitalia in affected males.

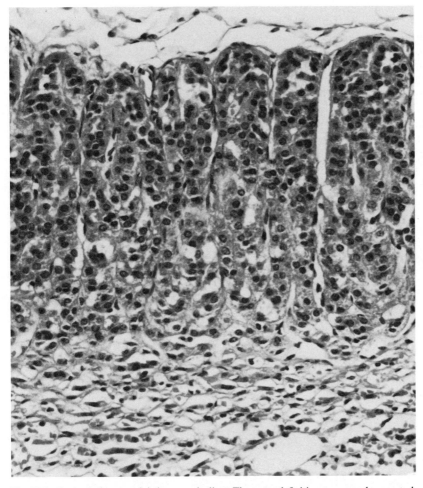

Fig. 20.2. Congenital tropoprivic hypocorticalism. The outer definitive zone may be seen to be of a normal appearance. Only a vestigial fetal zone is present in this cortex from an anencephalic. (H + E × 400)

Pathology

Gross appearance   In many cases of anencephalia the adrenals are of normal size up to about the 20th week of gestation (Benirschke 1956). In later stages, however, there is a progressive deficit in gland weight (Fig. 9.1) and at birth they typically weigh 0.5–1 g each. In some instances they may be even smaller and have occasionally escaped detection within the retroperitoneal fat, although they are probably never completely absent. There is, however, no consistent relationship between the size of the anterior pituitary and the adrenal in such monsters (Angevine 1938) as it is probably the functional drive to the former from the hypothalamus rather than the absence of pituitary tissue per se that governs the extent of hypocorticalism.

Hypoplasia of the cortex in hydrocephalics is, when present, usually less profound than in anencephalics, probably because of the later onset of neurological disturbances.

Microscopic appearance   Histologically it is apparent that the weight deficit in the adrenal glands of anencephalics is accounted for primarily by the failure of the provisional (fetal) cortex to enlarge normally (Figs. 20.1 and 20.2). Bernirschke (1956) has described what appear to be involutional changes in some premature anencephalic adrenals, and it may be that some degree of atrophy as well as absence of hyperplasia occurs during the last trimester. At term, therefore, the fetal zone of the anencephalic cortex usually occupies less than 25 % of its width (Benirschke 1956; Van Hale and Turkel 1979) compared with over 75 % in the normal fetus (Fig. 6.1). Thus, although such glands generally resemble those of the young infant after involution (the so-called 'miniature' glands originally described by Thomas and Elliot in 1911), they usually contain at least some fetal-type cells (Dhöm 1965). The definitive (adult) cortex in anencephalic adrenals may appear somewhat thicker than normal in sections; this is, however, probably due to the reduced circumference of the gland and in absolute terms there may be slight atrophy of this zone as well (Benirschke 1956). Cytomegaly is not a feature of the anencephalic adrenal cortex (Kerenyi 1961), except in very rare instances (Aterman et al. 1972).

Part D
OTHER PATHOLOGICAL CHANGES

Chapter 21
Haemorrhage and Necrosis

The first description of adrenal haemorrhage is credited to Griselius. In 1900, Arnaud was able to collect and review 79 cases. In the earlier literature, the association of adrenal haemorrhage with septicaemia, particularly that due to the meningococcus, was the most frequently recognised association. There have been many comprehensive reviews of this condition including those by Waterhouse (1911) and Friderichsen (1955) after whom this particular syndrome is now generally known. Adrenal haemorrhage is, however, also found in the absence of infective disorders of this type.

Incidence

Adrenal haemorrhage with necrosis is a relatively rare entity which may be found in neonates, children and adults. It may be unilateral or bilateral; when unilateral, the right gland is more frequently involved, particularly in neonates (Black and Williams 1973). In the adult, so-called 'spontaneous' haemorrhage is commoner in males than females and is particularly prevalent (70% of cases) after the age of 50 years with 30% of cases stated to occur in adults over the age of 70 years (Greendyke 1965). Examples of the Waterhouse-Friderichsen syndrome, on the other hand, occur particularly during the first two years of life and haemorrhage in the newborn may sometimes precede delivery (Pinck et al. 1979).

Although the incidence of adrenal haemorrhage is said to lie between 0.14% and 0.6% of all autopsies (Lawson et al. 1969), Xarli et al. (1978) found bilateral adrenal haemorrhages in 1.1% of their consecutive autopsy series of 2000 adult cases. 0.5%–1% of all neonatal autopsies are stated to show adrenal haemorrhage (Brown et al. 1962); recent evidence, however, indicates that many neonates may survive such haemorrhage (Black and Williams 1973) so that as in adults the true incidence of haemorrhage may be higher than the figures quoted above.

Signs and Symptoms

Clinical recognition is difficult, varying with the age of the patient and the cause and extent of the haemorrhage and any associated disorder. It is extremely rare to find adrenal haemorrhage affecting the healthy (Lawson et al. 1969). Generally it occurs during the acute phase of a life-threatening disorder presenting as an abdominal mass with weakness, lethargy and sometimes pain or with signs and symptoms suggesting shock and blood loss (Sober and Hirsch 1965) when it is often misdiagnosed, although surgical intervention may be curative (Nakamura et al. 1973). Nonetheless, cases associated even with extensive and bilateral haemorrhage still come to autopsy without having evoked overt clinical signs and symptoms (Sommerschild 1970). The extent of the adrenal haemorrhage and necrosis, therefore, seldom seems to bear any relationship to the clinical manifestations. The multiple afferent and efferent vascular supply to the gland must serve to protect it from total destruction.

Pathology

Several patterns of adrenal haemorrhage have been recorded (Symington 1969; DeSa and Nicholls 1972; Russell 1972; Fox 1976), and each would appear to be a different morphological manifestation of a pathological continuum.

Adrenal haemorrhage may vary from microscopic dimensions to a large palpable lesion of the order of 15 cm diameter and containing up to two litres of blood. One type takes the form of a central haematoma which pushes the adrenal medulla, or fetal cortex in the neonate, to one side, and extends and stretches the overlying cortex (Fig. 21.1). However, a peripheral viable rim of cortex usually remains. In other instances this centrally placed haemorrhage may extend into the cortex and even breach the cortical capsule to produce extracapsular foci of haemorrhage.

In other instances, the adrenal glands are swollen but tend to retain their overall shape. Such changes are due to haemorrhage and congestion in the gland occurring focally or diffusely in the cortex and/or medulla. Frequently congestion and haemorrhage are most marked throughout the zona reticularis and extend in a focal finger-like manner into the outer cortical layers (Symington 1969). In the vast majority of such cases there is associated necrosis, although the immediate subcapsular cortical cells are usually spared. These are the appearances together with polymorph infiltration classically associated with the Waterhouse-Friderichsen syndrome. In the neonate, the foci of haemorrhage and necrosis tend to involve the fetal cortex although they may also extend into the adult outer zones.

Areas of infarction may also be noted in the cortex. In the adult, they may be focal, rounded or wedge-shaped and can also involve the medulla. Such adult adrenal glands also show evidence of various responses to stress, and interestingly nodules, which become increasingly prominent in an ageing population, may also be the seat of haemorrhage and necrosis (Kaufman 1974). In the neonatal gland, such infarcts tend to be most frequent in the alae of the gland and involve the fetal cortex preferentially leaving a narrow rim of viable outer cortex (DeSa and Nicholls 1972). Such lesions by contrast with the adult, may be due to thrombi in the capsular adrenal arteries.

Adrenal vein thrombosis frequently accompanies adrenal haemorrhage and necrosis (Fox 1976). However, only if the emissary and capsular veins are also occluded by thrombi do areas of necrosis and haemorrhage develop. If there is central vein thrombosis but the emissary and capsular veins remain patent then necrosis and haemorrhage are not observed. Many previous studies have failed to recognise the primacy of adrenal vein thrombosis in the causation of necrosis and haemorrhage. This may in part be due to the thrombosis being patchy in its distribution so that many histological sections need to be examined to detect or exclude its presence. The related capsular and intra-adrenal arteries do not show any occlusion in most cases of adult haemorrhage or necrosis although they may be lined by fibrinous deposits or exhibit a so-called fibrinous vasculosis with fibrin in the medial coat (Fox 1976).

Aetiology

Experimental studies have shown that ACTH-induced adrenal changes include hyperaemia, which may predispose to adrenal haemorrhage (Grant et al. 1957a; Levin and Cluff 1965). Consequently it is not surprising to find in adults and children,

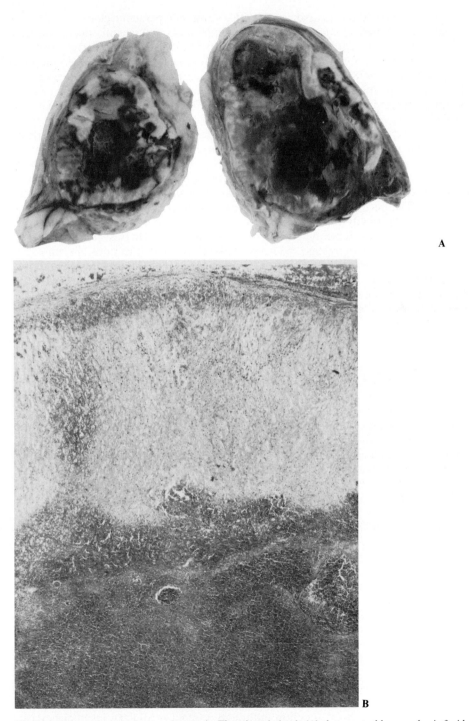

Fig. 21.1. Adrenal haemorrhage and necrosis. The adrenal glands (**A**) show central haemorrhagic foci but have retained their overall shape. The presence of haemorrhage is confirmed microscopically together with its extension out towards the capsule. There is also cortical necrosis.
Courtesy of Dr. B. Fox (London) (**A** × 2; **B** H + E × 40)

haemorrhage and necrosis in association with a stressed hyperaemic gland. Conditions associated with haemorrhage and necrosis include sepsis, septicaemia due to various organisms, burns, myocardial infarction, congestive cardiac failure, hypertensive heart disease, haemorrhage into other organs, acute tubular necrosis and hypothermia (Fox 1976; Xarli et al. 1978). Anticoagulants, often given prophylactically or therapeutically for many of the above disorders, may also precipitate adrenal haemorrhage in some instances and increase its severity in others (O'Connell and Aston 1974; Xarli et al. 1978).

In many of the above disorders, hypotensive episodes occur and may alter adrenal vascular dynamics to precipitate adrenal vein thrombosis. In neonates, fetal distress with bradycardia may be the commonest mode of precipitating haemorrhage (DeSa and Nicholls 1972) and may occur before labour in association with antepartum haemorrhage, placenta praevia, during labour or as part of the respiratory distress syndrome. The resulting hypoxia and ischaemia may induce relative stasis and congestion in the highly vascular neonatal gland with resulting thrombosis.

However, not all cases in adults or neonates may be induced in this manner. Focal or sequential adrenal haemorrhage and necrosis associated with infections, disseminated thromboembolic phenomena, pathological pregnancies including eclampsia and pre-eclampsia (Attia et al. 1970), compromised arteriovenous circulation involving the adrenal gland, trauma and haemorrhagic diatheses may arise by primary local damage to the cortical vascular endothelium (Kaufman 1974; Szabo et al. 1980).

Prognosis

In the adult and child, adrenal haemorrhage occurs mostly during the acute phase of a life-threatening disorder and appears usually to contribute indirectly, but not through functional acute adrenal insufficiency, to the patient's demise. Neonatal adrenal haemorrhage on the other hand may be an incidental phenomenon that is not, in the vast majority of cases, life-threatening. It is recognised now with increasing frequency as non-invasive diagnostic techniques are improved. Surgical intervention is therefore less important unless a massive haematoma is involved with intraperitoneal leakage (Nakamura et al. 1973) provided supportive measures are instituted (Black and Williams 1973; Smith and Middleton 1979). Steroid therapy is seldom essential but is often given.

In the neonatal gland the areas of haemorrhage undergo organisation and subsequently foci of calcification often develop. This process occurs very rapidly and may be detected within 14 days of the haemorrhage and necrosis (Black and Williams 1973). Indeed, the calcification has been detected radiographically in a one-day-old adrenal gland (Pinck et al. 1979) thereby showing that haemorrhage and necrosis may occur prior to birth.

This calcification commences peripherally and then slowly contracts into an area the size and shape of the original adrenal gland (Black and Williams 1973) which subsequently develops from the residual outer cortex. Such foci may also be the source of osseous metaplasia in the adrenal. Differential diagnosis of neonatal or childhood adrenal calcification involves primarily its discrimination from calcified adrenal tumours such as neuroblastomas (Jarvis and Seaman 1959). It has recently been convincingly shown by Hoeldtke et al. (1980) that such areas of calcification do not compromise adrenocortical function, although adrenal medullary insufficiency can develop. Indeed calcification of the adrenal gland has been followed by bilateral hyperplasia causing Cushing's syndrome in one instance (Price and Farmer 1969).

Chapter 22
Congenital Defects of Adrenal Development

Malformations and Heterotopias

Severe congenital morphological anomalies of adrenal development are rare (Warkany 1971). They occur mainly in cases of serious vertebral malformations and deformities of the lower half of the body. Thus, midline fusions giving a single 'butterfly' or 'horseshoe' gland above the aorta occur in some embryos and neonates with central nervous system defects such as spina bifida or meningomyelocoele (Koenig 1972; Bell 1979). Histology of these glands is essentially normal, except where CNS defects include anencephalia, when the gland is hypoplastic (p. 272).

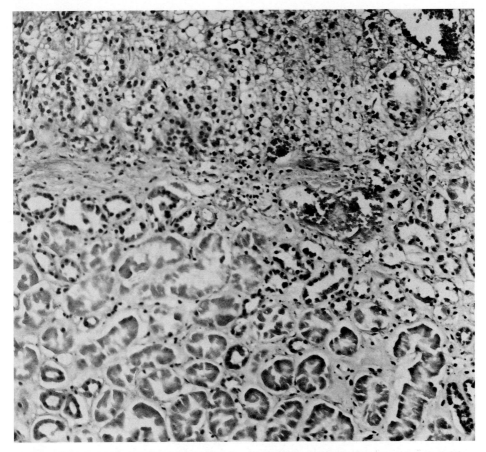

Fig. 22.1. Adrenorenal fusion. The (*upper*) adrenal cortex and (*lower*) kidney are separated on the left by a capsule but on the right show contiguity of the parenchymal cells. (H + E × 120)

Also rarely reported, but probably more frequent, are the cases of innocuous adrenorenal and adrenohepatic unions. Reported frequencies range from 0.4% for bilateral union to 3% of unselected autopsies with a unilateral defect (Dolan and Janowski 1968). In cases of fusion there is complete or partial absence of an intervening capsule with contiguity of parenchymal cells (Fig. 22.1). In adrenorenal or adrenohepatic adhesion the organs share a common capsule without intermingling of parenchymal elements. In both cases the defect probably stems from failure of the periadrenal capsular mesenchyme to complete the individuation of the gland at the appropriate time in early embryogenesis (p. 13) (Honoré and O'Hara 1976). One rare clinical problem that may be caused by true adrenal heterotopia is the inadvertent removal of a gland during, for example, nephrectomy, or hepatic lobectomy. Although occasional tumours have been noted (e.g. Wilkins and Ravitch 1952) such heterotopic glands are not, however, unduly prone to neoplasia.

Unilateral aplasia of the adrenal gland occurs in approximately 1 in 10 000 individuals (Ashley and Mostofi 1960). Renal agenesis, however, is not commonly associated with adrenal aplasia. Thus, only 21/374 cases of renal agenesis and dysgenesis reviewed by Ashley and Mostofi (1960) showed adrenal abnormalities.

Adrenal Rests and Accessory Adrenal Glands

Incidence and Distribution

The presence of accessory adrenal glands or rests of adrenocortical tissue outside the glands proper is common. They cannot, therefore be considered strictly pathological. They do, however, have some interesting pathological consequences as a potential source of hyperplastic and neoplastic lesions.

In contrast to true heteropias, adrenocortical rests and accessory glands are, by definition, always accompanied by an orthotopic adrenal. Such aberrant adrenal tissue probably originates at the time that the adrenal primordium is invaded and disrupted by the nerve tracts that pave the way for the neural crest cells ultimately destined to form the medulla (p. 13). This takes place prior to the encapsulation of the gland. Distribution of such accessory elements may therefore be widespread. Most have been found in immediately adjacent or pelvic structures, such as the coeliac plexus, the broad ligament (as originally described by Marchand in 1883) and other paraovarian sites, spermatic and ovarian vessels, the inferior pole of the kidney, uterus and within the scrotum or in hernial sacs. Other abdominal viscera may be less common sites of accessory cortical tissue, including the pancreas, transverse colon, gallbladder, liver and mesentery. In very rare cases supradiaphragmatic organs including the lung, spinal nerves and even the brain may contain displaced adrenal elements. The larger rests and those nearest the orthotopic gland are the most likely to contain medulla as well as cortex with normal patterns of cortical zonation in the larger rests (Falls 1955). More distant foci usually consist only of cortical tissue.

It has long been accepted that adrenocortical rests are common in infants, especially in the vicinity of the gonads (<50% of cases). Their incidence in adults has, however, been subject to widely ranging estimates. The most careful studies indicate that they are probably as frequent as in infants, although their bulk may be reduced. Thus, systematic examination of just two potential sites, the coeliac plexus (Graham 1953) and the broad ligament (Falls 1955) gave histologically verified frequencies of 32% and 23% of individuals respectively, with most nodules of accessory tissue being 1–3 mm diameter.

Two potential sites of adrenal rest tissue, the ovary and the testis are of particular pathophysiological significance, because tumours arising from them may be histologically impossible to distinguish from those originating from orthotopic steroidogenic cells of the gonads. The proximity of the developing adrenal and gonadal primordia (p. 11) lends itself to a potential intermingling of the two cell types. Nevertheless, although accessory cortical tissue can be found along the track of the caudal displacement of the gonads during development, the presence of recognisable cortical-type cells within the substance of the ovary and the testis has, surprisingly, seldom been reported. Only the report of Symonds and Driscoll (1973) has provided evidence of an adrenal rest *within* the ovary. No such rests have been convincingly identified within the testis although Mikuz et al. (1975) have described, within a cryptorchid testis, cells with some of the ultrastructural characteristics of adrenocortical cells, but which also contained Reinke crystalloids. Dahl and Bahn (1962) contend that adrenal rests are to be found only in paratesticular locations such as the spermatic vessel, the epididymis and the tunica albuginea. However, histological and ultrastructural criteria, may simply fail to discriminate between cortical and Leydig cells in this context (Newell et al. 1977).

Hyperplasia and Tumours of Accessory Adrenocortical Tissue

Incidence and distribution   Some of the strongest evidence for the presence of adrenal-type cells (or cells capable of differentiating into adrenal-like cells) in the vicinity of the gonads, and possibly within their substance, comes from the functional properties of some tumours and hyperplastic lesions found in paragonadal sites. All cortical rest tissues are, however, sites of potential neoplastic and hyperplastic lesions. Although both benign and maligant cortical neoplasms have been reported at extra-adrenal and extragonadal locations (Ney et al. 1966; Leger et al. 1975), ectopia per se does not appear to markedly predispose these cells to neoplastic conversion, as the numbers reported have been very small. In so far as can be ascertained from their limited incidence, the histological and functional properties of these ectopic tumours resemble those of corresponding tumours arising from orthotopic adrenal tissue. Some care should, however, be taken before any extra-adrenal and extragonadal tumour composed of lipid-rich vacuolated cells (spongiocytes) is accepted as an adrenal-rest tumour (thus see Hamperl 1970). Functional studies must be considered mandatory before this diagnosis can be accepted, and few, if any, of the older reports meet these stringent criteria.

Testicular 'tumours' in congenital adrenal hyperplasia and Nelson's syndrome   The so-called testicular 'tumours' that occur in some patients in whom ACTH levels are chronically elevated belong to an essentially different category. There is no evidence, in the vast majority of cases, that these lesions are autonomous neoplasms. Over 30 such cases have now been documented in detail (Burke et al. 1973); most take the form of multiple hilar nodules. Many have been observed in patients with congenital adrenal hyperplasia (CAH) due to enzymatic defects in glucocorticoid biosynthesis (p. 155). In fact, virtually all male CAH cases show microscopic paratesticular nodules (Shanklin et al. 1963) which are usually bilateral, although a palpable 'tumour' may appear unilaterally in some cases (Newell et al. 1977). Functional studies have shown that the testicular lesions possess all the attributes of the abnormal adrenal cortex in these cases (Kirkland et al. 1977). Thus, although intrinsically deficient in glucocorticoid secretion, some can still form steroids such as cortisol in reduced amounts (Fore et al. 1972; Radfar et al. 1977). Histologically they are composed of compact-type cells typical of the hyperplastic adrenals, and devoid of testicular interstitial cell features such as crystalloids of Reinke.

Similar nodules have been noted in the testis in cases of Nelson's syndrome (Krieger et al. 1978) and have been stated to be responsible for the recurrence of Cushing's syndrome after adrenalectomy (Hamwi et al. 1963). In these cases considerable amounts of cortisol may be produced as there are no intrinsic defects of adrenal biosynthesis. Again compact-type cells with prominent lipofuscin composed the testicular nodules.

Ovarian 'tumours' in congenital adrenal hyperplasia and Nelson's syndrome
Corresponding lesions to those described above in the testis have recently been reported in association with the ovary. Thus, Völpel (1971) noted microscopic hilar cell nodules in a newborn girl with congenital adrenal hyperplasia, and Mötlik and Starka (1973) have described an ovarian 'tumour' composed of lipfuscin-rich compact-type cells found in a 9-year-old girl some time after removal of hyperplastic adrenal glands, and in whom a diagnosis of adrenogenital syndrome had been reported; although the lesion caused recurrent virilisation, in vitro studies clearly demonstrated that it could also form cortisol and corticosterone in limited amounts. Baranetsky et al. (1979) reported an interesting case of a woman with Nelson's syndrome developing after adrenalectomy for Cushing's syndrome, who then became virilised. At surgery paraovarian nodules composed of dark compact-type cells were detected; these cells converted steroid precursors to testosterone in vitro. Glucocorticoids were not detected in this case. Nevertheless, the androgen output in vivo was clearly stimulated by ACTH indicating some adrenal-like behaviour by these cells. Whether their origin was adrenal rest cells or metaplasia of some true ovarian component under prolonged ACTH stimulation cannot unfortunately be determined.

Autonomous primary neoplasms of adrenal type in the gonads   Well authenticated cases of true autonomous primary neoplasms of adrenal-type cells arising in the gonads are extremely rare, and adequate functional characterisation has seldom been performed in these cases. Many benign and malignant so-called adrenal-rest (lipoid cell) tumours of the ovary, associated with masculinisation, show no real functional evidence of specific adrenal attributes either in the form of glucocorticoid synthesis or ACTH responsiveness (Koss et al. 1969; Sobrihno and Kase 1970; Parker et al. 1974). Most may in fact arise from true ovarian stromal cells (Lipsett et al. 1970).

Other recent candidates have included a malignant ovarian tumour causing primary aldosteronism (Todesco et al. 1975). This tumour contained cells similar in appearance to those with relatively lipid-poor cytoplasm, a high nuclear:cytoplasmic ratio and dense chromatin also found in malignant aldosteronomas arising in the adrenal (p. 218). Although such histological appearances can be deceptive, this ovarian tumour did, however, appear to form aldosterone in vitro (see also Ehrlich et al. 1963). Another reported case comprised a purportedly malignant scrotal tumour associated with Cushing's syndrome and what were described as retroperitoneal secondaries (Morimoto et al. 1971). Other indisputable glucocorticoid-producing primary tumours arising in the testis have been described (Besch et al. 1963) and must be deemed evidence of adrenal cell rests therein.

Ectopic Tissues Within the Adrenal Cortex

Gonadal cells

As the corollary of ectopic adrenocortical tissue located in distant organs, the possibility of gonadal cells, or cells capable of differentiating into gonadal cells, being incorporated within the adrenal gland must be considered, especially as a potential source of neoplasms with apparently anomalous functional attributes.

Wong and Warner (1971) and Fidler (1977) have described so-called 'ovarian thecal metaplasia' within the adrenals of middle-aged women. Such foci of apparent ectopic ovarian stromal elements are generally attached to the adrenal capsule. They consist of interlacing bundles or whorls of basophilic spindle cells with prominent reticulin fibres simulating the ovarian theca. They have been found by serial sectioning in the adrenals of approximately 4% of 39–65-year-old females (Fidler 1977) but were not visible macroscopically; in other respects the adrenals were normal. We have seen similar appearances in single sections of only one gland in over 200 similar cases examined (Fig. 22.2).

The theca-granulosa tumour described by Orselli and Bassler (1973) in the adrenal gland of a postmenopausal woman may have arisen from such elements. Likewise, the HCG-responsive virilising tumours arising in the adrenals of some older women (p. 171) may also stem from cells with gonadal rather than adrenal properties, and it may be that the post-menopausal hormonal milieu facilitates metaplasia and ectopic neoplasia of this type.

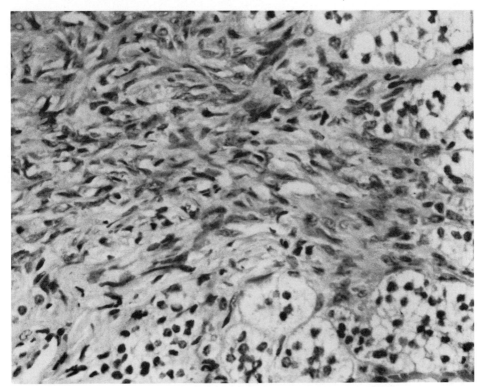

Fig. 22.2. Ovarian thecal metaplasia. A focus of so called 'ectopic ovarian stromal elements' is noted in the substance of the cortex from a 60-year-old woman, but close to the capsule. (H + E × 280)

There is less evidence of corresponding gonadal-type cells in male adrenal glands, perhaps because of the difficulty in distinguishing histologically between adrenocortical and testicular steroidogenic cells. An old report (Allen and Vespignani 1938) did note an active seminiferous tubule embedded in the capsule of an otherwise normal adrenal gland, but this remains a unique observation. Scully and Cohen (1961) have described cells morphologically identical to testicular hilar cells within a medullary ganglioneuroma, distinguished by their contents of eosinophilic paracrystalline Reinke crystalloids. This case could be interpreted as indicating the presence of some cells with, or capable of acquiring, testicular properties in at least some adrenal glands. This proposition has received recent support from the observations of Horvath et al. (1980) who noted Leydig-type cells with Reinke crystalloids associated with non-myelinated sympathetic nerve fibres in both the cortex and medulla of a hyperplastic gland removed from a premenopausal female patient with the 'ectopic ACTH' syndrome.

Other Tissues

There have been few reports of other tissues within the cortex, in contrast to the wide distribution of accessory cortical elements outwith the gland. Heterotopic renal tissue has been noted within an otherwise normal gland (Milliser et al. 1969) an evidently very rare association without apparent pathophysiological significance.

Congenital Adrenocortical Cytomegaly

Adrenal cytomegaly is characterised by the presence within the cortex of large ($>150\ \mu$m) eosinophilic cells with giant ($>40\ \mu$m) nuclei with vacuoles, eosinophilic inclusion bodies and a dense, hyperchromatic chromatin network (Figs. 22.3, 22.4). The nuclei of normal cortical cells measure 7–8 μm diameter and the presence of significantly enlarged nuclei of this type may be considered the definitive criterion of adrenal cytomegaly, in the absence of neoplastic, inflammatory or other degenerative changes. Other characteristics include deformed, often eccentrically located nuclei surrounded by coarse cytoplasmic granules, and occasional cytoplasmic vacuolation. At the electron-microscopical level, the cytomegalic elements are unremarkable and show large quantities of smooth endoplasmic reticulum, characteristic of normal fetal zone adrenocortical cells (Borit and Kosek 1969; Oppenheimer 1970).

'Idiopathic' Congenital Cytomegaly

Cells with these features were first described in the first trimester fetal adrenal cortex by Kampmeier (1927). They have also been detected in 3%–5% of the stillborn and perinatal mortalities, (Craig and Landing 1951; Bech 1971; Aterman et al. 1972). Their incidence declines in postnatal adrenals as the gland involutes; they are rarely seen in adult glands.

Although adrenocortical cytomegaly has been observed in newborns dying from a variety of causes, it is reportedly common in cases of Rh-incompatability (Dhöm 1965; Aterman et al. 1972), situations which presumably impose considerable stress on the fetus. Cytomegaly is not normally found in other tissues in these cases. Many undoubtedly stressed fetal adrenals do not, however, show cytomegalic change.

In the later fetal and perinatal adrenals, cytomegalic cells are found only in the fetal

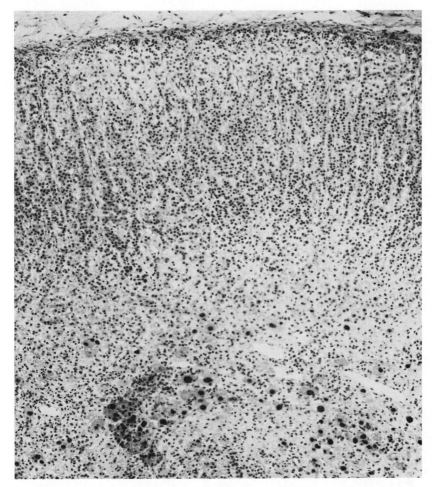

Fig. 22.3. Congenital adrenal cytomegaly. Numerous enlarged hyperchromatic cells are present focally in the fetal cortex of this neonatal adrenal gland. (H + E × 100)

zone and they are often confined to the inner-third of the gland. They may be diffusely distributed with a gradual transition to normal cells (Fig. 22.4) or they may occur in sharply demarcated foci which may take the form of wedge-shaped segments or nodules compressing the surrounding normal cells (Fig. 22.3).

Contrary to some suggestions (e.g. Craig and Landing 1951), there is no good evidence that cytomegaly is a precursor of childhood adrenal tumours in the vast majority of cases, and such cells certainly do not represent carcinoma 'in situ'.

The condition should not be confused with 'cytomegalic inclusion disease' (generalised salivary gland virus infection). This condition is most frequently observed in infants but it does occasionally result in a form of cytomegaly in adult adrenal glands (Delvaux 1957; Lebreuil et al. 1971). Cytologically the virally infected cells show basophilic (rather than eosinophilic) cytoplasm and the large intranuclear inclusion bodies are amphophilic and surrounded by a clear halo, an appearance quite distinct from the inclusion bodies in idiopathic adrenal cytomegaly, and illustrated by Frenkel (1960). Widely distributed necrotic foci are a feature of cytomegalic inclusion disease, rimmed by the cytomegalic elements.

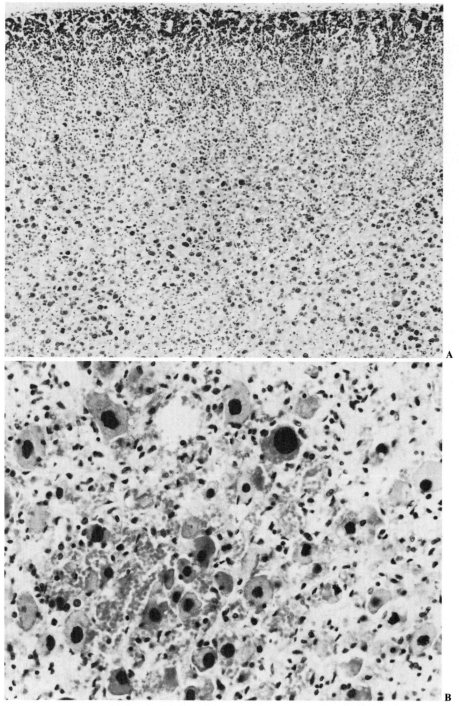

Fig. 22.4. Congenital adrenal cytomegaly. The cytomegalíc cells were distributed diffusely throughout the fetal zone of this second trimester adrenal gland obtained from an otherwise normal abortus (**A**). The cells are enlarged, pleomorphic in shape and size and have hyperchromatic bizarre enlarged nuclei (**B**). (H + E **A** ×80; **B** ×300)

In the fetal and neonatal cases of cytomegaly referred to above no viruses have been found in the cells (Oppenheimer 1970) and the nuclear inclusion bodies are simply cytoplasmic invaginations (Borit and Kosek 1969). It seems likely that the unusual appearance of the cells is due to endomitosis and polyploidy (Aterman et al. 1972). The possible roles of pituitary hormones, secreted adrenal steroids, or toxic factors in this process remain obscure. Polyploidy is not, incidentally, a significant feature of the adult human adrenal cortex (Gilbert and Pfitzer 1977).

Cytomegaly in the Beckwith-Weidemann Syndrome

The Beckwith-Weidemann or exomphalos:macroglossia:gigantism (EMG) syndrome is a congenital condition first reported in 1963 (Beckwith 1963) and found in approximately 1:14000 births (Thorburn et al. 1970). It presents as gigantism with the other eponymous defects and with hypoglycaemia, and is probably inherited as an autosomal dominant condition with incomplete penetrance (Kosseff et al. 1972). One feature of the syndrome is fetal visceromegaly, a feature it shares with congenital hemihypertrophy (p. 116). The adrenal glands in the Beckwith-Weidemann syndrome may be moderately enlarged ($>50\%$) in some cases although they are often of apparently normal weight at autopsy (Roe et al. 1973). Diffuse adrenocortical cytomegaly cytologically identical to that seen in a small number of otherwise normal glands, and confined to the fetal zone is a consistent feature of all these infants autopsied in the neonatal period (Cohen 1971). Cystic change may also be seen. In infants who survive longer, cytomegaly may be obscured by the normal involution of the gland (Reddy et al. 1972).

Although the ubiquity of cytomegalic changes in this condition also precludes their classification as a form of carcinoma in situ, adrenocortical carcinomas have been associated with the Beckwith-Weidemann syndrome, as have other intra-abdominal malignancies. The reported cases indicate that up to 10% of surviving infants may develop lesions of this type.

Chapter 23
Myelolipoma and Related Changes

Incidence and Symptoms

The term myelolipoma was first coined by Oberling (1929) to denote a rare benign lesion of the adrenal gland which consists of admixtures of adipose, bone marrow and lymphocyte-like elements, whose first description is usually credited to Gierke in 1905. Nearly 200 examples of this rare entity have now been described in the world literature, and the review and analysis by Plaut (1958) is by far the most comprehensive. There does not appear to be either sex or side predilection and there is no correlation with anaemia in the adult, unlike extra-adrenal myelolipomas. Although normal fatty marrow will aromatise androgens to oestrogens (Frisch et al. 1980), these lesions are not associated with detectable aberrations of steroidogenesis or haematopoeisis in the vast majority of cases and hence present as 'non-functioning' tumours. Most are asymptomatic and are detected as incidental autopsy findings. However, some of the larger lesions may cause pain, haematuria or present as abdominal masses. With recent advances in radiological technology and sonography (Gee et al. 1975; Behan et al. 1977) an increasing number have been detected during life and removed successfully at operation (Newman and Silen 1968; Whittaker 1968; Olsson et al. 1973; Desai et al. 1979) the first successful example being recorded by Dyckman and Freedman (1957). According to Desai et al. (1979), an adrenal myelolipoma should be suspected when a biochemically non-functioning radiolucent, solid adrenal mass without neovascularity on angiography is detected.

Almost all myelolipomas are located in relation to one or other adrenal gland; most are single and generally they are unilateral although the smaller lesions may be multiple. They have also been reported to occur in accessory adrenal tissues (Cerny 1970; Murayama et al. 1979) and have recently been reported bilaterally at the site of total and subtotal adrenalectomies for Cushing's disease (Bennett et al. 1980), when the large myelolipomas contained sufficient functioning cortical tissue for Cushing's syndrome to recur, a report thus far unique within the literature.

The recorded frequency of myelolipomas has varied greatly from one autopsy series to the next. Estimates of between 0.08 % and 0.2 % have been made (McDonnell 1956; Olsson et al. 1973). The latter figure is almost certainly too high. However, they occur more frequently after the fifth decade and estimates of 0.01 % have been made in one autopsy series of subjects between the ages of 36 and 65 years with an estimated incidence of 0.002 % for all age groups (Plaut 1958). Although their frequency increases with age examples have been described from the ages of 17 years onwards (Plaut 1958). They are not, however, found in children. Many patients with large myelolipomas are obese and some degree of hypertension may be present (Olsson et al. 1973; Desai et al. 1979).

Pathology

Gross appearance   The majority of myelolipomas are of microscopic dimensions to
0.5 to 2.0 cm in diameter, and are incidental autopsy findings detected on sectioning
the adrenal gland (Symington 1969; Dean 1971). However, larger lesions are not
uncommon and sizes of up to 25–34 cm diameter and >1 kg weight have been
recorded in the literature (Dyckman and Freedman 1957; Parsons and Thompson
1959; Lopez et al. 1967; Tulcinsky et al. 1970; Desai et al. 1979). The largest lesions
reported to date weighed 1590 g (Bennett et al. 1980) and 5900 g (Boudreaux et al.
1979) respectively.

The adrenal distrubution of many myelolipomas mirrors that of the so-called 'non-
functioning' nodules being located intraglandularly and found only on sectioning the
gland, at one pole or in a closely applied extracapsular position. When microscopic
they tend to occur within the zona fasciculata (Snearly and Ram 1978). Foci of
necrosis, haemorrhage and calcification may be present, especially in association with
larger lesions and ectopic bone may also occur. Their shape is variable but most have
irregularly rounded contours. Often the smaller lesions are visibly multiple and the less
regular shapes of some larger lesions may indicate multicentric origin. Their cut
surface varies from greyish-red to yellow/white depending upon the relative amounts
of myeloid and adipose tissue. Those lesions which are intracapsular may compress the
related gland, although there is sometimes no sharp macroscopic dividing line
separating them from the related tissues.

Myelolipomas situated within the adrenal gland are unencapsulated; those in
apparent extra-capsular positions, however, have a peripheral fibrous capsule derived
from that of the adrenal gland. Little, if any, compression of the related adrenal cells is
noted. Some authors have stated that the medulla is absent in cases of myelolipoma.
This is not our experience and may well reflect solely the occurrence of the lesion in the
alae or tail of the gland where medullary elements are not normally present.

Microscopic appearance   Microscopically, myelolipomas consist of admixtures of
adipose, bone marrow-type elements and lymphocyte-like cells (Fig. 23.1). Their
proportions vary from lesion to lesion and even within one lesion.

In paraffin sections, the adipose cells, which tend to predominate in most lesions,
especially in the central areas, present as large vacuolated cells occurring singly or
forming bands, networks and islands. They possess centrally placed irregularly shaped
single nuclei. Their characteristic punched-out appearance referred to as 'lochkern'
(nucleus with a hole) is due to a lipid inclusion which indents the nucleus and is
continuous with the remainder of the adipose cytoplasm (Plaut 1958). Such fat cells do
not resemble the clear lipid-laden cells of the zona fasciculata or those of congenital
lipoid hyperplasia (Fig. 13.11).

The cellular foci between the fat cells tend to be located towards the periphery of the
lesion and consist most often of collections of lymphocyte-like cells. In addition
erythroblasts, cells of the myeloid series with granular Giemsa-positive cytoplasm and
occasional megakaryocytes may be present.

The above description has referred to a distinct clearly definable tumour-like entity.
Similar changes in part or in whole may, however, be detected as minute microscopic
foci in many adrenal glands (Symington 1969). The accumulation of small groups or
islands of adipose cells is referred to as *fatty metaplasia* (Fig. 7.2) while that of
lymphocyte and myeloid-type cells is called *myeloid metaplasia*. While they may occur
separately, they are more commonly found together and when multiple foci are noted
may be referred to as *myelolipomatosis*. Such minute foci occur most frequently
between the columns of zona fasciculata cells, in the zona reticularis, medulla and in

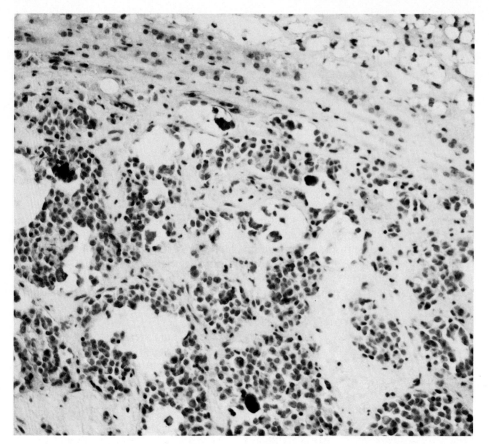

Fig. 23.1. Myelolipoma of the adrenal. A 30-cm lesion was found at autopsy of a 60-year-old male subject with metastatic prostatic carcinoma. The lesion contained numerous adipose cells, lymphocytes and marrow elements with evidence of active haemopoeisis. (H + E × 120)

cortical nodules. Their frequency rises, as does that of myelolipomas, with increasing age. The effects of stress or raised plasma ACTH levels as in bilateral hyperplasia in Cushing's syndrome are also associated with frequent myelolipomatosis (Fig. 12.6). This change is, however, rare in children and was never detected in a series of adrenal glands from healthy younger persons who died suddenly (e.g. road traffic accidents) (Plaut 1958). Conversely, in severely stressed (burned) subjects these changes were frequent (Delarue and Monsaingeon 1950).

Aetiology

The adrenal gland probably contains reticulum or mesenchymal stem cells in association with the vasculature and stromal network. These are probably the progenitors of myelolipomatosis. Metaplasia of cortical parenchymal cells seems most unlikely as no transitions between the two cell types have been noted. It would appear that stress and raised ACTH levels play a part in the evolution of these changes. In experimental systems, Selye and Stone (1950) with injection of necrotic tumour extracts and with pituitary extracts, testosterone and thyroxine in the rat induced similar changes. Some workers (e.g. Olsson et al. 1973) consider that necrosis, rather than hormonal overstimulation, is the most probable cause. A combination of the two seems to us the most likely factor. No convincing evidence for or against the role of steroids in this process has yet been adduced. However, what induces such foci of myelolipomatosis to undergo further local growth intensification and form a frank, myelolipoma, if indeed this is the progression that occurs, remains unknown. Despite the reports of myelolipomas having been found in the absence of adrenocortical nodules a number of examples have been recorded in association with 'adenomas' (in reality macronodules) (Murayama et al. 1979). Our own experience would tend to draw attention to their similar distribution with limited occurrence in young persons, and association with hypertension and obesity. Moreover, myelolipomatous changes are undoubtedly frequent within nodules themselves, especially those of nodular hyperplasia in Cushing's syndrome. It may well be that most myelolipomas commence in and eventually replace the adrenal tissue of such nodules and thus represent one end stage in their life history. As such they may be regarded as part of the ageing process as it affects the adrenal glands.

Chapter 24
Cysts

Incidence and Symptoms

Cysts of the adrenal gland are rare. To date about 250 individual examples have been reported and they usually pose greater problems to the radiologist and urologist than pathologist. Many are incidental findings. They occur in approximately 1 in 1500 unselected autopsies (0.06 %) (Wahl 1951) with an equal frequency in the right and left glands. Cysts are bilateral in 10 %–15 % of cases and occur in women twice as often as men with a peak incidence between the third and fifth decades (Kearny and Mahony 1977) with fewer than 5 % occurring in children (Van der Water and Fonkalsrud 1966).

Large non-neoplastic adrenal cysts may cause symptoms resulting from displacement of other viscera but most are asymptomatic. In at least one reported case a cyst has simulated metastatic disease with pressure resulting in local osseous resorption (Levin et al. 1974). They are not associated with adrenal insufficiency except in very rare cases in the newborn. The fluid contents of pseudocysts (vide infra) usually contain high concentrations of cholesterol, often in crystalline form which imparts a characteristic turbid appearance to the liquid. Its steroid content is more or less the same as that of the normal cortical tissue, with levels intermediate between tissue and plasma concentrations (Faarvang et al. 1969; Jacobi et al. 1978). Although the vast majority of adrenal cysts occur without endocrine symptoms, cases have been reported associated with hypertension which was cured by its removal (e.g. Lynn 1965; Fontaine et al. 1969; Gigax et al. 1972; Uretsky et al. 1978). Compression of the renal vein is probably the causative factor. However, phaeochromocytomas and functioning adrenal carcinomas should always be excluded by appropriate biochemical studies prior to surgery.

Pathology

Gross appearance Adrenal cysts exhibit a wide size range from microscopic to giant forms containing several litres of fluid. So-called microcysts (0.1–1 mm diameter) occur frequently in the definitive cortex of older fetuses (Gruenwald 1946), perinates and infants (Oppenheimer 1969; Rodin et al. 1976). Their precise aetiology is unknown; both infection and perinatal stress have been tentatively implicated. Studies with twins indicate that microcystic change in the newborn is probably reversible (Damjanov and Janculjak 1974), and it seems doubtful if a true pathological process is involved. In our experience they seem common in abortuses.

Microscopic appearance Various classifications of the larger adrenal cysts occurring mainly in adults have been proposed, based on their histological features. Aetiologically, three basic types can be recognised. Least frequent (<10 % in non-tropical zones), are the parasitic (usually echinococcal) cysts. Somewhat less than half of the remainder are lined by recognisable endothelial cells. Some of these cysts are

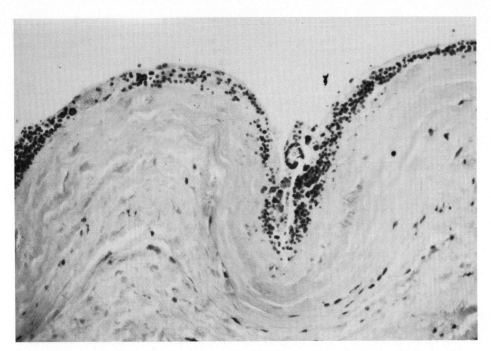

Fig. 24.1. Adrenal cyst. The thick-walled connective tissue capsule had no apparent endothelial lining in this 10-cm diameter 'pseudo-cyst' which was an incidental autopsy finding. The luminal aspect shows numerous small areas of calcification. (H + E × 120)

small and they may be multilocular. It has been proposed (Abeshouse et al. 1959) that they are of lymphangiomatous, or more rarely, angiomatous origin, arising respectively from maldevelopment of lymphatics associated with the capsule and blood vessels and parenchymal capillary sinusoids. Although cysts lined with what have been described as epithelial cells have been illustrated (Ghandur-Mnaymneh et al. 1979) it is difficult to envisage from which component of the normal gland these cells could be derived.

The majority (~ 60 %) of adrenal cysts are not lined by recognisable endothelial (or epithelial) cells. These have probably originated from haemorrhage into otherwise normal glands with subsequent liquefaction, resorption of necrotic elements and gradual enlargement of the fluid contents; they are the so-called parenchymal cysts or 'pseudocysts'. Compressed cortical cells line the cavity of some of these lesions or more commonly form small islands within the fibrous capsule. Pigment-laden macrophages may also be found on the inner surface of the fibrous tissue that usually lines the cystic cavity (Fig. 24.1). Multiple calcified foci are common in the capsule of these larger cysts and form an important radiological feature (peripheral curvilinear calcification) in differential diagnosis, with calcification in various neoplasms, familial xanthomatoses (Wolman's disease), tuberculosis etc. appearing, with rare exceptions (Twersky and Levin 1975), as amorphous masses within the gland or lesion.

Cystic changes in cortical tumours, not infrequent in the larger carcinomas, are sometimes also included in the pseudocyst category.

Chapter 25
Miscellaneous Changes

Erythroblastosis Fetalis

Mention has already been made of the tendency of fetal adrenal cytomegaly to be apparently associated with Rh-incompatibility of the newborn (p. 286) with perhaps 10% of such cases showing this feature (Burne and Langley 1956). Other changes found with this condition include intra-adrenal haemopoeitic foci in about half the cases with their frequency increasing with the severity of the anaemia (Burne and Langley 1956). Newborn and stillborn adrenal weights are slightly ($\sim 20\%$) increased in this disease, possibly as a consequence of oedema, although the cortical cells themselves are somewhat hypertrophied with an increased cytoplasmic volume (Naeye 1967). The most striking adrenal change in erythroblastosis fetalis is, however, a marked cytoplasmic vacuolation in the fetal zone. This is reportedly seen in $>80\%$ of such glands and involves the entire fetal zone in nearly half the cases studied (Bartman and Driscoll 1969). Similar vacuolation, which appears to be due in part at least to lipid accumulation, is also seen in α-thalassaemia (Pearson et al. 1965) a non-immunological haemolytic anaemia. Care should be taken not to confuse this condition with congenital lipoid hyperplasia due to enzymatic defects (p. 167) where the secretion of steroid hormones by the gland is virtually abolished.

Haemochromatosis

In haemochromatosis it is common to find deposits of iron pigment in cells of the zona glomerulosa and the outer zona fasciculata where it abuts onto the capsule (Fig. 25.1). Although a tendency to hyperpigmentation and hypotension has been noted in patients with haemochromatosis (see Milder et al. 1980 for review) this is almost certainly not due to any form of adrenal insufficiency (Charbonnel et al. 1980) but probably stems from extra-adrenal changes associated with this disease.

Syphilis

Syphilitic lesions of the adrenal gland (gummata) are now encountered rarely. Even in the era in which they were commoner almost no proved case of adrenocortical insufficency due to this disorder was noted (Guttman 1930).

Malacoplakia

Malacoplakia is an inflammatory process typified by the accumulation of histiocytes containing laminated calcospherites and PAS-positive granules (Michaelis-Gutmann bodies). It occurs most frequently in the urinary tract and bladder, other pelvic organs

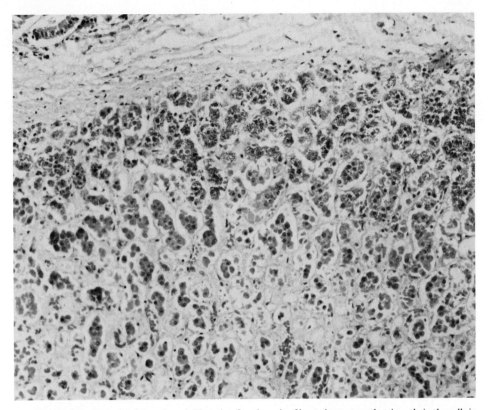

Fig. 25.1. Haemosiderosis of the adrenal. There is a fine deposit of iron pigment predominantly in the cells in the subcapsular zone of the gland but also extending inwards in a series of tongue-like protrusions. (H + E × 120)

and the testis. One case in a 6-week-old infant has been recorded (Sinclair-Smith et al. 1975) where most of the adrenal gland was replaced by an orange-yellow mass consisting of macrophages, surrounded by a thin rim of yellow cortical tissue. There was no evidence of adrenal insufficiency. A second case has recently been reported in an adult, where the lesion (4 × 5 × 3 cm) mimicked a neoplasm (Benjamin and Fox 1981).

Wolman's Disease

This form of hereditary xanthomatosis usually causes death in early infancy (Wolman et al. 1961). The adrenal glands may be enlarged with a broadened bright yellow cortex consisting of clear cells with cholesterol clefts. Notably there is necrosis, amorphous or punctate calcification and fibrosis of the inner cortex, a feature apparently pathognomonic of this disorder and distinguishing it from classical Niemann-Pick disease. No cases of hypoadrenocorticism have been noted in this condition, however (Marshall et al. 1969); it is due to acid esterase deficiency and abnormal accumulation of cholesterol and triglycerides (Raafat et al. 1973).

Post-irradiation Fibrosis

The human adrenal cortex is relatively radioresistant compared with many other endocrine glands. Nevertheless, high-dose X-irradiation (>5000 roentgens) to the abdominal, pelvic or lumbar region has been reported to cause hyaline fibrosis of the zona reticularis (Sommers and Carter 1975). This effect is probably caused by damage to the more sensitive capillary plexus. The adrenocortical cells remain essentially undamaged and no adrenal insufficiency seems to ensue.

Appendix A
Plasma Steroids

Typical normal mean plasma levels of adrenocortical steroids and steroids to which the adrenal cortex makes a significant contribution. Values given are for adult males.[1]

Steroid	μg(ng)/100 ml[2]	nmol/(pmol)/litre
Dehydroepiandrosterone sulphate	150 μg	3500 nmol
Cortisol (F) (total)	14 μg	400 nmol
Cortisol (unbound)	1.5 μg	43 nmol
Cortisone (E)	1.6 μg	45 nmol
Dehydroepiandrosterone (DHA)	400 ng	14 nmol
Corticosterone (B)	400 ng	11 nmol
11-Deoxycortisol (S)	200 ng	6 nmol
11β-Hydroxyandrostenedione	200 ng	7 nmol
Androstenedione	120 ng	4 nmol
17-Hydroxyprogesterone	100 ng	3 nmol
Δ^5-Androstenediol	100 ng	3.5 nmol
Δ^5-Pregnenolone	75 ng	2 nmol
16α-Hydroxyprogesterone	70 ng	2 nmol
17-Hydroxypregnenolone	70 ng	2 nmol
16β-Hydroxy DHA	30 ng	1 nmol
Progesterone	20 ng	570 pmol
18-Hydroxycorticosterone	17 ng	480 pmol
Aldosterone (upright)	15 ng	430 pmol
(recumbent)	8 ng	230 pmol
18-Hydroxydeoxycorticosterone	10 ng	280 pmol
Deoxycorticosterone (DOC)	6 ng	170 pmol
16β-Hydroxy DHA sulphate	6 ng	150 pmol

[1]Values collated from various published sources are shown, representing mean daytime results measured by radioimmunoassay; see Gray and James (1979) for further details of normal values and pathological variations.
[2]Coefficients of variation (standard deviation/mean $\times$ 100) are 30%–50% in most cases.

Appendix B
Urinary Steroids

Typical normal values for urinary steroid excretion in adults (mg/μg per day, $\pm$S.D.).

Steroid	Males		Females
17-Ketosteroids[1]	5–28 mg		3–20 mg
17-Hydroxysteroids:			
i) 17-Ketogenic steroids[2]	5–21 mg		4–16 mg
ii) Porter-Silber chromogens[3]	5–14 mg		4–12 mg
11-Hydroxycorticosteroids[4]	230$\pm$66 μg		174$\pm$53 μg
Cortisol (free)		50$\pm$20 μg	
Cortisol (glucuronide)		16–100 μg	
Cortisone (glucuronide)		55–120 μg	
Tetrahydrocortisol (THF)		1.4–2.4 mg	
Tetrahydrocortisone (THE)		1.1–1.6 mg	
Tetrahydrodeoxycortisol (THS)		10–65 μg	
Tetrahydrodeoxycorticosterone (THDOC)		30$\pm$15 μg	
Aldosterone (free)		5–15 μg	
Aldosterone (total)		$\sim$100 μg	
18-Hydroxycorticosterone		4.0$\pm$1.5 μg	
+Pregnanediol	0.2–1.2 mg		0.1–1.2 mg (F)
			1.2–9.5 mg (L)
+Pregnanetriol (5β-pregnane-3α,17α,20α-triol)	0.5–2.0 mg		0.5–2.0 mg
+Androsterone	2.0–5.0 mg		0.5–3.0 mg
+Aetiocholanolone	1.4–5.0 mg		0.8–4.0 mg
+Dehydroepiandrosterone[5]	0.2–2.0 mg		0.2–1.8 mg
+Δ^5-Pregnenetriol	N.D.		0.2–0.9 mg
+11-Ketoandrosterone	0.2–1.0 mg		0.2–0.8 mg
+11-Ketoaetiocholanolone	0.2–1.0 mg		0.2–0.8 mg
+11β-Hydroxyandrosterone	0.1–0.8 mg		0–0.5 mg
+11β-Hydroxyaetiocholanolone	0.2–0.6 mg		0.1–1.1 mg
+11-Ketopregnanetriol	N.D.		0–0.3 mg
Oestrogens (total)	5–18 μg		4–25 μg (F)
			22–105 μg (L)

[1]Zimmerman reaction (Lancet i, 1415, 1963).
[2]Norymberski method (Lancet i, 1415, 1963).
[3]Does not include 21-deoxysteroids.
[4]Mattingly fluorometric method.
[5]Values higher using colorimetric methods.
+Measured by gas-liquid chromatography (Tietz, N.W. Fundamentals of clinical chemistry. Saunders: Philadelphia (1970) p. 529).
F: Follicular phase.
L: Luteal phase.
N.D. Not determined.

References

Aarskog D, Tverteraas E (1968) McCune-Albright's syndrome following adrenalectomy for Cushing's syndrome in infancy. J Pediatr 73:89

Abeshouse GA, Goldstein RB, Abeshouse BS (1959) Adrenal cysts: Review of the literature and report of three cases. J Urol 81:711

Abraham GE, Maroulis GB (1975) Effect of exogenous estrogen on serum pregnenolone, cortisol, and androgens in postmenopausal women. Obstet Gynecol 45:271

Adam WR, Funder JW, Mercer J, Ulick S (1978) Amplification of the action of aldosterone by 5α-dihydrocortisol. Endocrinology 103:465

Adams EW (1903) Results of organotherapy in Addison's disease. Practitioner 71:472

Adams E, Baxter M (1949) Lipid fractions of human adrenal glands. Arch Pathol 48:13

Adams JB, Edwards AM (1968) Enzymic synthesis of steroid sulphates. VII. Association-dissociation equilibria in the steroid alcohol sulphotransferase of human adrenal gland extracts. Biochim Biophys Acta 167:122

Adams JB, McDonald D (1979) Enzymic synthesis of steroid sulphates. XII. Isolation of dehydroepiandrosterone sulphotransferase from human adrenals by affinity chromatography. Biochim Biophys Acta 567:144

Addison T (1855) On the constitutional and local effects of disease of the suprarenal capsules. Highley, London

Agate FJ, Hudson PB, Podberezec M (1953) Concentration of ascorbic acid in human adrenal cortex before and after ACTH stimulation. Proc Soc Exp Biol Med 84:109

Aguilera G, Catt KJ (1978) Regulation of aldosterone secretion by the renin-angiotensin system during sodium restriction in man. Proc Natl Acad Sci USA 75:4057

Aguilera G, Catt KJ (1979) Loci of action of regulators of aldosterone biosynthesis in isolated glomerulosa cells. Endocrinology 104:1046

Aguilera G, Marusic ET (1971) Role of the renin-angiotensin system in the biosynthesis of aldosterone. Endocrinology 89:1524

Aguilera G, Menard RH, Catt KJ (1980) Regulatory actions of angiotensin II on receptors and steroidogenic enzymes in adrenal glomerulosa cells. Endocrinology 107:55

Aguilera G, Hauger RL, Catt KJ (1978) Control of aldosterone secretion during sodium restriction: Adrenal receptor regulation and increased adrenal sensitivity to angiotensin II. Proc Natl Acad Sci USA 75:975

Aimone V, Campagnoli C (1970) Severe adrenal hypoplasia in a live-born normocephalic infant with neurohypophyseal aplasia. Am J Obstet Gynecol 107:327

Aitchison J, Brown JJ, Ferriss JB, Fraser R, Kay AW, Lever AF, Neville AM, Symington T, Robertson JIS (1971) Quadric analysis in the preoperative distinction between patients with and without adrenocortical tumors in hypertension with aldosterone excess and low plasma renin. Am Heart J 82:660

Akhtar M, Gonsalbez T, Young I (1974) Ultrastructural study of androgen-producing adrenocortical adenoma. Cancer 34:322

Albano JDM, Brown BL, Ekins RP, Tait SAS, Tait JF (1974) The effects of potassium, 5-hydroxytryptamine, adrenocorticotrophin and angiotensin II on the concentration of adenosine 3':5'-cyclic monophosphate in suspensions of dispersed rat adrenal zona glomerulosa and zona fasciculata cells. Biochem J 142:391

Albright F (1943) Cushing's syndrome. Harvey Lect 38:123

Albright F (1947) Osteoporosis. Ann Intern Med 27:861

Al-Dujaili EAS, Hope J, Estivariz FE, Lowry PJ, Edwards CRW (1981) Circulating human pituitary pro-γ-melanotropin enhances the adrenal response to ACTH. Nature 291:156

Allbrook D (1956) Size of adrenal cortex in East African males. Lancet II:606

Allen E, Vespignani PM (1938) Active testicular epithelium in the connective tissue surrounding a human suprarenal gland. Anat Rec 72:293

Alterman SL, Dominguez C, Lopez-Gomez A, Lieber AL (1969) Primary adrenocortical carcinoma causing aldosteronism. Cancer 24:602

Ames RP, Borkowski AJ, Sicinski AM, Laragh JH (1965) Prolonged infusions of angiotensin II and norepinephrine and blood pressure, electrolyte balance and aldosterone and cortisol secretion in normal man and in cirrhosis with ascites. J Clin Invest 44:1171

Anderson ABM, Laurence KM, Turnbull AC (1969) The relationship in anencephaly between the size of the adrenal cortex and the length of gestation. J Obstet Gynaecol Br Cwlth 76:196

Anderson DC (1980) The adrenal androgen-stimulating hormone does not exist. Lancet II:454

Anderson DC, Yen SSC (1976) Effects of estrogens on adrenal 3β-hydroxysteroid dehydrogenase in ovariectomized women. J Clin Endocrinol Metab 43:561

Anderson DC, Child DF, Sutcliffe CH, Buckley CH, Davies D, Longson D (1978) Cushing's syndrome, nodular adrenal hyperplasia and virilizing carcinoma. Clin Endocrinol (Oxf) 9:1

Anderson E, Haymaker W (1937) Prolonged survival of adrenalectomized rats treated with sera from Cushing's disease. Science 86:545

Anderson JR, Goudie RB, Gray KG, Timbury GC (1957) Auto-antibodies in Addison's disease. Lancet I:1123

Andrada JA, Bigazzi PL, Andrada E, Milgrom F, Witebsky E (1968) Serological investigation on Addison's disease. JAMA 206:1535

Andrada JA, Murray FT, Andrada EC, Ezrin C (1979) Cushing's syndrome and autoimmunity. Arch Pathol 103:244

Angevine DM (1938) Pathologic anatomy of hypophysis and adrenals in anencephaly. Arch Pathol 26:507

Arce B, Licea M, Hung S, Padron R (1978) Familial Cushing's syndrome. Acta Endocrinol (Copenh) 87:139

Armato U, Andreis PG, Draghi E (1977) Dose related persistent proliferogenic action of corticotrophin 1-24 in normal adult human adrenocortical cells in primary tissue culture. J. Endocrinol 72:97

Armato U, Nussdorfer GG, Andreis PG, Mazzocchi G, Draghi E (1975a) Primary tissue culture of human adult adrenocortical cells: Methodology and electron microscopic observations on ACTH-deprived and ACTH-treated cortical cells. Cell Tissue Res 155:155

Armato U, Nussdorfer GG, Mazzocchi G, Andreis PG, Draghi E (1975b) Cyclic AMP induces ultrastructural differentiation of normal adult human adrenocortical cells cultured in vitro. Am J Anat 142:533

Arnaud F (1900) Les hemorrhages des surrenales. Arch Gen Med 4:5

Arnold F (1831) Der Kopfteil des vegatativen Nervensystems. Salzburger Medizinische Zeitung 1831:301

Arnold J (1866) Ein Beitrag zu der feiner Struktur und dem Chemismus der Nebennieren. Virchows Arch 35:64

Artigas JLR, Niclewicz ED, Silva APG, Ribas DB, Athayde SL (1976) Congenital adrenal cortical carcinoma. J Pediatr Surg 11:247

Ascoli G, Legnani T (1912) Die Folgen der Exstirpation der Hypophyse. MMW 10:518

Ashley DJB, Mostofi FK (1960) Renal agenesis and dysgenesis. J Urol 83:211

Aterman K, Kerenyi N, Lee M (1972) Adrenal cytomegaly. Virchows Arch [Pathol Anat] 355:105

Attia O, Fadel HE, Mahran M, Sabour MS, Mahallawy MN (1970) Lesions of the suprarenal glands in pre-eclampsia and eclampsia demonstrated in biopsy material. Am J Obstet Gynecol 107:889

Atwill WH, Ensor RD, Glenn JF (1970) Massive pregnanetriol excretion due to virilizing adrenal tumour. J Endocrinol 46:547

Aubert ML, Grumbach MM, Kaplan SL (1974) Heterologous radioimmunoassay for plasma human prolactin (hPRL); values in normal subjects, puberty, pregnancy and in pituitary disorders. Acta Endocrinol (Copenh) 77:460

August GP, Hung W, Mayes DM (1975) Plasma androgens in premature pubarche: Value of 17α-hydroxyprogesterone in differentiation from congenital adrenal hyperplasia. J Pediatr 87:246

Aupetit B, Duchier J, Legrand JC (1978) Action des spironolactones sur la synthèse de l'aldostérone et sur la métabolism surrénalien. Ann Endocrinol (Paris) 39:355

Axelrad BJ, Luetscher JA (1954) Adrenal cortical activity in normal men on diets of low sodium content. J Clin Invest 33:916

Axelrod LR, Goldzieher JW, Woodhead DM (1969) Steroid biosynthesis in a feminizing adrenal carcinoma. J Clin Endocrinol Metab 29:1481

Ayers PJ, Garrod O, Tait SAS, Tait JF (1958) Primary aldosteronism (Conn's syndrome). In: Muller AF, O'Connor CM (eds) An international symposium on aldosterone. Churchill, London p. 143

Bacon GE, Lowrey GH (1965) Feminizing adrenal tumor in a six-year-old boy. J Clin Endocrinol Metab 25:1403

Baer L, Sommers SC, Krakoff LR, Newton MA, Laragh JH (1970) Pseudoprimary aldosteronism. An entity distinct from pure primary aldosteronism. Circ Res 26/27 [Suppl 1]:203

Bahu RM, Battifora H, Shambaugh G (1974) Functional black adenoma of the adrenal gland. Arch Pathol 98:139

Bailey RE (1971) Periodic homonogenesis – a new phenomenon. Periodicity in function of a hormone-producing tumor in man. J Clin Endocrinol Metab 32:317

Bailey RE, Slade CI, Lieberman AH, Luetscher JA Jr (1960) Steroid production by human adrenal adenomata and nontumorous adrenal tissue in vitro. J Clin Endocrinol Metab 20:457

Baird DT, Uno A, Melby JC (1969) Adrenal secretion of androgens and oestrogens. J Endocrinol 45:135

Baker MR (1938) A pigmented adenoma of the adrenal. Arch Pathol 26:845

Baker W de C, Wise G, Mezger ML (1967) Cytomegalic adrenal hypoplasia in a 4 and one-half-year-old boy. Am J Dis Child 114:180

Balfour FM (1878) Monograph on the development of the Elasmobranch fishes. London

Baranetsky NG, Zipser RD, Goebelsmann U, Kurman RJ, March CM, Morimoto I, Stanczyk FZ (1979) Adrenocorticotropin-dependent virilizing paraovarian tumors in Nelson's syndrome. J Clin Endocrinol Metab 49:381

Barbieri RL, Osathanondh R, Canick JA, Stillman RJ, Ryan KJ (1980) Danazol inhibits human adrenal 21- and 11β-hydroxylation in vitro. Steroids 35:251

Bardin CW, Lipsett MB, French A (1968) Testosterone and androstenedione production rates in patients with metastatic adrenal cortical carcinoma. J Clin Endocrinol Metab 28:215

Barker NW (1928) The pathologic anatomy in twenty-eight cases of Addison's disease. Arch Pathol 8:432

Barragry JM, Mason AS, Seamark DA, Trafford DJH, Makin HLJ (1980) Defective cortisol binding globulin affinity in association with adrenal hyperfunction: A case report. Acta Endocrinol (Copenh) 95:194

Bartholinus C (1611) Anatomicae Institutiones Corporis Humani. Wittenberg

Bartman J, Driscoll SG (1969) Fetal adrenal cortex in erythroblastosis fetalis. Arch Pathol 87:343

Bartter FC (1977) Bartter's syndrome. Urol Clin North Am 4:253

Bartter FC, Pronove P, Gill JR, MacCardle RC (1962) Hyperplasia of the juxtaglomerular complex with hyperaldosteronism and hypokalemic alkalosis: A new syndrome. Am J Med 33:811

Bartter FC, Henkin RI, Bryan GT (1968) Aldosterone hypersecretion in 'non-salt-losing' congenital adrenal hyperplasia. J Clin Invest 47:1742

Barzilai D, Dickstein G, Kanter Y, Plavnik Y, Schramek A (1980) Complete remission of Cushing's disease by total bilateral adrenalectomy and adrenal autotransplantation. J Clin Endocrinol Metab 50:853

Bassi F, Guisti G, Borsi L, Cattaneo S, Giannotti P, Forti G, Pazzagli M, Vigiani C, Serio M (1977) Plasma androgens in women with hyperprolactinaemic amenorrhea. Clin Endocrinol (Oxf) 6:5

Bauer J (1936) Was ist Cushingsche Krankheit? Schweiz Med Wochenschr 39:938

Baumann G, Loriaux DL (1976) The effect of endogenous prolactin on renal salt and water excretion and adrenal function in man. J Clin Endocrinol Metab 43:643

Baumber JS, Davis JO, Johnson JA, Witty RT (1971) Increased adrenocortical potassium in association with increased biosynthesis of aldosterone. Am J Physiol 220:1094

Bayard F, Ances IG, Tapper AJ, Weldon VV, Kowarski A, Migeon CJ (1970) Transplacental passage and fetal secretion of aldosterone. J Clin Invest 49:1389

Beall D (1939) Isolation of oestrone from adrenal glands. Nature 144:76

Bech K (1971) Cytomegaly of the foetal adrenal cortex. Acta Pathol Microbiol Scand[A] 79:279

Beckwith JB (1963) Extreme cytomegaly of the fetal adrenal cortex, omphalocele, hyperplasia of kidneys and pancreas, and Leydig cell hyperplasia. Another syndrome? Presented at the Annual Meeting of Western Society for Pediatric Research Los Angeles, California, November 11

Begue R-J, Brun J-M, Desgres J, Padieu P (1976) Steroids urinaires dans un corticosurrénalome virilisant. J Steroid Biochem 7:583

Behan M, Martin EC, Muecke EC, Kazam E (1977) Myelolipoma of the adrenal: two cases with ultrasound and CT findings. Am J Roentgenol 129:993

Bell JE (1979) Fused suprarenal glands in association with central nervous system defects in the first half of foetal life. J Pathol 127:191

Bell PH (1954) Purification and structure of β-corticotropin. J Am Chem Soc 76:5565

Bell JBG, Gould RP, Hyatt PJ, Tait JF, Tait SAS (1978) Properties of rat adrenal zona reticularis cells: Preparation by gravitational sedimentation. J Endocrinol 77:25

Benaily M, Schweisguth O, Job J-C (1975) Les tumeurs cortico-surrenales de l'enfant. Arch Fr Pediatr 32:441

Benirschke K (1956) Adrenals in anencephaly and hydrocephaly. Obstet Gynecol 8:412

Benjamin E, Fox H (1981) Malakoplakia of the adrenal gland. J Clin Pathol 34:606

Benner MC (1940) Studies on the involution of the fetal cortex of the adrenal glands. Am J Pathol 16:787

Bennett AH, Harrison JH, Thorn GW (1971) Neoplasms of the adrenal gland. J Urol 106:607

Bennett BD, McKenna TJ, Hough AJ, Dean R, Page DL (1980) Adrenal myelolipoma associated with Cushing's disease. Am J Clin Pathol 73:443

Bergenstal DM, Lipsett MB, Moy RH, Hertz R (1959) Regression of adrenal cancer and suppression of adrenal function in man by o,p'-DDD. Trans Assoc Am Physicians 72:341

Bergenstal DM, Hertz R, Lipsett M, Moy RH (1960) Chemotherapy of adrenocortical cancer with o,p'-DDD. Ann Intern Med 53:672

Bermudez JA, Lipsett MB (1972) Early adrenal response to ACTH: Plasma concentrations of pregnenolone, 17-hydroxypregnenolone, progesterone, and 17-hydroxyprogesterone. J Clin Endocrinol Metab 34:241

Berson SA, Yalow RS (1968) Radioimmunoassay of ACTH in plasma. J Clin Invest 47:2725

Besch PK, Watson DJ, Barry RD, Hamwi GJ, Mostow J, Gwinup G (1963) In vitro cortisol biosynthesis by a testicular tumor. Steroids 1:644

Beskid M, Borowicz J, Kobuszewska-Faryna M, Kwiatkowska J (1978) Histochemical investigation of aldosterone-secreting cells adenoma of the adrenal cortex. Endokrinologie 72:57

Besser GM, Landon J (1968) Plasma levels of immunoreactive corticotrophin in patients with Cushing's syndrome. Br Med J iv:552

Besser GM, Cullen DR, Irvine WJ, Ratcliffe JG, Landon J (1971) Immunoreactive corticotrophin levels in adrenocortical insufficiency. Br Med J i:374

Bhettay E, Bonnici F (1977) Pure oestrogen-secreting feminizing adrenocortical adenoma. Arch Dis Child 52:241

Biglieri EG, Hane S, Slaton PE, Forsham PH (1963) In vivo and in vitro studies of adrenal secretions in Cushing's syndrome and primary aldosteronism. J Clin Invest 42:516

Biglieri EG, Herron MA, Brust N (1966) 17-Hydroxylation deficiency in man. J Clin Invest 45:1946

Biglieri EG, Slaton PE, Schambelan M, Kronfield SJ (1968) Hypermineralocorticoidism. Am J Med 45:170

Biglieri EG, Stockigt JR, Schambelan M (1972) Adrenal mineralocorticoids causing hypertension. Am J Med 52:623

Bittorf A (1919) Nebennierentumor und Geschledtsdrusenausfall beim Mann. Ber Klin Wochenschr 56:776

Black J, Williams DI (1973) Natural history of adrenal haemorrhage in the newborn. Arch Dis Child 48:183

Blacklock JWS, Williams JRB (1961) The localization of tuberculous infection at the site of injury. J Pathol Bacteriol 74:119

Blackman SS Jr (1946) Concerning the function and origin of the reticular zone of the adrenal cortex. Hyperplasia in the adrenogenital syndrome. Bull Johns Hopkins Hosp 78:180

Blair-West JR, Coghlan JP, Denton JA, Goding JR, Munroe JA, Peterson RE, Wintour M (1962) Humoral stimulation of adrenal cortical secretion. J Clin Invest 41:1606

Blankstein J, Fujieda K, Reyes FI, Faiman C, Winter JSD (1980a) Aldosterone and corticosterone in amniotic fluid during various stages of pregnancy. Steroids 36:161

Blankstein J, Faiman C, Reyes FI, Schroeder ML, Winter JSD (1980b) Adult-onset familial adrenal 21-hydroxylase deficiency. Am J Med 68:441

Blau N, Miller WE, Miller ER, Cervi-Skinner SJ (1975) Spontaneous remission of Cushing's syndrome in a patient with an adrenal adenoma. J Clin Endocrinol Metab 40:659

Blaw ME (1970) Melanodermic type leucodystrophy (adreno-leucodystrophy). In: Vinken PG, Bruyn GW (eds) Handbook of clinical neurology, vol 10. Elsevier, New York, p 128

Bledsoe T, Island DP, Ney RL, Liddle GW (1964) An effect of o,p'-DDD on the extra-adrenal metabolism of cortisol in man. J Clin Endocrinol Metab 24:1303

Blichert-Toft M, Vejlsted H, Kehlet H, Abrechsten R (1975) Virilizing adrenocortical adenoma responsive to gonadotropin. Acta Endocrinol (Copenh) 78:77

Blizzard RM, Chee D, Davis W (1967) The incidence of adrenal and other antibodies in the sera of patients with idiopathic adrenal insufficiency (Addison's disease). Clin Exp Immunol 2:19

Bloch E, Benirschke K (1959) Synthesis in vitro of steroids by human fetal adrenal gland slices. J Biol Chem 234:1085

Bloch E, Benirschke K (1962) Steroidogenic capacity of foetal adrenals in vitro. In: Currie AR, Symington T, Grant JK (eds) The human adrenal cortex. Livingstone, Edinburgh p 589

Böhm N, Schuchmann L, Schreiber R (1972) Angeborene sekundare Nebennierenhypoplasie mit Hypoglykämie. Congenital secondary adrenal hypoplasia with hypoglycemia. Verh Dtsch Ges Pathol 56:151

Boiti C, Yalow RS (1978) Corticosteroid response of rabbits and rats to exogenous ACTH. Endocr Res Commun 5:21

Bolté E, Coudert S, Lefebrve Y (1974) Steroid production from plasma cholesterol. II. In vivo conversion of plasma cholesterol to ovarian progesterone and adrenal C_{19} and C_{21} steroids in humans. J Clin Endocrinol Metab 38:394

Bongiovanni AM (1961) Unusual steroid pattern in congenital adrenal hyperplasia: Deficiency of 3β-hydroxy dehydrogenase. J Clin Endocrinol Metab 21:860

Bongiovanni AM (1962) The adrenogenital syndrome with deficiency of 3β-hydroxysteroid dehydrogenase. J Clin Invest 41:2086

Borit A, Kosek J (1969) Cytomegaly of the adrenal cortex. Electron microscopy in Beckwith's syndrome. Arch Pathol 88:58

Borkowski A, Delcroix C, Levin S (1972) Metabolism of adrenal cholesterol in man. I. In vivo studies. J Clin Invest 51:1664

Böstrom H, Franksson C, Wengle B (1964) Studies on ester sulphates 22. Sulphate conjugation in adult human adrenal extracts. Act Endocrinol (Copenh) 47:633

Bottomley RH, Condit PT (1968) Cancer families. Cancer Bull 20:22

Boudreaux D, Waisman J, Skinner DG, Low R (1979) Giant adrenal myelolipoma and testicular interstitial cell tumor in a man with congenital 21-hydroxylase deficiency. Am J Surg Pathol 3:109

Boyar RM, Hellman L (1974) Syndrome of benign nodular hyperplasia associated with feminization and hyperprolactinemia. Ann Intern Med 80:389

Boyar RM, Nogeire C, Fukushima D, Hellman L, Fishman J (1977) Studies of the diurnal pattern of plasma corticosteroids and gonadotropins in two cases of feminizing adrenal carcinoma: Measurements of estrogen and corticosteroid production. J Clin Endocrinol Metab 44:39

Boyns AR, Cole EN, Golder MP, Danutra V, Harper ME, Brownsey B, Cowley T, Jones GE, Griffiths K (1972) Prolactin studies with the prostate. In: Boyns AR, Griffiths K (eds) Prolactin and carcinogenesis. Alpha-Omega-Alpha. Cardiff, p 207

Bradley EL (1975) Primary and adjunctive therapy in carcinoma of the adrenal cortex. Surg Gynecol Obstet 141:507

Braley LM, Williams GH (1979) The effects of angiotensin II and saralasin on 18-hydroxy-11-deoxycorticosterone production by isolated human adrenal glomerulosa cells. J Clin Endocrinol Metab 49:600

Branchaud CT, Goodyer CG, Hall CS, Arato JS, Silman RE, Giroud CJ (1978) Steroidogenic activity of hACTH and related peptides on the human neocortex and fetal adrenal cortex in organ culture. Steroids 31:57

Brautbar C, Rosler A, Landau H, Cohen I, Nelken D, Cohen T, Levine C, Sack J, Benderli A, Moses S, Lieberman E, Dupont B, Levine LS, New MI (1979) No linkage between HLA and congenital adrenal hyperplasia due to 11-hydroxylase deficiency. N Engl J Med 300:205

Bravo EL, Saito I, Zanella T, Sen S, Bumpus FM (1980) In vitro steroidogenic properties of a new hypertension-producing compound isolated from normal human urine. J Clin Endocrinol Metab 51:176

Breustedt HJ, Nolde S, Tamm J (1977) Ein mit HCG stimulierbares, feminisierendes Nebennierenrindenadenom mit Cushing Syndrom. Verh Dtsch Ges Inn Med 83:1340

Brewer DB (1957) Congenital absence of the pituitary gland and its consequences. J Pathol Bacteriol 73:59

Brien TG (1980) Free cortisol in human plasma. Horm Metab Res 12:643

Britton KE (1979) Radionuclide imaging in adrenal disease. In: James VHT (ed) The adrenal gland. Raven Press. New York, p 309

Brook CGD, Bambach M, Zachmann M, Prader A (1973) Familial congenital adrenal hypoplasia. Helv Paediatr Acta 28:277

Brooks RV, Felix-Davies D, Lee MR, Robertson PW (1972) Hyperaldosteronism from adrenal carcinoma. Br Med J i:220

Brorson I (1964) Syndrome of mineralocorticoid excess illustrated by a case history of two tumours of the adrenal cortex in one patient. Acta Chir Scand 128:316

Brown AK, Zuelzer WW (1958) Studies on the neonatal development of the glucuronide conjugating system. J Clin Invest 37:332

Brown BS, Dunbar JS, MacEwan DW (1962) The radiologic features of acute massive adrenal hemorrhage of the newborn. J Can Assoc Radiol 13:100

Brown G, Douglas J, Bravo E (1980) Angiotensin II receptors and in vitro aldosterone-producing adenomas, adjacent non-tumorous tissue, and normal human adrenal glomerulosa. J Clin Endocrinol Metab 51:718

Brown JJ, Davies DL, Lever AF, Robertson JIS (1964) Influence of sodium deprivation and loading on plasma renin in man. J Physiol (Lond) 173:408

Brown JJ, Ferriss JB, Fraser R, Lever AF, Love DR, Robertson JIS, Wilson A (1972a) Apparently isolated excess deoxycorticosterone in hypertension. A variant of the mineralcorticoid-excess syndrome. Lancet II:243

Brown JJ, Fraser R, Lever AF, Robertson JIS (1972b) Aldosterone: Physiological and pathophysiological variations in man. Clin Endocrinol Metab 1:397

Brown JJ, Chinn RH, Fraser R, Lever AF, Morton JJ, Robertson JIS, Tree M, Waite MA, Park DM (1973) Recurrent hyperkalaemia due to selective aldosterone deficiency: correction by angiotensin infusion. Br Med J i:650

Brown RD, Strott CA (1971) Plasma deoxycorticosterone in man. J Clin Endocrinol Metab 32:744

Brown RD, Van Loon GR, Orth DN (1973) Cushing's disease with periodic hormonogenesis: one explanation for paradoxical response to dexamethasone. J Clin Endocrinol Metab 36:445

Brown RD, Nicholson WE, Chick WT, Strott CA (1973) Effect of o,p'-DDD on human adrenal steroid 11 β-hydroxylation activity. J Clin Endocrinol Metab 36:730

Brown-Séquard E (1856) Recherches expérimentales sur la physiologie et la pathologie des capsules surrénales Arch Gén Méd 8:385

Brunner HR, Baer L, Sealy JE, Ledingham JGG, Laragh JH (1970) The influence of potassium administration and of potassium deprivation on plasma renin in normal and hypertensive subjects. J Clin Invest 49:2128

Bryson MJ, Young RB, Reynolds WA, Sweat ML (1968) Biosynthesis of steroid hormones in a human feminizing adrenal carcinoma. Cancer 21:501

Bulger AR, Correa RJ (1977) Experience with adrenal cortical carcinoma. Urology 10:12

Bulloch W, Sequeira JH (1905) On the relation of the suprarenal capsules to the sexual organs. Trans Path Soc Lond 56:189

Burke EF, Gilbert E, Uehling DT (1973) Adrenal rest tumors of the testes. J Urol 109:649

Burne JC, Langley FA (1956) The changes in the adrenal cortex in haemolytic disease of the newborn. J Pathol Bacteriol 72:47

Burr IM, Sullivan J, Graham T, Hartman WH, O'Neill J (1973) A testosterone-secreting tumour of the adrenal producing virilisation in a female infant. Lancet II:643

Burrington JD, Stephens CA (1969) Virilising tumors of the adrenal gland in childhood: report of eight cases. J Pediatr Surg 4:291

Burstein S, Kimball HL, Gut M (1970) Transformation of labeled cholesterol, 20α-hydroxycholesterol, (22R)-22-hydroxycholesterol and (22R)-20α-22-dihydroxycholesterol by adrenal acetone-dried preparations from guinea pigs, cattle and man II Kinetic studies. Steroids 15:809

Bush IE, Sandberg AA (1953) Adrenocortical hormones in human plasma. J Biol Chem 205:783

Cain DR, Van der Velde RL, Shapiro SJ (1974) Spironolactone inclusions in an aldosteronoma. Am J Clin Pathol 61:412

Cain JP, Tuck ML, Williams GH, Dluhy RG, Rosenoff SH (1972) The regulation of aldosterone secretion in primary aldosteronism. Am J Med 53:627

Camacho AM, Kowarski A, Migeon CJ, Brough AJ (1968) Congenital adrenal hyperplasia due to a deficiency of one of the enzymes involved in the biosynthesis of pregnenolone. J Clin Endocrinol Metab 28:153

Cameron EHD, Beynon MA, Griffiths K (1968) The role of progesterone in the biosynthesis of cortisol in human adrenal tissue. J Endocrinol 41:319

Cameron EHD, Jones T, Jones D, Anderson ABM, Griffiths K (1969) Further studies on the relationship between C_{19}- and C_{21}-steroid synthesis in the human adrenal gland. J Endocrinol 45:215

Cameron EHD, Hammerstein J, Jones D, Morris S, Griffiths K (1970) Steroid synthesis in a human virilising adrenal carcinoma – some unusual features. Acta Endocrinol (Copenh) 65:133

Canlorbe P, Bader J-C, Job J-C (1971) Problèmes diagnostiques posés par une tumeur virilisante maligne de la corticosurrénale. Ann Pediatr 18:593

Cannon PJ, Ames RP, Laragh JH (1966) Relation between potassium balance and aldosterone secretion in normal subjects and in patients with hypertensive or renal tubular disease. J Clin Invest 45:865

Caplan RH, Virata RL (1974) Functional black adenoma of the adrenal cortex. A rare cause of primary aldosteronism. Am J Clin Pathol 62:97

Carballeira A, Cheng SC, Fishman LM (1974) Metabolism of (4-^{14}C)cholesterol by human adrenal glands in vitro and its inhibition by metyrapone. Acta Endocrinol (Copenh) 76:689

Carey RM, Vaughan ED, Peach MJ, Ayers CR (1978) Activity of des-Asp^1-angiotensin II and angiotensin II in man. Differences in blood pressure and adrenocortical responses during normal and low sodium intake. J Clin Invest 61:20

Carpenter CCJ, Solomon N, Silverberg SG, Bledsoe T, Northcutt RC, Klinenberg JR, Bennett IL, Harvey AM (1964) Schmidt's syndrome (thyroid and adrenal insufficiency): A review of the literature and report of fifteen new cases including ten instances of co-existent diabetes mellitus. Medicine 43:153

Carr BR, MacDonald PC, Simpson ER (1980a) The regulation of de novo synthesis of cholesterol in the human fetal adrenal gland by low density lipoprotein and adrenocorticotropin. Endocrinology 107:1000

Carr BR, Parker CR, Porter JC, MacDonald PC, Simpson ER (1980b) Regulation of steroid secretion by adrenal tissue of a human anencephalic fetus. J Clin Endocrinol Metab 50:870

Carr BR, Parker CR, Milewich L, Porter JC, MacDonald PC, Simpson ER (1980c) Steroid secretion by ACTH-stimulated human fetal adrenal tissue during the first week in organ culture. Steroids 36:563

Carr BR, Porter JC, MacDonald PC, Simpson ER (1980d) Metabolism of low density lipoprotein by human fetal adrenal tissue. Endocrinology 107:1034

Carr I (1959) The human adrenal cortex at the time of death. J Pathol Bacteriol 78:533

Carr I (1960) The ultrastructure of the human adrenal cortex before and after stimulation with ACTH. J Pathol Bacteriol 81:101

Carter JN, Tyson JE, Warne GL, McNeilly AS, Faiman C, Friesen HG (1977) Adrenocortical function in hyperprolactinemic women. J Clin Endocrinol Metab 45:973

Cassan P, Baglin A, Coulbois J, Saigot T, Kuhn I-M, Betourne C (1978) Cortico-surrénalomes malins non-sécrétants révélés par une fièvre prolongée. Quatre cas. Nouv Presse Med 7:2153

Cathelineau G, Poizat R (1976) Tumeur feminisante de la surrénale avec hyperaldostéronisme primaire et hypertension arterielle maligne. Ann Endocrinol (Paris) 37:59

Cathelineau G, Brerault J-L, Fiet J, Julien R, Dreux C, Canivet J (1980) Adrenocortical 11β-hydroxylation defect in adult women with post-menarchial onset of symptoms. J Clin Endocrinol Metab 51:287

Cedermark BJ, Sjöberg HE (1981) The clinical significance of metastases to the adrenal glands. Surg Gynecol Obstet 152:607

Cerny E (1970) Subendometriale Lokalization einer akzessorischen Nebennierenrinde bei einer altan Frau. Zentralbl Allg Pathol 113:552

Chajek T, Romanoff H (1976) Cushing's syndrome with cyclical edema and periodic secretion of corticosteroids. Arch Intern Med 136:441

Chakmakjian ZH, Abraham GE (1975) Peripheral steroid levels in a patient with virilizing adenoma. Obstet Gynecol 46:544

Challis JRG, Torosis JD (1977) Is α-MSH atrophic hormone to adrenal function in the foetus? Nature 269:818

Challis JRG, Jones CT, Robinson JS, Thorburn GD (1977) Development of fetal pituitary-adrenal function. J Steroid Biochem 8:471

Charbonnel B, Chupin M, Lucas B, Chupin F, Guillon J (1980) Adrenocortical function in idiopathic haemochromatosis. Acta Endocrinol (Copenh) 95:67–70

Charreau EH, Dufau ML, Villee DB, Villee CA (1968) Synthesis of 5α-pregnane-3,20-dione by fetal and adult human adrenals. J Clin Endocrinol Metab 28:629

Charro AL, Hofeldt FD, Becker N, Levin SR, Forsham PH (1973) Adrenocortical function in acromegaly. Am J Med Sci 266:211

Check JH, Goldfarb AF, Rakoff AE, Jackson L (1977) Sexual infantilism related to adrenogenital syndrome in conjunction with a chromosomal defect. Am J Obstet Gynecol 129:919

Cheng SC, Suzuki K, Sadee W, Harding BW (1976) Effects of spironolactone, canrenone and canrenoate-K on cytochrome P450, and 11β- and 18-hydroxylation in bovine and human adrenal cortical mitochondria. Endocrinology 99:1097

Chester Jones I (1955) The adrenal cortex in reproduction. Br Med Bull 11:156

Chester Jones I (1957) The adrenal cortex. University Press, Cambridge

Chester Jones I, Henderson IW (1976) General, comparative and clinical endocrinology of the adrenal cortex, vol 1. Academic Press, London New York San Francisco

Chester Jones I, Henderson IW (1978) General, comparative and clinical endocrinology of the adrenal cortex, vol 2. Academic Press, London New York San Francisco

Chester Jones I, Henderson IW (1980) General, comparative and clinical endocrinology of the adrenal cortex, vol 3. Academic Press, London New York San Francisco

Child DF, Bul'lock DE, Anderson DC (1979) Adrenal steroidogenesis in heterozygotes for 21-hydroxylase deficiency. Clin Endocrinol (Oxf) 11:391

Childs B, Grumbach MM, Van Wyk JJ (1956) Virilizing adrenal hyperplasia: A genetic and hormonal study. J Clin Invest 35:213

Choi Y, Werk EE, Sholiton IJ (1970) Cushing's syndrome with dual pituitary adrenal control. Arch Intern Med 125:1045

Chute AL, Robinson GC, Donohue WL (1949) Cushing's syndrome in children. J Pediatr 34:20

Coghlan JP, Denton DA, Fan JSK, McDougall JG, Scoggins BA (1976) Hypertensive effect of 17α,20α-dihydroxyprogesterone and 17α-hydroxyprogesterone in the sheep. Nature 263:608

Cohen RB (1966) Observations on cortical nodules in human adrenal glands: Their relationship to neoplasia. Cancer 19:552

Cohen MM (1971) Macroglossia, omphalocele, visceromegaly, cytomegaly of the adrenal cortex and neonatal hypoglycemia. Birth Defects 7:266

Cohen T, Theodor R, Rösler A (1977) Selective hypoaldosteronism in Iranian Jews: An autosomal recessive trait. Clin Genet 11:25

Collip JB, Anderson EM, Thomson DL (1933) The adrenotropic hormone of the anterior pituitary lobe. Lancet II:347

Collu R, Ducharme JR (1978) Role of adrenal steroids in the initiation of pubertal mechanisms. In: James VHT, Serio M, Giusti G, Martini L (eds) The endocrine function of the human adrenal cortex. Academic Press, London New York San Francisco, p 547

Coneybeare JJ, Millis GC (1924) Observations on twenty-nine cases of Addison's disease treated in Guy's Hospital between 1904 and 1923. Guy's Hosp Rep 74:369

Conn JW (1955) Presidential address. Part I: Painting the background. Part II: Primary aldosteronism: A new clinical syndrome. J Lab Clin Med 45:3

Conn JW, Hinerman DL (1977) Spironolactone-induced inhibition of aldosterone biosynthesis in primary aldosteronism: Morphological and functional studies. Metabolism 26:1293

Conn JW, Knopf RF, Nesbit RM (1964) Clinical characteristics of primary aldosteronism from an analysis of 145 cases. Am J Surg 107:159

Conn JW, Beirwaltes WH, Lieberman LM, Ansari AN, Cohen EL, Bookstein JJ, Herwig KR (1971) Primary aldosteronism: Preoperative tumor visualization by scintillation scanning. J Clin Endocrinol Metab 33:713

Conn JW, Morita R, Cohen EL (1972) Primary aldosteronism. Photoscanning of tumors after administration of [131]-I-19-iodocholesterol. Arch Intern Med 129:417

Conn JW, Cohen EL, Herwig KR (1977) Primary aldosteronism: A noninvasive procedure for tumor localization as well as for distinction from bilateral hyperplasia. Adv Nephrol 7:137

Cooke BA, Taylor PD (1971) Site of dehydroepiandrosterone sulphate biosynthesis in the adrenal gland of the previable fetus. J Endocrinol 51:547

Cooke BA, Vanha-Perttula T, Klopper A (1968) Steroid biosynthesis in vitro by 6–8 week human foetal adrenal glands. Scand J Clin Lab Invest 21 [Suppl 101]:30

Cooke BA, Cowan RA, Taylor PD (1970) Pathways of dehydroepiandrosterone sulphate biosynthesis in the human foetal adrenal gland. J Endocrinol 47:295

Cooke BA, Shirley IM, Dobbie J, Taylor PD (1971) Metabolism of pregnenolone and dehydroepiandrosterone by homogenized tissue from the separated zones and whole adrenal glands from newborn anencephalic infants. J Endocrinol 51:533

Coombes RC, Powles TJ, Ford HT, Gazet J-C, Gehrke CW, Keyser JW, Mitchell PEG, Patel S, Stimson WH, Abbott M, Worwood M, Neville AM (1980) The value of sequential marker estimations following mastectomy for breast cancer. In: Mouridsen HT, Palshof T (eds) Breast cancer: Experimental and clinical aspects. Pergamon, Oxford, p 25

Copeland KC, Paunier L, Sizonenko PC (1977) The secretion of adrenal androgens and growth patterns of patients with hypogonadotropic hypogonadism and idiopathic delayed puberty. J Pediatr 91:985

Corrall RJM, Stewart GW, Ratcliffe JG (1979) Acute adrenal insufficiency due to isolated corticotrophin deficiency. J R Soc Med 72:530

Costin G, Goebelsmann U, Kogut MD (1977) Sexual precocity due to a testosterone-producing adrenal tumor. J Clin Endocrinol Metab 45:912

Coupland RE (1961) The distribution of cholinesterase and other enzymes in the adrenal glands of the ox and man and in a human phaeochromocytoma. In: Cytology of nervous tissue. Taylor & Francis, London, p 28 (Anatomical Society of Great Britain Symposium)

Coupland RE (1975) Blood supply of the adrenal gland. In: Greep RO, Astwood EB (eds) Handbook of physiology: vol VI, Adrenal gland. American Physiological Society, Washington, p 283

Cowan JS, Kinson GA, Poznanski WJ (1977) Effect of corticotrophin on cortisol and testosterone secretion in suspensions of normal and abnormal human adrenal cells. J Endocrinol 72:247

Craig JM, Landing BH (1951) Anaplastic cells of fetal adrenal cortex. Am J Clin Pathol 21:940

Crivello JF, Jefcoate CR (1980) Intracellular movement of cholesterol in rat adrenal cells. Kinetics and effects of inhibitors. J Biol Chem 255:8144

Crowder RE (1957) The development of the adrenal gland in man, with special reference to origin and ultimate location of cell types and evidence in favor of the cell migration theory. Carnegie Contrib Embryol 36:193

Currie AR, Symington T, Grant JK (1962) The human adrenal cortex. Livingstone, Edinburgh London

Cushing H (1932) The basophil adenomas of the pituitary body and their clinical manifestations (Pituitary basophilism). Bull Johns Hopkins Hosp 50:137

Cutler CB, Glenn M, Bush M, Hodgen GD, Graham CE, Loriaux DL (1978) Adrenarche: A survey of rodents, domestic animals, and primates. Endocrinology 103:2112

Cuvier G (1805) Leçons d'anatomie comparée. Paris

Daeschner GL (1965) Adrenal cortical adenoma arising in a girl with congenital adrenogenital syndrome. Pediatrics 36:140

Dahl EV, Bahn RC (1962) Aberrant adrenal cortical tissue near the testis in human infants. Am J Pathol 40:587

Dahl V, Scattini CM, Lantos CP (1976) Comparative biosynthetic studies in a case of primary aldosteronism. J Steroid Biochem 7:715

Dale SL, Melby JC (1973) Isolation and identification of 16α, 18-dihydroxydeoxycorticosterone from human adrenal gland incubations. Steroids 21:617

Dallman MF, Engeland WC, Holzwarth MA, Scholz PM (1980) Adrenocorticotropin inhibits compensatory adrenal growth after unilateral adrenalectomy. Endocrinology 107:1397

Damjanov I, Janculjak I (1974) Microzystische Veränderungen der äusseren fetalen Nebennierenrinde bei Zwillingen. Zentralbl Allg Pathol 118:494

Danon M, Robboy SJ, Kim S, Scully R, Crawford JD (1975) Cushing syndrome, sexual precocity, and polyostotic fibrous dysplasia (Albright syndrome) in infancy. J Pediatr 87:917

Danowski TS, Fisher ER, Stephan T, Nolan S, Clare DW, Khurana RC (1973) 17(OH)corticosteroid and oestrogen excretion with virilizing adrenal tumors. Horm Res 4:34

Daughaday WM (1978) Cushing's disease and basophilic microadenomas. N Engl J Med 298:793

David R, Golan S, Drucker W (1968) Familial aldosterone deficiency: Enzyme defect, diagnosis and clinical course. Pediatrics 41:403

Davies D, Kelly WF, Laing I, O'Hare MJ, Loizou, S (1981) DOC-oma: An adrenal carcinoma secreting deoxycorticosterone but not aldosterone. Acta Endocrinol (Copenh) Suppl 243:133

Davies DL, Beevers DG, Brown JJ, Cumming AMM, Fraser R, Lever AF, Mason PA, Morton JJ, Robertson JIS, Titterington M, Tree M (1979) Aldosterone and its stimuli in normal and hypertensive man: Are essential hypertension and primary hyperaldosteronism without tumour the same condition? J Endocrinol 81:79P

Davis DA, Medline NM (1970) Spironolactone (Aldactone) bodies: concentric lamellar formations in the adrenal cortices of patients treated with spironolactone. Am J Clin Pathol 54:22

Davis JO (1975) Regulation of aldosterone secretion. In: Greep RO, Astwood EB (eds) Handbook of physiology: vol VI, Adrenal gland. Am Physiol Soc Washington, D.C. p 77

Davis JO, Yankopoulos NA, Lieberman F, Holman J, Bahn RC (1960) The role of the anterior pituitary in the control of aldosterone secretion in experimental secondary hyperaldosteronism. J Clin Invest 39:765

Davis JO, Urquhart J, Higgins JT (1963) The effects of alterations in plasma sodium and potassium concentration on aldosterone secretion. J Clin Invest 42:597

Davis WW, Newsome HH, Wright LD, Hammond WR, Easton J, Bartter FC (1967) Bilateral adrenal hyperplasia as a cause of primary aldosteronism with hypertension, hypokalemia and suppressed renin activity. Am J Med 42:642

deAlvare LR, Kimura T, Singhakowinta A, Honn KV, Chavin W (1977) Mitochondrial redox components of human adrenocortical steroid hydroxylases under physiological conditions and in focal hyperplasia of the zona fasciculata. Acta Endocrinol (Copenh) 84:780

Dean G (1971) Myelolipoma of the adrenal gland. Scott Med J 16:513

Deane HW (1962) The anatomy, chemistry and physiology of adrenocortical tissue. In: Eichler O, Farah A (eds) Handbuch der experimentellen Pharmakologie. Springer, Berlin Gottingen Heidelberg, p 1

deAsis Jr DN, Samaan NA (1978) Feminizing adrenocortical carcinoma with Cushing's syndrome and pseudohyperparathyroidism. Arch Intern Med 138:301

DeCourt J, Anoussakis C (1969) Les tumeurs virilisantes de la corticosurrénale chez l'enfant avant l'age de la puberté. Sem Hop Paris 45:817

DeCrecchio L (1865) Sopra un caso di apparenze virile in una donna. Il Morgangi 7:151

Degenhart HJ, Visser HKA, Wilmink R, Croughs W (1965) Aldosterone and cortisol secretion rates in infants and children with congenital adrenal hyperplasia suggesting different 21-hydroxylation defects in 'salt-losers' and 'non salt-losers'. Acta Endocrinol (Copenh) 48:587

Degenhart HJ, Frankena L, Visser HKA, Cost WS, Van Seters AP (1966) Further investigation of a new hereditary defect in the biosynthesis of aldosterone. Evidence for a defect in 18-hydroxylation of corticosterone. Acta Physiol Pharmacol Neerl. 14:88

Degenhart HJ, Visser HKA, Boon H, O'Doherty NJ (1972) Evidence for deficient 20α-cholesterol-hydroxylase activity in adrenal tissue of a patient with lipoid adrenal hyperplasia. Acta Endocrinol (Copenh) 71:512

DeLange WE, Pratt JJ, Doorenbos H (1980) A gonadotrophin responsive testosterone producing adrenocortical adenoma and high gonadotrophin levels in an elderly woman. Clin Endocrinol (Oxf) 12:21

Delarue J, Monsaingeon A (1950) Métaplasies myeloides dans la corticosurrénale des brûles. C R Soc Biol (Paris) 144:777

Dell'Acqua S, Lucisano A, Tortorolo G, Zuppa A, Arno E (1978) Adrenal function in the foetus. In: James VHT et al. (ed) The endocrine function of the human adrenal cortex. Academic Press, London New York San Francisco, p 529

Del Negro G, Melo EHL, Rodbard D, Melo MR, Layton J, Wachslicht-Rodbard H (1980) Limited adrenal reserve in paracoccidoidomycosis: Cortisol and aldosterone responses to 1–24 ACTH. Clin Endocrinol (Oxf) 13:553

Delvaux TC (1957) Viral lesions complicating lymphoma in an adult. Localized cytomegalic inclusion disease and a second viral infection. Am J Clin Pathol 28:286

Dempsey H, Hill SR (1963) Studies in man on gonadotropin-responsive feminizing adrenal cortical neoplasia. J Clin Endocrinol Metab 23:173

DeSa DJ, Nicholls S (1972) Haemorrhagic necrosis of the adrenal gland in perinatal infants: A clinico-pathological study. J Pathol 106:133

Desai SB, Dourmashkin L, Kabakow BR, Leiter E (1979) Myelolipoma of the adrenal gland: Case report, literature review and analysis of diagnostic features. Mt Sinai J Med (NY) 46:155

Dexter RN, Fishman LM, Ney RL, Liddle GW (1967) Inhibition of adrenal corticosteroids by aminoglutethimide: studies of the mechanism of action. J Clin Endocrinol Metab 27:473

Dhöm G (1965) Die Nebennierenrinde im Kindesalter. Springer, Berlin Heidelberg New York

Dhöm G (1973) The prepuberal and puberal growth of the adrenal (adrenarche). Beitr Pathol 150:357

Dhöm G, Ross W, Widok K (1958) Die Nebennieren des Feten und des Neugeborenen. Ein quantitative und qualitative Analyse. Beitr Pathol Anat 119:177

Diczfalusy E, Pion R, Schwers J (1965) Steroid biogenesis and metabolism in the human foeto-placental unit at mid-pregnancy. Arch Anat Microsc Morphol Exp 54:67

Dluhy RG, Barlow JJ, Mahoney EM, Shirley RL, Williams GH (1971) Profile and possible origin of an adrenocortical carcinoma. J Clin Endocrinol Metab 33:312

Dluhy RG, Axelrod L, Underwood RH, Williams GH (1972) Studies of the control of plasma aldosterone concentration in normal man. J Clin Invest 51:1950

Dobbie JW (1969) Adrenocortical nodular hyperplasia: The ageing adrenal. J Pathol 99:1

Dobbie JW, MacKay AM, Symington T (1967) The structure and functional zonation of the human adrenal cortex. Mem Soc Endocrinol 17:103

Doberne Y, Levine LS, New MI (1975) Elevated urinary testosterone and androstanediol in precocious adrenarche. Pediatr Res 9:794

Dohan FC, Rose E, Eiman JW, Richardson EM, Zintel H (1953) Increased urinary estrogen excretion associated with adrenal tumors: Report of four cases. J Clin Endocrinol Metab 13:415

Dolan MF, Janovski NA (1968) Adreno-hepatic union. Arch Pathol 86:22

Dominguez OV, Samuels LT (1963) Mechanism of inhibition of adrenal steroid 11β-hydroxylase by methopyrapone (metopirone). Endocrinology 73:304

Dominguez OV, Valencia-Sanchez A, Rangel-Cabiedes L (1970) Accion de la corticotrofina sobre la esteroide-sulfatasa en la corticosuprarrenal humana y su participacion en la biosintesis de corticoides. Gac Med Mex 100:861

Dominguez OV, Valencia SA, Loza AC (1975) On the role of steroid sulfates in hormone biosynthesis. J Steroid Biochem 6:301

Donaldson MDC, Grant DB, O'Hare MJ, Shackleton CHL (1981) Familial congenital Cushing's syndrome due to bilateral nodular adrenal hyperplasia. Clin Endocr 14:519

Drayer, NM, Roberts KD, Bandi L, Lieberman S (1964) The isolation of cholesterol sulfate from bovine adrenals. J Biol Chem 239:3112

Drop SLS, Bruining GJ, Visser HKA, Sippell WG (1981) Prolonged galactorrhoea in a 6-year-old girl with isosexual precocious puberty due to a feminizing adrenal tumour. Clin Endocr (Oxf) 15:37

Dubin B, Maclennan WJ, Hamilton JC (1978) Adrenal function and ascorbic acid concentrations in elderly women. Gerontology 24:473

Ducharme JR, Leboeuf G, Sandor T (1970) C21 steroid metabolism and conjugation in the human premature neonate. I. Urinary excretion and the response to ACTH. J Clin Endocrinol Metab 30:96

Dufau ML, Villee DB (1969) Aldosterone biosynthesis by human fetal adrenal in vitro. Biochim Biophys Acta 176:637

Dunnick NR, Schaner EG, Doppman JL, Strott CA, Gill JR, Javadpour N (1979) Computed tomography in adrenal tumors. Am J Roentgenol 132:43

Dupont B, Oberfield SE, Smithwick EM, Lee TD, Levine LS (1977) Close genetic linkage between HLA and congenital adrenal hyperplasia (21-hydroxylase deficiency). Lancet II: 1309

Dyckman J, Freedman D (1957) Myelolipoma of the adrenal with clinical features and surgical excision. Mt Sinai J Med (NY) 24:793

Easterling WR, Simmer HH, Dignam WJ, Frankland MV, Naftolin F (1966) Neutral C19 Steroids and steroid sulfates in human pregnancy. II. Dehydroepiandrosterone sulfate, 16α hydroxy-dehydroepiandrosterone, and 16α hydroxy-dehydroepiandrosterone sulfate in maternal and fetal blood of pregnancies with anencephalic and normal fetuses. Steroids 8:157

Eastman AR, Neville AM (1977) 5-Ene-3β-hydroxysteroid dehydrogenase of human and bovine adrenocortical endoplasmic reticulum: Solubilization and fractionation. J Endocrinol 72:225

Eberlein WR (1965) Steroids and sterols in umbilical cord blood. J Clin Endocrinol Metab 25:1101

Eberlein WR, Bongiovanni AM (1955) Congenital adrenal hyperplasia with hypertension: Unusual steroid pattern in blood and urine. J Clin Endocrinol Metab 15:1531

Eberlein WR, Bongiovanni AM (1958) Steroid metabolism in 'salt losing' form of congenital adrenal hyperplasia. J Clin Invest 37:889

Ecker A (1846) Der feinere Bau der Nebennieren beim Menschen und den vier Wirbeltheirclassen. Braunschweig

Egdahl RH, Melby JC (1967) Recurrent Cushing's disease and intermittent functional adrenal cortical insufficiency following subtotal adrenalectomy. Ann Surg 166:586

Ehrlich EN, Dominguez OV, Samuels LT, Lynch D, Oberhelman H, Warner NE (1963) Aldosteronism and precocious puberty due to an ovarian androblastoma (Sertoli cell tumor). J Clin Endocrinol Metab 23:358

Ehrlich EN, Straus FH, Hunter RL, Weist WG (1969) Cytomegalic adrenocortical hypoplasia and increased plasma 20α-hydroxypregn-4-en-3-one in a man exhibiting the features of selective mineralocorticoid deficiency. J Clin Endocrinol Metab 29:523

Eisenstein AB (ed) (1967) The adrenal cortex. Little Brown, Boston

Elias H, Pauly JE (1956) The structure of the human adrenal cortex. Endocrinology 58:714

Elliot TR, Armour RG (1911) The development of the cortex in the human suprarenal gland and its condition in hemicephaly. J Pathol Bacteriol 15:481

Emanuel RL, Cain JP, Williams GH (1973) Double antibody radioimmunoassay of renin activity and angiotensin II in human peripheral plasma. J Lab Clin Med 81:632

Engeland WC, Dallman MF (1975) Compensatory adrenal growth is neurally mediated. Neuroendocrinology 19:352

Engeland WC, Shinsako J, Dallman MF (1975) Corticosteroids and ACTH are not required for compensatory adrenal growth. Am J Physiol 229:1461

Escobar V, Brandt IK, Bixler D (1977) Unusual association of Saethre-Chotzen syndrome and congenital adrenal hyperplasia. Clin Genet 11:365

Ewing LL, Chubb CE, Robaire B (1976) Macromolecules, steroid binding and testosterone secretion by rabbit testes. Nature 264:84

Eymontt MJ, Gwinup G, Kruger FA, Maynard DE, Hamwi GJ (1965) Cushing's syndrome with hypoglycemia caused by adrenocortical carcinoma. J Clin Endocrinol Metab 25:46

Faarvang HJ, Francis D, Buus O (1969) Content of some adrenal steroids in the cyst fluid from a lymphangiomatous adrenal cyst. Acta Endocrinol (Copenh) 60:486

Falls JL (1955) Accessory adrenal cortex in the broad ligament. Incidence and functional significance. Cancer 8:143

Fang VS (1977) Establishment and characterization of a strain of human adrenal tumor cells that secrete estrogens. Proc Natl Acad Sci USA 74:1067

Fang VS, Furuhashi N, Gomez O (1978) Human prolactin stimulates estrogen production by feminizing adrenal neoplastic cells. Proc Soc Exp Biol Med 157:159

Fantl V, Booth M, Gray CH (1973) Urinary pregn-5-ene-3α,6α,20α-triol in adrenal dysfunction. J Endocrinol 57:135

Farese RV, Sabir AM (1980) Polyphosphoinositides: Stimulator of mitochondrial side-chain cleavage and possible identification as an adrenocorticotropin-induced, cycloheximide-sensitive, cytosolic, steroidogenic factor. Endocrinology 106:1869

Farrell G (1960) Adrenoglomerulotropin. Circulation 21:1009

Favara BE, Franciosi RA, Miles V (1972) Idiopathic adrenal hypoplasia in children. Am J Clin Pathol 57:287

Fellerman H, Dalakos TG, Streeten DHP (1970) Remission of Cushing's syndrome after unilateral adrenal phlebography. Ann Intern Med 73:585

Fencl M, Osathanondh R, Tulchinsky D (1976) Plasma cortisol and cortisone in pregnancies with normal and anencephalic fetuses. J Clin Endocrinol Metab 43:80

Fencl M, Stillman RJ, Cohen J, Tulchinsky D (1980) Direct evidence of sudden rise in fetal glucocorticoids late in human gestation. Nature 287:225

Ferriss JB, Neville AM, Brown JJ, O'Muircheartaigh IG, Fraser R, Robertson JIS, Kay AW, Symington T, Lever AF (1970) Hypertension with aldosterone excess and low plasma-renin: Preoperative distinction between patients with and without adrenocortical tumour. Lancet II:995

Ferriss JB, Brown JJ, Fraser R, Haywood E, Davies DI, Kay AW, Lever AF, Robertson JIS, Owen K, Peart WS (1975) Results of adrenal surgery in patients with hypertension, aldosterone excess, and low plasma renin concentration. Br Med J i:135

Ferriss JB, Beevers DG, Brown JJ, Fraser R, Lever AF, Padfield PL, Robertson JIS (1978) Low-renin ('primary') hyperaldosteronism. Am Heart J 95:641

Feyrter R, Holczabek W (1978a) Nebennierenstudien II: Die Complexus cortico-neurales. Exp Pathol (Jena) 15:17

Feyrter R, Holczabek W (1978b) Nebennierenstudien III: Über abwegige Veränderungen der Lymphgefässe in perisuprarenalen Raum des Menschen. Exp Pathol (Jena) 15:26

Fichman MP, Littenburg G, Brooker G (1972) Effect of prostaglandin A1 on renal and adrenal function in man. Circ Res 31 [Suppl 2]:19

Fidler WJ (1977) Ovarian thecal metaplasia in adrenal glands. Am J Clin Pathol 67:318

Field S, Saxton H (1974) Venous anomalies complicating left adrenal catheterization. Br J Radiol 47:219

Filipecki S, Feltynowski T, Poplawska W, Lapinska K, Krus S, Wocial B, Januszewicz W (1972) Carcinoma of the adrenal cortex with hyperaldosteronism. J Clin Endocrinol Metab 35:225

Finkelstein MJ, Goldberg S (1957) A test for qualitative and quantitative estimation of pregnane-3α, 17α, 20α-triol-11-one in urine, and its significance in adrenal disturbances. J Clin Endocrinol Metab 17:1063

Fisher ER, Danowski TS (1973) Ultrastructural study of virilizing adrenocortical adenoma. Am J Clin Pathol 59:480

Flanagan MJ, McDonald JH (1967) Heterotopic adrenocortical adenoma producing primary aldosteronism. J Urol 98:133

Fontaine R, Babin S, Warter P, Kuhn A (1969) L'hypertension arteriélle des kystes ou faux-kystes de la surrénale. J Urol Nephrol (Paris) 75:47

Fore WW, Bledsoe T, Weber DM, Akers R, Brooks RT (1972) Cortisol production by testicular tumors in adrenogenital syndrome. Arch Intern Med 130:59

Forest MG, Lecornu M, Peretti E (1980) Familial male pseudohemaphroditism due to 17-20-desmolase deficiency. I. In vivo endocrine studies. J Clin Endocrinol Metab 50:826

Fox B (1976) Venous infarction of the adrenal glands. J Pathol 119:65

Foye LV, Feichtmeir TV (1955) Adrenal cortical carcinoma producing solely mineralocorticoid effect. Am J Med 19:966

Franckson JRM, Lejeune-Lenain C, Wolter R (1980) Basal level and responsiveness of 11β-hydroxyandrostenedione secretion in normal pubertal children. In: Genazzani AR, Thijssen JHH, Siterii PK (eds) Adrenal androgens. Raven, New York, p 167

Frandsen VA, Stakemann G (1964) The site of production of oestrogenic hormones in human pregnancy.

III. Further observations on the hormone excretion in pregnancy with anencephalic foetus. Acta Endocrinol (Copenh) 47:265

Frank RT (1937) Test for adrenal carcinoma. JAMA 109:1121

Franks RC, Nance WE (1970) Hereditary adrenocortical unresponsiveness to ACTH. Pediatrics 45:43

Fraser R, Lantos CP (1978) 18-Hydroxycorticosterone: A review. J Steroid Biochem 9:273

Fraser R, James VHT, Landon J, Peart WD, Rawson A, Giles CA, MacKay AM (1968) Clinical and biochemical studies of a patient with a corticosterone-secreting adrenocortical tumour. Lancet II:1116

Fraumeni JF, Miller RW (1967) Adrenocortical neoplasms with hemihypertrophy, brain tumors, and other disorders. J Pediatr 70:129

Fredlund P, Saltman S, Kondo T, Douglas J, Catt KJ (1977) Aldosterone production by isolated glomerulosa cells: Modulation of sensitivity to angiotensin II and ACTH by extracellular potassium concentration. Endocrinology 100:481

Frenkel JK (1960) Pathogenesis of infections of the adrenal gland leading to Addison's disease in man: The role of corticoids in adrenal and generalized infection. Ann NY Acad Sci 84:391

Friderichsen C (1955) Waterhouse-Friderichsen syndrome. Acta Endocrinol (Copenh) 18:482

Frisch RE, Canick JA, Tulchinsky D (1980) Human fatty marrow aromatizes androgen to estrogen. J Clin Endocrinol Metab 51:394

Fujita H, Ihara T (1973) Electron-microscopic observations on the cytodifferentiation of adrenocortical cells of the human embryo. Z Anat Entwickl-Gesch 142:267

Fukushima DK, Gallagher TF (1963) Steroid production in 'nonfunctioning' adrenal cortical tumor. J Clin Endocrinol Metab 23:923

Gabrilove JL (1958) Spermatogenic maturation arrest and the male adrenogenital syndrome. Lancet II:904

Gabrilove JL, Sharma DC, Wotiz HH, Dorfman RI (1965) Feminizing adrenocortical tumors in the male. A review of 52 cases including a case report. Medicine 44:37

Gabrilove JL, Nicolis GL, Hausknecht RU, Wotiz HH (1970) Feminizing adrenocortical carcinoma in a man. Cancer 25:153

Gabrilove JL, Nicolis GL, Sohval AR (1973) Non-tumorous feminizing adrenogenital syndrome in the male subject. J Urol 110:710

Gabrilove JL, Nicolis GL, Mitty HA (1976) Virilizing adrenocortical adenoma studied by selective adrenal venography. Am J Obstet Gynecol 125:180

Gagnon R (1956) The venous drainage of the human adrenal gland. Rev Can Biol 14:350

Gagnon R (1957) The arterial supply of the human adrenal gland. Rev Can Biol 16:421

Gallais A (1912a) Le syndrome genitosurrénal: Etude anatomio-clinique. Theses de Paris 225

Gallais A (1912b) Les troubles nerveux et mentaux dans trois observations personelles de tumeur primitive de la glande surrénale. Le virilisme surrénal Encephale 1:368

Gallant S, Brownie AC (1973) The in vivo effect of indomethacin and prostaglandin E_2 on ACTH and DBcAMP-induced steroidogenesis in hypophysectomised rats. Biochem Biophys Res Commun 55:831

Ganguly A, Weinberger MH (1979) Preoperative distinction of adenoma from hyperplasia in primary aldosteronism. Lancet I:826

Ganguly A, Melada GA, Luetscher JA, Dowdy AJ (1973) Control of plasma aldosterone in primary aldosteronism: Distinction between adenoma and hyperplasia. J Clin Endocrinol Metab 37:765

Gann DS, DeLea CS, Gill JR, Thomas JP, Bartter FC (1964) Control of aldosterone secretion by change of body potassium in normal man. Am J Physiol 207:104

Garcia-Alvarez F (1970) Estudio ultraestructural sobre la inervacion de la corteza suprarenal. Anal Anat (Zarragosa) 47:267

Garret R, Ames RP (1973) Black-pigmented adenoma of the adrenal gland. Arch Pathol 95:349

Gaunt R (1975) History of the adrenal cortex. In: Greep RO, Astwood EB (eds) Handbook of physiology, Section 7, Vol VI, Adrenal gland. American Physiological Society, Washington DC, p 1

Gee WF, Chikos PM, Greaves JP, Ikemoto N, Tremann JA (1975) Adrenal myelolipoma. Urology 5:562

Gelfman NA (1964) Morphologic changes of adrenal cortex in disease. Yale J Biol Med 37:31

Genazzani AR, Thijssen JHH, Siiteri PK (1980) Adrenal androgens. Raven Press, New York

Genest J, Nowaczynski W, Koiw E, Sandor T, Biron P (1960) Adrenocortical function in essential hypertension. In: Bock KD, Cottier PT (eds) Essential hypertension. Springer, Berlin, p 126

Gewirtz G, Yalow RS (1974) Ectopic ACTH production in carcinoma of lung. J Clin Invest 53:1022

Ghandur-Mnaymneh L, Slim M, Muakassa K (1979) Adrenal cysts: Pathogenesis and histological identification with a report of 6 cases. J Urol 122:87

Giebink GS, Gotlin RW, Biglieri EG, Katz FH (1973) A kindred with familial glucocorticoid-suppressible aldosteronism. J Clin Endocrinol Metab 36:715

Gierke E (1905) Über Knochenmarkesgewebe in der Nebennieres. Beitr Pathol Anat [Suppl] 7:311

Gigax JH, Bucy JG, Troxler G, Chunn SP (1972) Cystic hamartoma of the adrenal gland associated with hypertension. J Urol 107:161

Gilbert P, Pfitzer P (1977) Facultative polyploidy in endocrine tissues. Virchows Arch [Cell Pathol] 25:233

Gill GN (1976) ACTH regulation of the adrenal cortex. Pharmacol Ther B 2:313

Gill GN, Ill CR, Simonian MH (1977) Angiotensin stimulation of bovine adrenocortical cell growth. Proc Natl Acad Sci USA 74:5569

Gill JR, Fröhlich JC, Bowden RE, Taylor AA, Keiser HR, Seyberth HW, Oates JA, Bartter FC (1976) Bartter's syndrome: A disorder characterized by high urinary prostaglandins and a dependence of hyperreninemia on prostaglandin synthesis. Am J Med 61:43

Girard J, Bauman JB, Bühler U, Zuppinger K, Haas HG, Staub JJ, Wyss HI (1978) Cyproterone acetate and ACTH adrenal function. J Clin Endocrinol Metab 47:581

Givens JR, Andersen RN, Wiser WL, Coleman SA, Fish SA (1974) A gonadotropin-responsive adrenocortical adenoma. J Clin Endocrinol Metab 38:126

Glickman JR, Carson GD, Challis JRG (1979) Differential effects of synthetic adrenocorticotropin$^{1-24}$ and α-melanocyte-stimulating hormone on adrenal function in human and sheep fetuses. Endocrinology 104:34

Glossman H, Baukal AJ, Catt KJ (1974) Properties of angiotensin II receptors in the bovine and rat adrenal cortex. J Biol Chem 249:825

Glynn P, Cooper DMF, Schulster D (1979) The regulation of adenylate cyclase of the adrenal cortex. Mol Cell Endocrinol 13:99

Goldblatt E, Snaith AH (1958) A case of Cushing's syndrome in an infant. Arch Dis Child 33:540

Golden MP, Lippe BM, Kaplan SA (1977) Congenital adrenal hypoplasia and hypogonadotropic hypogonadism. Am J Dis Child 131:1117

Goldman AS, Yakovac WC, Bongiovanni AM (1966) Development of activity of 3β-hydroxysteroid dehydrogenase in human fetal tissues and two anencephalic newborns. J Clin Endocrinol Metab 26:14

Gomez-Sanchez C, Holland OB, Hall CE, Ayachi S (1976) On the mineralocorticoid and hypertensogenic properties of 16β-hydroxydehydroepiandrosterone. Expierentia 32:1067

Gomez-Sanchez CE, Holland OB, Murry BA, Lloyd HA, Milewich L (1979) 19-Nor-deoxycorticosterone: A potent mineralocorticoid isolated from the urine of rats with regenerating adrenals. Endocrinology 105:708

Goodman DS, Arigan J, Wilson H (1962) The in vitro metabolism of desmosterol with adrenal and liver preparations. J Clin Invest 41:2135

Goodyer CG, Hall CSG Branchaud C, Giroud CJP (1977) Exploration of the human fetal pituitary adrenal axis: Stimulation of cortisol and dehydroepiandrosterone sulfate biosynthesis by homologous pituitary in organ culture. Steroids 29:407

Gorgas K, Böck P, Wuketich S (1976) Fine structure of a virilizing adrenocortical adenoma. Beitr Pathol 159:371

Gottschau M (1883) Structur und embryonale Entwickelung der Nebennieren bei Saugethieren. Arch Anat Physiol Lpz. Anatom Abt 412

Goudie RB, McDonald E, Anderson JR, Gray K (1968) Immunological features of idiopathic Addison's disease: Characterization of the adrenocortical antigens. Clin Exp Immunol 3:119

Gower DB, Stern MI (1969) Steroid excretion and biosynthesis, with special reference to androst-16-enes in a woman with virilising adrenocortical carcinoma. Acta Endocrinol (Copenh) 60:265

Graham IS (1953) Celiac accessory adrenal glands. Cancer 6:149

Granger P, Genest J (1970) Autopsy study of adrenals in unselected normotensive and hypertensive patients. Can Med Assoc J 103:34

Granoff AB, Abraham GE (1979) Peripheral and adrenal venous levels of steroids in a patient with virilizing adrenal adenoma. Obstet Gynecol 53:111

Grant JK (1960) The biosynthesis of the adrenocortical steroids. Biochem Soc Symp 18:24

Grant JK (1978) An introductory review of adrenocortical steroid biosynthesis. In: James VHT, Serio M, Giusti G, Martini L (eds) The endocrine function of the human adrenal cortex. Academic Press, London New York San Francisco, p 1

Grant JK, Griffiths K (1962) Steroid secretion by slices of tissue of the human adrenal cortex. In: Currie AR, Symington T, Grant J (eds) The human adrenal cortex. Livingstone, Edinburgh, p 26

Grant JK, Forrest APM, Symington T (1957a) The secretion of cortisol and corticosterone by the human adrenal cortex. Acta Endocrinol (Copenh) 26:195

Grant JK, Symington T, Duguid WP (1975b) Effect of adrenocorticotropic therapy on the in vitro 11β-hydroxylation of deoxycorticosterone by human adrenal homogenates. J Clin Endocrinol Metab 17:933

Grant JK, Griffiths K, Lowe M (1968) Biochemical investigations of the actions of corticotrophins on the adrenal cortex. In: James VHT, Landon J (eds). The investigation of hypothalamic-pituitary adrenal function. University Press, Cambridge, p 113

Graves PE, Salhanick HA (1979) Stereospecific inhibition of aromatase by enantiomers of aminoglutethimide. Endocrinology 105:52

Grawitz P (1883) Die sogenannten Lipome der Niere. Virchows Arch 93:39

Gray CH, James VHT (1979) Hormones in blood, 3rd edn, vol 3. Academic Press, London New York San Francisco

Green JRB, Van't Hoff W (1975) Cushing's syndrome with fluctuation due to adrenal adenoma. J Clin Endocrinol Metab 41:235

Greenblatt RB, Colle ML, Mahesh VB (1976) Ovarian and adrenal steroid production in the post-menopausal woman. Obstet Gynecol 47:383

Greendyke RM (1965) Adrenal hemorrhage. Am J Clin Pathol 43:210

Gregory T, Gardner LI (1976) Hypertensive virilizing adrenal hyperplasia with minimal impairment of synthetic route to cortisol. J Clin Endocrinol Metab 43:769

Grekin RJ, Dale SL, Melby JC (1973) The role of 18-hydroxy-11-deoxycorticosterone as a precursor in human adrenal tissue in vitro. J Clin Endocrinol Metab 37:261

Griffin JW, Goren E, Schaumburg H, Engel WK, Loriaux L (1977) Adrenomyeloneuropathy: A probable variant of adrenoleukodystrophy. Neurology 27:1107

Griffiths K, Cameron EHD (1970) Steroid biosynthetic pathways in the human adrenal. In: Briggs MH (ed) Advances in steroid biochemistry and pharmacology. Vol 2 Academic Press, London New York, p 223

Griffiths K, Grant JK, Symington T (1963) A biochemical investigation of the functional zonation of the adrenal cortex in man. Endocrinology 23:776

Grim CE, McBryde AC, Glenn JF, Gunnells JC Jr (1967) Childhood primary aldosteronism with bilateral adrenocortical hyperplasia: Plasma renin activity as an aid to diagnosis. J Pediatr 71:377

Gross F (1960) Adrenocortical function and renal pressor mechanisms in experimental hypertension. In: Bock KD, Cottier PT (eds) Essential hypertension. Springer, Berlin, p 92

Gruber KA, O'Brien LV, Gerstner R (1976) Vitamin A: Not required for adrenal steroidogenesis in rats. Science 191:472

Gruenwald P (1946) Embryonic and postnatal development of the adrenal cortex, particularly the zona glomerulosa and accessory nodules. Anat Rec 95:391

Grumbach MM, Richards GE, Conte FA, Kaplan SL (1978) Clinical disorders of adrenal function and puberty: An assessment of the role of the adrenal cortex in normal and abnormal puberty in man and evidence for an ACTH-like pituitary adrenal androgen stimulating hormone. In: James VHT, Serio M, Giusti G, Martini L (eds). The endocrine function of the human adrenal cortex. Academic Press, London New York San Francisco, p 583

Guieysse A (1901) La capsule surrénale du cobaye-histologie et fonctoinnement. J Anat (Paris) 37:312

Guinet P, Putelat R, Bret P, Béthoux R, Revol A (1959) Les tumeurs cortico-surrénales virilisantes chez la femme. Rev Lyon Med 8:97

Gutman Y, Shamir Y, Glushevitsky D, Hochman S (1972) Angiotensin increases microsomal (Na^+-K^+)-ATPase activity in several tissues. Biochim Biophys Acta 273:401

Guttman PH (1930) Addison's disease: A statistical analysis of 566 cases and a study of the pathology. Arch Pathol 10:742

Gyorkey F, Min KW, Krisko I, Gyorkey P (1975) The usefulness of electron microscopy in the diagnosis of human tumors. Hum Pathol 6:421

Haicken BN, Schulman NH, Schneider KM (1973) Adrenocortical carcinoma and congenital hemihypertrophy. J Pediatr 83:284

Hajjar RA, Hickey RC, Samaan NA (1975) Adrenal cortical carcinoma. A study of 32 patients. Cancer 35:549

Hall CE, Gomez-Sanchez CE, Holland OB, Nasseth D (1979) Influence of 19-nor-deoxycorticosterone on blood pressure, saline consumption, and serum electrolytes, corticosterone and renin activity. Endocrinology 105:600

Halmi KA, Lascari AD (1971) Conversion of virilization to feminization in a young girl with adrena cortical carcinoma. Cancer 27:931

Hamperl H (1970) On the 'adrenal rest-tumors' (hypernephromas) of the liver. Z Krebsforsch 74:310

Hamwi GJ, Gwinup G, Mostow JH, Besch PK (1963) Activation of testicular adrenal rest tissue by prolonged excessive ACTH production. J Clin Endocrinol Metab 23:861

Haning R, Tait SAS, Tait JF (1970) In vitro effects of ACTH, angiotensins, serotonin and potassium on steroid output and conversion of corticosterone to aldosterone by isolated adrenal cells. Endocrinology 87:1147

Hardy J (1971) Transphenoidal hypophysectomy. J Neurosurg 34:582

Harley G (1858) The histology of the suprarenal capsules. Lancet:511

Harrop GA, Weinstein A (1932) Addison's disease treated with suprarenal cortical hormone (Swingle-Pfiffner). JAMA 98:1525

Hartemann P, Leclere, J, Groussin M, Valdenaire JC, Mizrahi R (1978) Tumeurs virilisantes cortico-surrénaliens à forme d'hirsutisme isolé. Ann Med Nancy 17:565

Hartman FA, Brownell KA, Hartman WE, Dean GA, MacArthur CG (1928) The hormone of the adrenal cortex. Am J Physiol 86:353

Hasegawa K, Moriwaki K, Igarashi T, Sugase T, Kawakami F, Itoh Y, Nishikawa M (1975) Studies on the responsiveness of human adrenocortical tumors to ACTH. The clinical and experimental observations. Folia Endocrinol Jpn 51:749

Hashida, Y, Yunis EJ (1972) Ultrastructure of the adrenal zona glomerulosa in children with renovascular hypertension. Hum Pathol 3:301

Hay ID (1977) Pubertal failure in congenital adrenocortical hypoplasia. Lancet II:1035

Haymaker W, Anderson E (1938) The syndrome arising from hyperfunction of the adrenal cortex: The adrenogenital and Cushing's syndromes – a review. Int Clinics 4:244

Hayslett JP, Cohn GL (1967) Spontaneous remission of Cushing's disease: Report of a case. N Engl J Med 276:968

Hechter O (1951) The biogenesis of adrenal cortical steroids. In: Ralli EP (ed) Transactions of the Third Conference on the Adrenal Cortex. Josiah Macy Jr Foundation, New York, p 115

Heinbecker P, O'Neal O, Ackerman LV (1957) Functioning and non-functioning adrenal cortical tumors. Surg Gynecol Obstet 105:21

Heinonen E, Krohn K (1977) Studies on an adrenal antigen common to man and different animals. Med biol 55:48

Heinonen E, Krohn K, Perheentupa J, Aro A, Pelkonen R (1976) Association of precipitating anti-adrenal antibodies with moniliasis-polyendocrinopathy syndrome. Ann Clin Res 8:262

Hench PS, Kendall EC, Slocumb CH, Pollye HF (1949) The effect of a hormone of the adrenal cortex (17-hydroxy-11-dehydrocorticosterone: Compound E) and of pituitary adrenocorticotropic hormone on rheumatoid arthritis: Preliminary report. Mayo Clin Proc 24:181

Henley WL (1973) Virilising adrenal carcinoma. Lancet II:1153

Herbeuval R, Boulangé M, Rauver G, Guerci O, Petitier H (1968) Corticosurrénalome malin avec hyperminéralocorticisme prédominant. Production anormale, par la tumeur, de cortexone et de cortexolone. Rev Fr Endocrinol Clin 9:489

Hertz R (1962). Pharmacological alteration of adrenal function and neoplasia in man. In: Currie AR, Symington T, Grant JK (eds) The human adrenal cortex. Livingstone, Edinburgh London, p 469

Hervonen A, Suoranta H (1972) Vascular supply of human foetal adrenals and the functional significance of the microvascular patterns. Z Anat Entwicklungsgesch 136:331

Hillman DA, Stachenko J, Giroud CJP (1962) In vitro studies of the human newborn adrenal cortex. In: Currie AR, Symington T, Grant JK (eds) The human adrenal cortex. Livingstone, Edinburgh, p 596

Hinshaw HT, Ney RL (1974) Abnormal hormone control in the neoplastic adrenal cortex. In: McKerns KW (ed) Hormones and cancer. Academic Press, New York, p 309

Hirano T, Seeler RA (1978) Congenital virilizing adrenal hyperplasia, segmental hypertrophy, macrodactyly, and cystic lymphangioma. J Pediatr 93:326

Hirschfeld AJ, Fleshman JL (1969) An unusually high incidence of salt-losing congenital adrenal hyperplasia in the Alaskan Eskimo. J Pediatr 75:492

Hoefnagel D, Van den Noort S, Ingbar SH (1962) Diffuse cerebral sclerosis with endocrine abnormalities in young males. Brain 85:553

Hoeldtke RD, Donald RA, Nicholls MG (1980) Functional significance of idiopathic adrenal calcification in the adult. Clin Endocrinol (Oxf) 12:319

Holdaway IM, Rees LH, Landon J (1973) Circulating corticotrophin levels in severe hypopituitarism and in the neonate. Lancet II: 1170

Holland OB, Gomez-Sanchez CE, Kem DC, Weinberger MH, Kramer NJ, Higgins JR (1977) Evidence against prolactin stimulation of aldosterone in normal human subjects and patients with primary aldosteronism, including a patient with primary aldosteronism and a prolactin-producing pituitary microadenoma. J Clin Endocrinol Metab 45:1064

Hollenberg NK, Chenitz WR, Adams DF, Williams GH (1974) Reciprocal influence of salt intake on adrenal glomerulosa and renal vascular responses to angiotensin II in normal man. J Clin Invest 54:34

Holmes RO, Moon HD, Rinehart JF (1951) A morphologic study of adrenal glands with correlations of body size and heart size. Am J Pathol 27:724

Honn KV, Chavin W (1976) Prostaglandin modulation of the mechanism of ACTH action in the human adrenal. Biochem Biophys Res Commun 73:164

Honn KV, Chavin W (1977) Effects of A and B series prostaglandins on cAMP, cortisol and aldosterone production by the human adrenal. Biochem Biophys Res Commun 76:977

Honn KV, Chavin W, Singhakowinta (1977) In vitro responses of focal hyperplastic tissue of the human adrenal zona fasciculata to ACTH. Acta Endocrinol (Copenh) 86:363

Honnebier WJ, Jobsis AC, Swaab DF (1974) The effect of hypophysial hormones and human chorionic gonadotrophin (HCG) on the anencephalic fetal adrenal cortex and on parturition in the human. J Obstet Gynaecol Br Cwlth 81:423

Honoré LH, O'Hara KE (1976) Combined adrenorenal fusion with adrenohepatic adhesion: A case report with review of the literature and discussion of pathogenesis. J Urol 115:323

Hornsby PJ (1980) Regulation of cytochrome P-450-supported 11β-hydroxylation of deoxycortisol by steroids, oxygen, and antioxidants in adrenocortical cell cultures. J Biol Chem 255:4020

Hornsby PJ, Gill GN (1977) Hormonal control of adrenocortical cell proliferation. Desensitisation to ACTH and interaction between ACTH and fibroblast growth factor in bovine adrenocortical cell cultures. J Clin Invest 60:342

Hornsby PJ, O'Hare MJ (1977) The roles of potassium and corticosteroids in determining the pattern of metabolism of (^{3}H) deoxycorticosterone by monolayer cultures of rat adrenal glomerulosa cells. Endocrinology 101:997

Hornsby PJ, O'Hare MJ, Neville AM (1974) Functional and morphological observations on rat adrenal zona glomerulosa cells in monolayer culture. Endocrinology 90:1240

Horton R, Finck E (1972) Diagnosis and localization in primary aldosteronism. Ann Intern Med 76:885

Horton R, Tait JF (1967) In vivo conversion of dehydroisoandrosterone to plasma androstenedione and testosterone in man. J Clin Endocrinol Metab 27:79

Houssay BA, Lewis JT (1923) The relative importance to life of cortex and medulla of the adrenal glands. Am J Physiol 64:512

Horvath E, Chalvardjian A, Kovacs K, Singer W (1980) Leydig-like cells in the adrenals of a woman with ectopic ACTH syndrome. Hum Pathol 11:284

Howard CP, Takahashi H, Hayles AB (1977) Feminizing adrenal adenoma in a boy. Case report and literature review. Mayo Clinic Proc 52:354

Hudson RW, Killinger DW (1972) The in vitro biosynthesis of 11β-hydroxyandrostenedione by human adrenal homogenates. J Clin Endocrinol Metab 34:215

Huguenin A, Leborgne P, Ferrand B, Logeais Y, Almange C, Murie N, Louvet JP, Ramee MP, Pierres J (1975) Syndrome de Conn du a un cortico-surrénalome avec metastases. Hyperaldostéronisme pur controle de l'aldostérone tumorale. Rev Fr Endocrinol Clin 16:237

Huhtaniemi I (1973) Identification and quantification of unconjugated neutral steroids in adrenal and liver tissue of early and mid-term human fetuses. Steroids 21:511

Huhtaniemi I (1974) Formation of neutral steroids from endogenous precursors in minced human fetal adrenals in vitro. Steroids 23:145

Huhtaniemi I (1977) Studies on steroidogenesis and its regulation in human fetal adrenal and testis. J Steroid Biochem 8:491

Huhtaniemi I, Luukkainen T, Vihko R (1970). Identification and determination of neutral steroid sulphates in human fetal adrenal and liver tissue. Acta Endocrinol (Copenh) 64:273

Huhtaniemi I, Kahri AI, Pelkonen R, Salmenperä M, Siluva A, Vihko R (1978) Ultrastructural and steroidogenic characteristics of an androgen-producing adrenocortical tumour. Clin Endocrinol (Oxf) 8:305

Hunt TK, Schambelan M, Biglieri EG (1975) Selection of patients and operative approach in primary aldosteronism. Ann Surg 182:353

Huq MS, Pfaff M, Jespersen D, Zucker IR, Kirschner MA (1976) Concurrence of aldosterone, androgen and cortisol secretion in adrenal venous effluents. J Clin Endocrinol Metab 42:230

Huschke E (1845) Capsules surrénales. In: Encyclopedia of anatomy. Paris, p 330

Hutter AM, Kayhoe DE (1966a) Adrenal cortical carcinoma. Clinical features of 138 patients. Am J Med 41:572

Hutter AM, Kayhoe DE (1966b) Adrenal cortical carcinoma. Results of treatment with o,p'-DDD in 138 patients. Am J Med 41:581

Huvos AG, Hajdu SI, Brasfield RD, Foote FW (1970) Adrenal cortical carcinoma – clinicopathologic study of 34 cases. Cancer 25:354

Hyodo T, Megyesi IK, Kahn CR, McLean JP, Friesen HG (1977) Adrenocortical carcinoma and hypoglycemia: Evidence for production of non-suppressible insulin-like activity by the tumor. J Clin Endocrinol Metab 44:1175

Idelman S (1978) The structure of the mammalian adrenal cortex. In: Chester Jones I, Henderson IW (eds) General, comparative and clinical endocrinology of the adrenal cortex, Vol 2. Academic Press, London New York San Francisco, p 2

Igarashi M, Schaumburg HH, Powers J (1976) Fatty acid abnormality in adrenoleukodystrophy. J Neurochem 26:851

Irvine WJ, Barnes EW (1972) Adrenocortical insufficiency. Clin Endocrinol Metab 1:549

Irvine WJ, Barnes EW (1974) Addison's disease and autoimmune ovarian failure. J Reprod Fertil [Suppl] 21:1

Irvine WJ, Stewart AG, Scarth L (1967) A clinical and immunological study of adrenocortical insufficiency (Addison's disease). Clin Exp Immunol 2:31

Irvine WJ, Chan MMW, Scarth L, Kolb FO, Hartog M, Bayliss RIS, Drury MI (1968) Immunological aspects of premature ovarian failure associated with idiopathic Addison's disease. Lancet II:883

Irvine WJ, Chan MMW, Scarth L (1969) The further characterization of autoantibodies reactive with extra-adrenal steroid producing cells in patients with adrenal disorders. Clin Exp Immunol 4:489

Irvine WJ, Toft AD, Feek CH (1979) Addison's disease. In: James VHT (ed) The adrenal gland. Raven, New York, p 131

Isherwood DM, Oakey RE (1976) Control of oestrogen production in human pregnancy: Effect of trophic hormones on steroid biosynthesis by the foetal adrenal gland in vitro. J Endocrinol 68:321

Israeli E, Levy J, Rosental E, Auslaender L, Peleg I, Barzilai D (1975) A human adrenocortical adenoma in tissue culture. Isr J Med Sci 11:1106

Jacobi JD, Carballeira A, Fishman LM (1978) Adrenal cysts: Hormonal contents and functional evaluation. Acta Endocrinol (Copenh) 88:347

Jaffe RB, Payne AH (1971) Gonadal steroid sulfates and sulfatase IV. Comparative studies on steroid sulfokinase in the human fetal testis and adrenal. J Clin Endocrinol Metab 33:392

Jaffe RB, Seron-Ferre M, Huhtaniemi I, Korenbrot C (1977) Regulation of the primate fetal adrenal gland and testis in vitro and in vivo. J Steroid Biochem 8:479

James VHT, Landon J, Fraser R (1968) Some observations on the control of corticosteroid secretion in man. Mem Soc Endocrinol 17:141

James VHT, Tunbridge RDG, Wilson GA (1976) Studies on the control of aldosterone secretion in man. J Steroid Biochem 7:941

James VHT, Serio M, Guisti G, Martini L (1978a) The endocrine function of the human adrenal cortex. Academic Press, London, New York San Francisco

James VHT, Tunbridge RDG, Wilson GA, Hutton J, Jacobs HS, Rippon AE (1978b) Steroid profiling: A technique for exploring adrenocortical physiology. In: James VHT, Serio M, Giusti G, Martini L (eds) The endocrine function of the human adrenal cortex. Academic Press, London New York San Francisco, p 179

Janigan DT (1963) Cytoplasmic bodies in the adrenal cortex of patients treated with spironolactone. Lancet I:850

Jara-Albarran A, Bayort J, Caballero A, Portillo J, Laborda L, Sampedro M, Cure C, Palacios Meteos JM (1979) Probable pituitary adenoma with adrenocorticotropin hypersecretion (corticotropinoma) secondary to Addison's disease. J Clin Endocrinol Metab 49:236

Jarvis JL, Seaman WB (1959) Idiopathic adrenal calcification in infants and children. Am J Roentgenol 82:510

Jean R, Legrand J-C, Meylan F, Rieu D, Astruc J (1969) Hypoaldostéronisme primaire par anomalie probable de la 18-hydroxylation. Arch Fr Pediatr 26:769

Jeffcoate WJ, Edwards CRW (1979) Cushing's syndrome: Pathogenesis diagnosis, and treatment. In: James VHT (ed) The adrenal gland. Raven Press, New York, p 165

Jenis EH, Hertzog RW (1969) Effect of spironolactone on the zona glomerulosa. Light and electron microscopy. Arch Pathol 88:530

Jenkins JS (1965). Metabolism of cortisol by the human adrenal cortex in vitro. J Clin Endocrinol Metab 25:649

Jessiman AG, Matson DD, Moore FD (1959) Hypophysectomy in the treatment of breast cancer. N Engl J Med 261:1199

Johannisson E (1968) The foetal adrenal cortex in the human. Its ultrastructure at different stages of development and in different functional states. Acta Endocrinol (Copenh) [Suppl] 130:1

Johnstone FRC (1957) The suprarenal veins. Am J Surg 94:615

Jones T, Groom M, Griffiths K (1970) Steroid biosynthesis by culture of normal human adrenal tissue. Biochem Biophys Res Commun 38:355

Jones CT, Roebuck MM (1980) ACTH peptides and the development of the fetal adrenal. J Steroid Biochem 12:77

Joseph TJ, Vogt PJ (1974) Disseminated herpes with hepatoadrenal necrosis in an adult. Am J Med 56:735

Josse RJ, Bear R, Kovacs K, Higgins HP (1980) Cushing's syndrome due to unilateral nodular adrenal hyperplasia: A new pathophysiological entity? Acta Endocrinol (Copenh) 93:495

Jost A (1975) The fetal adrenal cortex. In: Greep RO, Astwood EB (eds) Handbook of physiology Vol VI. Adrenal gland, Amer Physiol Soc, Washington, p 107

Kafrouni G, Oakes MD, Lurvey AN, DeQuattro V (1975) Aldosteronoma in a child with localization by adrenal vein aldosterone: Collective review of the literature. J Pediatr Surg 10:917

Kahn CR (1980) The riddle of tumour hypoglycaemia revisited. Clin Endocrinol Metab 9:335

Kahri AI, Pesonen S, Saure A (1970) Ultrastructure differentiation and progesterone-^{14}C metabolism in cultured cells of fetal rat adrenals under influence of ACTH. Steroidologia 1:25

Kahri AI, Huhtaniemi I, Salmenperä M (1976) Steroid formation and differentiation of cortical cells in tissue culture of human fetal adrenals in the presence and absence of ACTH. Endocrinology 98:33

Kahri AI, Voutilainen R, Salmenperä M (1979) Different biological action of corticosteroids, corticosterone and cortisol as a base of zonal function of adrenal cortex. Acta Endocrinol (Copenh) 91:329

Kaminsky N, Luse S, Hartroft P (1962) Ultrastructure of adrenal cortex of the dog during treatment with DDD. J Natl Cancer Inst 29:127

Kamp P, Platz P, Nerup J (1974) 'Steroid-cell' antibody in endocrine diseases. Acta Endocrinol (Copenh) 76:729

Kampmeier O (1927) Giant epithelial cells of the human fetal adrenal. Anat Rec 37:95

Kandeel FR, Rudd BT, Butt WR, Edwards RL, London DR (1978) Androgen and cortisol responses to ACTH stimulation in women with hyperprolactinaemia. Clin Endocrinol (Oxf) 9:123

Kano K, Sato S (1977) Fine structure of adrenal adenomata causing Cushing's syndrome. Virchows Arch [Pathol Anat] 374:157

Kano KI, Sato S, Hama H (1979) Adrenal adenomata causing primary aldosteronism. An ultrastructural study of twenty-five cases. Virchows Arch [Pathol Anat] 384:93

Kaplan NM (1967) The steroid content of adrenal adenomas and measurements of aldosterone production in patients with essential hypertension and primary hyperaldosteronism. J Clin Invest 46:728

Kaplan NM (1974) Adrenal causes of hypertension. Arch Intern Med 133:1001

Kaplan NM, Bartter FC (1962) The effect of ACTH, renin, angiotensin II, and various precursors on biosynthesis of aldosterone by adrenal slices. J Clin Invest 41:715

Katz FH, Romfh P, Smith JA (1972) Episodic secretion of aldosterone in supine man: Relationship to cortisol. J Clin Endocrinol Metab 35:178

Katz FH, Beck P, Makowski EL (1974) The renin-aldosterone system in mother and fetus at term. Am J Obstet Gynecol 118:51

Kaufman G (1974) Adrenal cortical necrosis. An autopsy study. Arch Pathol 97:395

Kay S (1976) Hyperplasia and neoplasia of the adrenal gland. Pathol Annu 11:103

Kearny GP, Mahoney EM (1977) Adrenal cysts. Urol Clin North Am 4:273

Keene MFL, Hewer EE (1927) Observations on the development of the human suprarenal gland. J Anat 61:302

Kelch RP, Kaplan SL, Biglieri EG, Daniels GH, Epstein CJ, Grumbach MM (1972) Hereditary adrenocortical unresponsiveness to adrenocorticotropic hormone. J Pediatr 81:726

Kelch RP, Connors MH, Kaplan SL, Biglieri EG, Grumbach MM (1973) A calcified aldosterone-producing tumor in a hypertensive, normokalemic, prepubertal girl. J Pediatr 83:432

Kelly WF, Joplin GF, Pearson GW (1977) Gonadotrophin deficiency and adrenocortical insufficiency in children: A new syndrome. Br Med J ii:98

Kelly WF, Barnes AJ, Cassar J, White M, Mashiter K, Loizou S, Welbourn RB, Joplin GF (1979) Cushing's syndrome due to adrenocortical carcinoma – a comprehensive clinical and biochemical study of patients treated by surgery and chemotherapy. Acta Endocrinol (Copenh) 91:303

Kem DC, Gomez-Sanchez C, Kramer NJ, Holland OB, Higgins JR (1975) Plasma aldosterone and renin activity response to ACTH infusion in dexamethasone-suppressed normal and sodium-depleted man. J Clin Endocrinol Metab 40:116

Kendall EC (1941) Function of adrenal cortex. JAMA 116:2394

Kendall EC, Mason HL, McKenzie BF, Myers CS, Koelsche GA (1934) Isolation in crystalline form of the hormone essential to life from the suprarenal cortex: Its chemical nature and physiologic properties. Mayo Clin Proc 9:245

Kendall JW, Sloop PR (1968) Dexamethasone-suppressible adrenocortical tumor. N Engl J Med 279:532

Kenny FM, Preeyasombat C, Migeon CJ (1966) Cortisol production rate. II Normal infants, children and adults. Pediatrics 37:34

Kenny FM, Hashida Y, Askari HA, Sieber WH, Fetterman GH (1968) Virilizing tumors of the adrenal cortex. Am J Dis Child 115:445

Kenny FM, Reynolds JW, Green OC (1971) Partial 3β-hydroxysteroid dehydrogenase (3β-HSD) deficiency in a family with congenital adrenal hyperplasia: evidence for increasing 3β-HSD activity with age. Pediatrics 48:756

Kerenyi N (1961) Congenital adrenal hypoplasia. Report of a case with extreme adrenal hypoplasia and neurohypophyseal aplasia, drawing attention to certain aspects of etiology and classification. Arch Pathol 71:336

Keymolen V, Dor P, Borkowski A (1976) Output of oestrogens, testosterone and their precursors by isolated human adrenal cells as compared with that of glucocorticosteroids. J Endocrinol 71:219

Khoury EL, Hammond L, Bottazzo GF, Doniach D (1981) Surface-reactive antibodies to human adrenal cells in Addison's disease. Clin Exp Immunol 45:48

Kielman N, Stachenko J, Giroud CJP (1966) Production rate of corticosterone sulfate in normal human adults. Steroids 8:993

King DR, Lack EE (1979) Adrenal cortical carcinoma. A clinical and pathologic study of 49 cases. Cancer 44:239

Kirkland RT, Kirkland JL, Librik L, Clayton GW (1972) The incidence of associated anomalies in 105 patients with congenital adrenal hyperplasia. Pediatrics 49:608

Kirkland RT, Kirkland JL, Johnson CM, Horning MG, Librik L, Clayton GW (1973) Congenital lipoid hyperplasia in an eight-year-old phenotypic female. J Clin Endocrinol Metab 36:488

Kirkland RT, Kirkland JL, Keenan BS, Bongiovanni AM, Rosenberg HS, Clayton GW (1977) Bilateral testicular tumors in congenital adrenal hyperplasia. J Clin Endocrinol Metab 44:369

Kirschner MA, Powell RD, Lipsett MB (1964) Cushings syndrome: nodular cortical hyperplasia of adrenal glands with clinical and pathological features suggesting adrenocortical tumor. J Clin Endocrinol Metab 24:947

Kirschner MA, Wiqvist N, Diczfalusy E (1966) Studies on oestriol synthesis from dehydroepiandrosterone sulphate in human pregnancy. Acta Endocrinol (Copenh) 53:584

Klein A, Curtius HC, Zachmann M (1974) Difference in 11β-hydroxylation of deoxycortisol and deoxycorticosterone by human adrenals. J Steroid Biochem 5:557

Klein GP, Giroud CJP (1967) Incorporation of 7α-³H-pregnenolone and 4-¹⁴C-progesterone into corticosteroids and some of their ester sulfates by human newborn adrenal slices. steroids 9:113

Klevit HD, Campbell RA, Blair HR, Bongiovanni AM (1966) Cushing's syndrome with nodular adrenal hyperplasia in infancy. J Pediatr 68:912

Koenig UD (1972) Besondere Fehlbildungen bei Nebennieren. Anat Anz 132:303

Koizumi S, Kyoya S, Miyawaki T, Kidani H, Funabashi T, Nakashima H, Nakanuma Y, Ohta G, Itagaki E, Katagiri M (1977) Cholesterol side-chain cleavage enzyme activity and cytochrome P-450 content in adrenal mitochondria of a patient with congenital lipoid adrenal hyperplasia (Prader disease). Clin Chim Acta 77:301

Kolanowski J, Crabbe J (1976) Characteristics of the response of human adrenocortical cells to ACTH. Mol Cell Endocrinol 5:255

Kolanowski J, Esselinckx W, Deuxchaisnes CN, Crabbe J (1977) Adrenocortical response upon repeated stimulation with corticotrophin in patients lacking endogenous corticotrophin secretion. Acta Endocrinol (Copenh) 85:595

Köllicker A von (1854) Mikroscopische Anatomie oder Gewebelehre des Menschen, Bd 2. Zweite Hälfte Leipzig, p 337

Komanicky P, Spark RF, Melby JC (1978) Treatment of Cushing's syndrome with trilostane (WIN 24,240), an inhibitor of adrenal steroid biosynthesis. J Clin Endocrinol Metab 47:1042

Kominami S, Ochi H, Kobayashi Y, Takemori S (1980) Studies on the steroid hydroxylation system in adrenal cortex microsomes. Purification and characterisation of cytochrome P-450 specific for steroid C-21 hydroxylation. J Biol Chem 255:3386

Kondo K, Saruta T, Saito I, Yoshida R, Maruyama H, Matsuki S (1976) Benign desoxycorticosterone-producing adrenal tumor. JAMA 236:1042

Kono T, Oseko F, Shimpo S, Nanno M, Endo J (1975) Biological activity of des-asp¹-angiotensin II (angiotensin III) in man. J Clin Endocrinol Metab 41:1174

Kornel L, Ezzeraimi E (1980) Cortisol-21-sulfate (FS) is secreted by the human adrenal gland. Proc VI Intern Congress Endocrinol, Melbourne Australia, Abstr 419

Koroscil TM, Gallant S (1980) On the mechanism of action of adrenocorticotropic hormone. The role of ACTH-stimulated phosphorylation and dephosphorylation of adrenal proteins. J Biol Chem 255:6276

Korth-Schutz S, Levine LS, New MI (1976a) Evidence for the adrenal source of androgens in precocious adrenarche. Acta Endocrinol (Copenh) 82:342

Korth-Schutz S, Levine LS, New MI (1976b) Dehydroepiandrosterone sulfate (DS) levels, a rapid test for abnormal adrenal androgen secretion. J Clin Endocrinol Metab 42:1005

Korth-Schutz S, Levine LS, Roth LA, Saenger P, New MI (1977) Virilizing adrenal tumor in a child suppressed with dexamethasone for three years. Effect of o,p'-DDD on serum and urinary androgens. J Clin Endocrinol Metab 44:433

Koss LG, Rothschild EO, Fleischer M, Francis JE (1969) Masculinizing tumor of the ovary, apparently with adrenocortical activity. Cancer 23:1245

Kosseff AL, Herrmann J, Optiz JM (1972) The Wiedemann-Beckwith syndrome: genetic considerations and a diagnostic sign. Lancet I:844

Kovacs K, Horvath E (1973) Ultrastructural features of corticomedullary cells in a human adrenocortical adenoma and in rat adrenal cortex. Anat Anz 134:387

Kovacs K, Horvath E, Singer W (1973) Fine structure and morphogenesis of spironolactone bodies in the zona glomerulosa of the human adrenal cortex. J Clin Pathol 26:949

Kovacs K, Horvath E, Delarue NC, Laidlaw JC (1974) Ultrastructural features of an aldosterone-secreting adrenocortical adenoma. Horm Res 5:47

Kovacs K, Horvath E, Feldman PS (1976) Pigmented adenoma of adrenal cortex associated with Cushing's syndrome. Light and electron microscopic study. Urology 7:641

Kowarski A, Lacerda L, Migeon CJ (1975) Integrated concentration of plasma aldosterone in normal subjects: correlation with cortisol. J Clin Endocrinol Metab 40:205

Kracht J (1971) Nebennierenpathologie des Cushing-Syndroms bei Kindern und Jugendlichen. Verh Dtsch Ges Pathol 55:142

Kramer RE, Gallant S, Brownie AC (1979) The role of cytochrome P-450 in the action of sodium depletion on aldosterone biosynthesis in rats. J Biol Chem 254:3953

Kramer RE, Gallant S, Brownie AC (1980) Actions of angiotensin II on aldosterone biosynthesis in the rat adrenal cortex. J Biol Chem 255:3442

Kreiner E, Dhöm G (1979) Altersveränderungen der menschlichen Nebenniere. Zbl Allg Pathol Anat 123:351

Krieger DT (1980) Plasma ACTH and corticosteroids. In: De Groot LJ et al. (eds) Endocrinology, vol 2. Grune and Stratton, New York, p 1139

Krieger DT, Allen W (1975) Relationship of bioassayable and immunoassayable plasma ACTH and cortisol concentrations in normal subjects and in patients with Cushing's disease. J Clin Endocrinol Metab 40:675

Krieger DT, Allen W, Rizzo F, Krieger HP (1971) Characterization of the normal temporal pattern of plasma corticosteroid levels. J Clin Endocrinol Metab 32:266

Krieger DT, Amorosa L, Linick F (1975) Cyproheptadine-induced remission of Cushing's disease. N Engl J Med 293:893

Krieger DT, Samojlik E, Bardin CW (1978) Cortisol and androgen secretion in a case of Nelson's syndrome with paratesticular tumors: response to cyproheptadine therapy. J Clin Endocrinol Metab 47:837

Krølner B, Larsen S, Nielsen MD (1979) Corticosterone secreting adrenal carcinoma and empty sella turcica: A case report. Acta Endocrinol (Copenh) 91:650

Krumrey WA, Buss IO (1969) Observations on the adrenal gland of the African elephant. J Mammal 50:90

Lancisius JM (1714) Tabulae anatomicae of Bartholomaeus Eustachius. Romae

Lanman JT (1956) Physiology of prematurity. Josiah Macy Foundation, New York p 29

Lanman JT (1961) The adrenal gland in the human fetus. An interpretation of its physiology and unusual developmental pattern. Pediatrics 27:140

Lanman JT (1962) Interpretation of human foetal adrenal structure and function. In: Currie AR, Symington T, Grant JK (eds) The human adrenal cortex. Livingstone, Edinburgh, p 547

Lanman JT, Silverman LM (1957) In vitro steroidogenesis in the human neonatal adrenal gland, including observations on human adult and monkey adrenal glands. Endocrinology 60:433

Laragh JH, Stoerk HC (1957) A study of the mechanism of secretion of the sodium-retaining hormone (aldosterone). J Clin Invest 36:383

Laragh JH, Ulick S, Januszcwicz V, Deming QB, Kelley WG, Liebermann S (1960) Aldosterone secretion in primary and malignant hypertension. J Clin Invest 39:1091

Laragh JH, Ledingham JGG, Sommers SC (1967) Secondary aldosteronism and reduced plasma renin in hypertensive disease. Trans Assoc Am Physicians 80:168

Larson BA, Vanderlaan WP, Judd HL, McCullough DL (1976) A testosterone-producing adrenal cortical adenoma in an elderly woman. J Clin Endocrinol Metab 42:882

Lauritzen C, Lehmann WD (1965) Ausscheidung von Dehydroepiandrosteron im Neugeborenenharn. Stimulierung durch Choriongonadotropin und ACTH. Arch Gynäkol 200:699

Lauritzen C, Lehmann WD (1967) Levels of chorionic gonadotrophin in the newborn infant and their relationship to adrenal dehydroepiandrosterone. J Endocrinol 39:173

Laverty CRA, Fortune DW, Beischer NA (1973) Congenital idiopathic adrenal hypoplasia. Obstet Gynecol 41:655

Lawson DW, Corry RJ, Patton AS, Daggett WM, Austen G (1969) Massive retroperitoneal adrenal hemorrhage. Surg Gynecol Obstet 129:989

Laychock SG, Franson RC, Weglicki WB, Rubin RP (1977) Identification and partial characterization of phospholipases in isolated adrenocortical cells: The effects of ACTH and calcium. Biochem J 164:753

Lazorthes G, Gaubert J, Poulhès J, Roulleau J, Martinez-Cobo C (1959) Note sur la vascularisation de la surrénale. CR Assoc Anat 45:489

Lebreuil G, Garbe L, Payan H (1971) Aspects anatomo – cliniques de la maladie cytomégalique de l'adulte. Arch Anat Cytol Pathol 19:247

Leditschke JF, Arden F (1964) Feminizing adrenal adenoma in a five year old boy. Aust Paediatr J 10:217

Lee PA, Kowarski A, Migeon CJ, Blizzard RM (1975) Lack of correlation between gonadotropin and adrenal androgen levels in agonadal children. J Clin Endocrinol Metab 40:664

Lee PA, Xenakis T, Winer J, Matsenbaugh S (1978) Independence of gonadotropin and adrenal androgen secretion. Andrologia 10:369

Leger L, Bouvresse M, DesLigneres S (1975) Cortico-surrénalome malin sur surrénale accessoire. J Chir (Paris) 110:7

Lehmann WD, Lauritzen C (1975) HCG + ACTH stimulation of in vitro dehydroepiandrosterone production in human fetal adrenals from precursor cholesterol and Δ^5-pregnenolone. J Perinat Med 3:231

Lejeune-Lenain C, Khodjasten Z, Copinschi G, Desir D, Franckson JRM (1980) Control of 11β-hydroxyandrostenedione secretion in normal adults. In: Genazzani AR, Thijssen JHH, Siiteri PK (eds) Adrenal androgens. Raven Press, New York, p 183

Letulle M (1889) Note sur la dégénerescence grasseuse de la capsule surrénale. Bull Mem Soc Anat Paris 3:264

Levin J, Cluff LE (1965) A study on endotoxemia and adrenal hemorrhage. A mechanism for the Waterhouse-Friderichsen syndrome. J Exp Med 121:247

Levin SE, Collins DL, Kaplan GW, Weller MH (1974) Neonatal adrenal pseudocyst mimicking metastatic disease. Ann Surg 179:186

Levine LS, Zachmann M, New MI, Prader A, Pollack MS, O'Neill GJ, Yang SY, Oberfield SE, Dupont B (1978) Genetic mapping of the 21-hydroxylase deficiency gene within the HLA linkage group. N Engl J Med 299:911

Levine LS, Dupont B, Lorenzen F, Pang S, Pollack M, Oberfield S, Kohn B, Lerner A, Cacciari E, Mantero F, Cassio A, Scaroni C, Chiumello G, Rondanini GF, Gargantini L, Giovannelli G, Virdis R, Bartolotta E, Migliori C, Pintor C, Tato L, Barboni F, New MI (1980a) Cryptic 21-hydroxylase deficiency in families of patients with classical congenital adrenal hyperplasia. J Clin Endocrinol Metab 51:1316

Levine LS, Rauh W, Gottesdiener K, Chow D, Gunczler P, Rapaport R, Pang S, Schneider B, New MI (1980b) New studies of the 11β-hydroxylase and 18-hydroxylase enzymes in the hypertensive form of congenital adrenal hyperplasia. J Clin Endocrinol Metab 50:258

Lewinsky BS, Grigor KM, Symington T, Neville AM (1974) The clinical and pathologic features of 'non-hormonal' adrenocortical tumors. Report of twenty new cases and review of the literature. Cancer 33:778

Lewis RA, Klein R, Wilkins L (1950) Congenital adrenal hyperplasia with pseudohermaphrodism and symptoms of Addison's disease. J. Clin Endocr Metab. 10:703

Leydig F (1852) Beitrage zur mikroskopische Anatomie und Entwicklungsgeschichte der Rochen und Haie. Leipzig

Li CH, Evans HM, Simpson ME (1943) Adrenocorticotropic hormone. J Biol Chem 149:413

Li FP, Fraumeni JF (1969) Soft-tissue sarcomas, breast cancer, and other neoplasms. A familial syndrome? Ann Intern Med 71:747

Liddle GW (1960) Tests of pituitary adrenal suppressibility in the diagnosis of Cushing's syndrome. J Clin Endocrinol Metab 20:1539

Liddle GW, Duncan LE, Bartter FC (1956) Dual mechanism regulating adrenocortical function in man. Am J Med 21:380

Liddle GW, Givens JR, Nicholson WE, Island DP (1965) The ectopic ACTH syndrome. Cancer Res 25:1057

Liddle GW, Sennett JA (1975) New mineralocorticoids in the syndrome of low-renin essential hypertension. J Steroid Biochem 6:751

Lightwood R (1932) Tumour of suprarenal cortex in an infant of 18 weeks. Arch Dis Child 7:35

Lieberman AH, Luetscher JA (1960) Some effects of abnormalities of pituitary, adrenal or thyroid function on excretion of aldosterone and the response to corticotropin or sodium deprivation. J Clin Endocrinol Metab 20:1004

Liggins GC (1976) Adrenocortical – related maturational events in the fetus. Am J Obstet Gynecol 126:931

Limjuco RA, Sherman L, Kolodny HD (1976) Isolated ACTH deficiency NY State J Med 76:439

Linde R, Coulam C, Battino R, Rhamy R, Gerlock J, Hollifield J (1979) Localization of aldosterone-producing adenoma by computed tomography. J Clin Endocrinol Metab 49:642

Lindholm, J, Kehlet H, Riishede J (1980) Urinary excretion of cortisol in acromegaly. J Clin Endocrinol Metab 50:796

Liotta A, Osathanondh R, Ryan KJ, Krieger DT (1977) Presence of corticotropin in human placenta: Demonstration of in vitro synthesis. Endocrinology 101:1552

Lipsett MB, Wilson H (1962) Adrenocortical cancer: Steroid biosynthesis and metabolism evaluated by urinary metabolites. J Clin Endocrinol Metab 22:906

Lipsett MB, Hertz R, Ross GT (1963) Clinical and pathophysiologic aspects of adrenocortical carcinoma. Am J Med 35:374

Lipsett MB, Kirschner MA, Wilson H, Bardin CW (1970) Malignant lipid cell tumor of the ovary: clinical, biochemical and etiologic considerations. J Clin Endocrinol Metab 30:336

Lisboa BP, Strassner M, Nocke-Finck L, Breuer H, Bayer JM (1978) Studies on the metabolism of steroid hormones in a virilizing adrenal cortex adenoma. Endokrinologie 72:311

Loeb RF (1932) Chemical changes in the blood in Addison's disease. Science 76:420

Long JA, Jones AL (1967) Observations on the fine structure of the adrenal cortex of man. Lab Invest 17:355

Lopez Engelking R, Ibarra Esparza N, Jimenez Velasco D, Maldonado E (1967) Myelolipoma of the adrenal gland and kidney adenocarcinoma: clinical case. J Urol 98:419

Lorenzen F, Pang S, New M, Pollack M, Oberfield S, Dupont B, Chow D, Schneider B, Levine L (1980) Studies of the C-21 and C-19 steroids and HLA genotyping in siblings and parents of patients with congenital adrenal hyperplasia due to 21-hydroxylase deficiency. J Clin Endocrinol Metab 50:572

Loriaux DL, Ruder HJ, Lipsett MB (1974) Plasma steroids in congenital adrenal hyperplasia. J Clin Endocrinol Metab 39:627

Loridan L, Senior B (1969) Cushing's syndrome in infancy. J Pediatr 9:62

Lubitz JA, Freeman L, Okun R (1973) Mitotane use in inoperable adrenal cortical carcinoma. JAMA 223:1109

Lucis OJ, Lucis R (1971) Comparison of steroidogenesis in adrenal tissue and adrenal adenoma from a case of primary aldosteronism. J Steroid Biochem 2:19

Luetscher JA, Axelrad BJ (1954) Increased aldosterone output during sodium deprivation in normal man. Proc Soc Exp Biol Med 87:650

Luetscher JA, Johnson BB (1954) Chromatographic separation of the sodium-retaining corticoid from the urine of children with nephrosis, compared with observations on normal children. J Clin Invest 33:276

Luetscher JA, Ganguly A, Melada GA, Dowdy AJ (1974) Preoperative differentiation of adrenal adenoma from ideopathic adrenal hyperplasia in primary aldosteronism. Circ Res [Suppl] 34 & 35:175

Lumb G, MacKenzie DH (1959) The incidence of metastases in adrenal glands and ovaries removed for carcinoma of the breast. Cancer 12:521

Luton JP, Mahoudeau JA, Bouchard P, Thieblot P, Hautcouverture M, Simon D, Laudat MH, Touitou Y, Bricaire H (1979) Treatment of Cushing's disease by o,p'-DDD. N Engl J Med 300:459

Lynn RB (1965) Cystic lymphangioma of the adrenal associated with arterial hypertension. Can J Surg 8:92

MacAdam RF (1970) Fine structure of a functional adrenal cortical adenoma. Cancer 26:1300

MacAdam RF (1971) Black adenoma of the human adrenal cortex. Cancer 27:116

MacKay AM (1969) Atlas of human adrenal cortex ultrastructure. In: Symington T (ed) Functional pathology of the human adrenal gland. Livingstone, Edinburgh, p 346

MacLaren NK, Migeon CJ, Raiti S (1975) Gynecomastia with congenital virilizing adrenal hyperplasia (11-β-hydroxylase deficiency). J Pediatr 86:579

MacNaughton MC, Taylor T, McNally EM, Coutts JRT (1977) The effect of synthetic ACTH on the metabolism of (4-^{14}C)-progesterone by the previable human fetus. J Steroid Biochem 8:499

Maeir F, Staehelin M (1968a) Adrenal hyperaemia caused by corticotrophin. Acta Endocrinol (Copenh) 58:613

Maeir R, Staehelin M (1968b) Adrenal responses to corticotrophin in the presence of an inhibitor of protein synthesis. Acta Endocrinol (Copenh) 58:619

Magalháes MC (1972) A new crystal-containing cell in human adrenal cortex. J Cell Biol 55:126

Mahloudji M, Ronaghy H, Dutz W (1971) Virilizing adrenal carcinoma in two sibs. J Med Genet 8:160

Maltini G, Arzilli F, Simonini N, Salvetti A (1973) The histopathology of Conn's adenoma and of attached adrenal cortex. Folia Endocrinol (Roma) 26:85

Mantero F, Scaroni C, Pasini CV, Fagiolo U (1980) No linkage between HLA and congenital adrenal hyperplasia due to 17-alpha-hydroxylase deficiency. N Engl J Med 303:530

Marchand F (1883) Uber accessorische Nebennieren im Ligamentum latum. Virchows Arch 92:11

Marek J, Mötlik K (1975) Ultrastructural changes of the adrenal cortex in Cushing's syndrome treated with aminoglutethimide (Elipten®, Ciba). Virchows Arch [Cell Pathol] 18:145

Marie J (1952) Le syndrome d'hyperplasie cérébriforme des surrénales de la périod néonatal (Syndrome de Debre-Fibiger). Arch Fr Ped 9:785

Marine D, Baumann EJ (1927) Duration of life after suprarenalectomy in cats and attempts to prolong it by injections of solutions containing sodium salts, glucose and glycerol. Am J Physiol 81:86

Marks TM, Thomas JM, Warkany J (1940) Adrenocortical obesity in children. Am J Dis Child 60:923

Maroulis GB, Abraham GE (1980) Concentration of androgens and cortisol in the zones of the adrenal cortex. In: Genazzani AR, Thijssen JHH, Siiteri PK (eds) Adrenal androgens. Raven Press, New York, p 49

Marquezy RA, Bricaire H, Laudat M-H, Courjaret J, Philbert M (1965) Adénocarcinome de la surrénale avec syndrome d'hyperandrogénie et syndrome d'hyperminéralocorticisme. Elimination urinaire du composé S et de la tetrahydro S, de la deoxycorticostérone e de la tétrahydrodesoxycorticostérone. Ann Endocrinol (Paris) 26:247

Marshall EK, Davis DM (1916) The influence of adrenals of the kidneys. J Pharmacol Exp Ther 8:525

Marshall JC, Anderson DC, Fraser TR, Harsoulis P (1973) Human luteinizing hormone in man: Studies of metabolism and biological action. J Endocrinol 56:431

Marshall WC, Ockenden BG, Fosbrooke AS, Cumings JN (1969) Wolman's disease. A rare lipidosis with adrenal calcification. Arch Dis Child 44:331

Marsiglia I, Pinto J (1966) Adrenal cortical insufficiency associated with paracoccidioidomycosis (South America blastomycosis). Report of four patients. J Clin Endocrinol Metab 26:1109

Marusic ET, Mulrow PJ (1967) Stimulation of aldosterone biosynthesis in adrenal mitochondria by sodium depletion. J Clin Invest 46:2101

Marusic ET, Mulrow PJ (1969) 18-Hydrocorticosterone biosynthesis in an aldosterone secreting tumor and in the surrounding nontumorous adrenal gland. Proc Soc Exp Biol Med 131:778

Marver D, Edelman IS (1978) Dihydrocortisol: A potential mineralocorticoid. J Steroid Biochem 9:1

Mason AS, Meade TW, Lee JAH, Morris JN (1968) Epidemiological and clinical picture of Addison's disease. Lancet II:744

Mason HL, Sprague RG (1948) Isolation of 17-hydroxycorticosterone from the urine in a case of Cushing's syndrome associated with severe diabetes mellitus. J Biol Chem 175:451

Mason PA, Lebel M, Fraser R (1975) A comparison of the dose-response relationships between ACTH and the corticosteroids, cortisol (F), 11-deoxycortisol (S), corticosterone (B), 11-deoxycorticosterone (DOC), 18-hydroxy-DOC (18-OH-DOC) and aldosterone in normal human subjects. Acta Endocrinol [Suppl] (Copenh) 199:364

Mason PA, Fraser R, Morton JJ, Semple PF, Wilson A (1976) The effect of angiotensin II infusion on plasma corticosteroid concentrations in normal man. J Steroid Biochem 7:859

Mason PA, Fraser R, Morton JJ, Semple PF, Wilson A (1977) The effect of sodium deprivation and of angiotensin II infusion on the peripheral plasma concentrations of 18-hydroxycorticosterone, aldosterone and other corticosteroids in man. J Steroid Biochem 8:799

Mason PA, Fraser R, Semple PF, Morton JJ (1979) The interaction of ACTH and angiotensin II in the control of corticosteroid plasma concentration in man. J Steroid Biochem 10:235

Mathur RS, Williamson HO, Moody LO, Diczfalusy E (1973) In vitro sterol and steroid biogenesis by a feminizing adrenocortical carcinoma. Acta Endocrinol (Copenh) 73:518

Matsukura S, Kakita T, Sueoka S, Yoshimi H, Hirata Y, Yokota M, Fujita T (1980) Multiple hormone receptors in the adenylate cylase of human adrenocortical tumors. Cancer Res 40:3768

Matsumoto K, Endo H, Yamane G, Kurachi K, Uozumi T (1968) 16α-Hydroxylation of pregnenolone by human fetus. Endocrinol Jpn 15:189

Matsuoka H, Mulrow PJ, Li CH (1980) β-Lipotropin: A new aldosterone stimulating factor. Science 209:307

Matsuoka H, Mulrow PJ, Franco-Saenz R, Li CH (1981) Stimulation of aldosterone production by β-melanotropin. Nature 291:155

Mäusle E (1971) Ultrastruktur des Involutionsprozesses der Cortex fetalis beim menschlichen Neugeborenen. Verh Dtsch Ges Pathol 55:147

Mäusle E (1972) Elektronmikroskopische Befunde an der menschlichen Neugeborenen-Nebenniere. Beitr Pathol 146:221

McArthur RG, Cloutier MD, Hayles AB, Sprague RG (1972) Cushing's disease in children. Findings in 13 cases. Mayo Clin Proc 47:318

McCaa RE, Young DB, Guyton AC, McCaa CS (1974) Evidence for a role of an unidentified pituitary factor in regulating aldosterone secretion during altered sodium balance. Circ Res [Suppl] 34–35:15

McCaa RE, Montalvo JM, McCaa SS (1978) Role of growth hormone in the regulation of aldosterone biosynthesis. J Clin Endocrinol Metab 46:247

McDonnell WV (1956) Myelolipoma of adrenal. Arch Pathol 61:416

McErlean DP, Doyle FH (1976) The pituitary fossa in Cushing's syndrome: A retrospective analysis of 93 patients. Br J Radiol 49:820

McKenna TJ, Miller RB, Liddle GW (1977) Plasma pregnenolone in patients with adrenal tumors, ACTH excess or idiopathic hirsutism. J Clin Endocrinol Metab 44:231

McKenna TJ, Island DP, Nicholson WE, Liddle GW (1978) Angiotensin stimulates cortisol biosynthesis in human adrenal cells in vitro. Steroids 32:127

McNutt NS, Jones AL (1970) Observations on the ultrastructure of cytodifferentiation in the human fetal adrenal cortex. Lab Invest 22:513

McQuarrie I, Johnson RM, Ziegler MR (1937) Plasma electrolyte disturbance in patient with hypercorticoadrenal syndrome contrasted with that found in Addison's disease. Endocrinology 21:762

Meador CK, Bowdoin B, Owen WC, Farmer TA Jr (1967) Primary adrenocortical nodular dysplasia: A rare cause of Cushing's syndrome. J Clin Endocrinol Metab 27:1255

Meckel JF (1806) Abhandlungen aus der menschlichen und vergleichenden Anatomie und Physiologie. Halle

Melby JC (1972) Identifying the adrenal lesion in primary aldosteronism. Ann Intern Med 76:1039

Melby JC, Dale SL, Grekin RJ, Gaunt R, Wilson TE (1972) 18-Hydroxy-11-deoxycorticosterone (18-OH-DOC) secretion in experimental and human hypertension. Recent Prog Horm Res 26:287

Menard RH, Bartter FC, Gillette JR (1976) Spironolactone and cytochrome P-450: Impairment of steroid 21-hydroxylation in the adrenal cortex. Arch Biochem Biophys 173:395

Menard RH, Guenthner TM, Kon H, Gillette JR (1979) Studies on the destruction of adrenal and testicular cytochrome P-450 by spironolactone. J Biol Chem 254:1726

Menkes JH, Corbo LM (1977) Adrenoleukodystrophy. Accumulation of cholesterol esters with very long chain fatty acids. Neurology 27:928

Merklin RJ (1962) Arterial supply of the suprarenal gland. Anat Rec 144:359

Merklin RJ (1966) Suprarenal gland lymphatic drainage. Am J Anat 119:359

Messerli FH, Nowaczynski W, Honda M, Genest J, Boucher R, Kuchel O, Rojo-Ortega JM (1977) Effects of angiotensin II on steroid metabolism and hepatic blood flow in man. Circ Res 40:204

Migeon CJ (1980) Diagnosis and treatment of adrenogenital disorders. In: De Groot LJ, Cahill GF, Odell WD, Martini L, Potts JT, Nelson DH, Steinberger E, Winegrad AI (eds) Endocrinology vol 2. Grune & Stratton, New York, p 1203

Migeon CJ, Kenny FM, Kowarski A, Snipes CA, Spaulding JS, Finkelstein JW, Blizzard RM (1968) The syndrome of congenital adrenocortical unresponsiveness to ACTH. Report of six cases. Pediatr Res 2:501

Migeon CJ, Kenny FM, Hung W, Voorness ML (1967) Study of adrenal function in children with meningitis. Pediatrics 40:163

Migeon CJ, Rosenwaks Z, Lee PA, Urban MD, Bias WB (1980) The attenuated form of congenital adrenal hyperplasia as an allelic form of 21-hydroxylase deficiency. J Clin Endocrinol Metab 51:647

Mikhail Y, Amin F (1969) Intrinsic innervation of the human adrenal gland. Acta Anat (Basel) 72:25

Mikuz G, Loewit K, Herbst M (1975) Über nebennierenindenartige Leydigsche Zwischenzellen. Virchows Arch [Cell Pathol] 19:359

Milder MS, Cook JD, Stray S, Finch CA (1980) Idiopathic hemochromatosis, an interim report. Medicine 59:34

Milla PJ, Trompeter R, Dillon MJ, Robins D, Shackleton C (1977) Salt-losing syndrome in 2 infants with defective 18-dehydrogenation in aldosterone biosynthesis. Arch Dis Child 52:580

Millington DS, Golder MP, Cowley T, London D, Roberts H, Butt WR, Griffiths K (1976) In vitro synthesis of steroids by a feminising adrenocortical carcinoma: Effect of prolactin and other protein hormones. Acta Endocrinol (Copenh) 82:561

Milliser RV, Greenberg SR, Neiman BH (1969) Heterotopic renal tissue in the human adrenal gland. J Urol 102:280

Mills IH (1964) Clinical aspects of adrenal function. Blackwell, Oxford

Mills IH, Cook RF, Galley JM, Edwards OM, Tait AD (1980) Corticosterone-secreting tumours: with and without renal artery stenosis. Clin Endocrinol (Oxf) 13:355

Minninberg DT, Levine LS, New MI (1979) Current concepts in congenital adrenal hyperplasia. Invest Urol 17:169

Mitchell FL, Shackleton CHL (1969) The investigation of steroid metabolism in early infancy. Adv Clin Chem 12:141

Mitchell GAG (1953) Anatomy of the autonomic nervous system. Livingstone, Edinburgh London

Mitschke H, Saeger W (1973) Zur Ultrastruktur der atrophischen Nebennierenrinde bei dissoziierter, sekundärer Nebennierenrindeninsuffizienz. Virchows Arch [Pathol Anat] 361:217

Mitschke H, Saeger W, Breustedt H-J (1973) Zur Ultrastruktur der Nebennierenrindentumoren beim Cushing-Syndrom. Virchows Arch [Pathol Anat] 360:253

Mitschke H, Saeger W, Breustedt H-J (1978) Feminizing adrenocortical tumor. Histological and ultrastructural study. Virchows Arch [Pathol Anat] 377:301

Mitsukuri K (1882) On the development of the suprarenal bodies in Mammalia. Q J Microsc Sci 22:17

Miura K, Yoshinaga K, Goto K, Katsushima I, Maebashi M, Demura H, Iino M, Demura R, Torikai T (1968) A case of glucocorticoid-responsive hyperaldosteronism. J Clin Endocrinol Metab 28:1807

Miyazaki G, Sasano N, Torikai T, Fukuchi S (1973) Adrenocortical carcinoma with an isolated mineralocorticoid excess and recurrency fourteen years after removal of the tumor. Tohoku J Exp Med 109:365

Modhi G, Bauman W, Nicolis G (1981) Adrenal failure associated with hypothalamic and adrenal metastases. A case report and review of the literature. Cancer 47:2098

Moncrieff MW, Hill DS, Archer J, Arthur LJH (1972) Congenital absence of pituitary gland and adrenal hypoplasia. Arch Dis Child 47:136

Monsaingeon A, Camus J-L, Ennuyer A (1963) Tumeur corticosurrénalienne féminisante chez une femme ménopausée Presse Med 44:2087

Mooppan MMU, Banerjee AK, Bhagwat AG, Gupta NM, Katariya RN, Talwar BL (1977) Large nonfunctioning adrenal cortical tumor: A case report. Am Surg 43:125

Moragas A, Ballabriga A (1969) Congenital lipoid hyperplasia of the fetal adrenal gland. Helv Paediatr Acta 24:226

Morgagni JB (1763) Opuscula miscellanea. Neapoli, Simoniana, p 62

Morgan MWE, O'Hare MJ (1979) Cytotoxic drugs and the human adrenal cortex: A cell culture study. Cancer 43:969

Morillo E, Gardner LI (1979) Genetics of acquired and congenital adrenal hyperplasia. Lancet II:202

Morimoto Y, Hiwada K, Nanahoshi M, Yano S, Kumagai A, Yamamura Y, Kotoh K, Uda H, Yamane G, Okano K (1971) Cushing's syndrome caused by malignant tumor in the scrotum: clinical, pathologic and biochemical studies. J Clin Endocrinol Metab 32:201

Mornex R, Gagnaire JC, Berthezene F, Stefanini P, Prost G (1972) Maladie de Cushing avec rétrocession spontanée pendant 30 ans et rechute. Sem Hop Paris 48:375

Mosier HD, Flynn PJ, Will DW, Turner RD (1960) Cushing's syndrome with multinodular adrenal glands. J Clin Endocrinol Metab 20:632

Mötlik K, Starka L (1973) Adrenocortical tumour of the ovary. Neoplasma 20:97

Mötlik K, Pinsker P, Starka L, Hradec E (1973) Effects of aminoglutethimide (Elipten-Ciba), a steroid biosynthesis blocking agent, on adrenal glands in Cushing's syndrome. Virchows Arch [Pathol Anat] 360:11

Müller J (1971) Regulation of aldosterone biosynthesis. Springer, Berlin Heidelberg New York

Murayama H, Kikuchi M, Imai T (1979) Myelolipoma in adenoma of accessory adrenal gland. Pathol Res Pract 164:207

Murphy BEP (1973) Does the human fetal adrenal play a role in parturition? Am J Obstet Gynecol 115:521

Murphy BEP (1974) Cortisol and cortisone levels in the cord blood at delivery of premature infants with and without the respiratory distress syndrome. Am J Obstet Gynecol 119:1112

Murphy BEP (1977) Chorionic membrane as an extra-adrenal source of foetal cortisol in human amniotic fluid. Nature 266:179

Murphy BEP, D'Aux RCD (1972) Steroid levels in the human fetus: cortisol and cortisone. J Clin Endocrinol Metab 35:678

Murphy BEP, Sebenick M, Patchell ME (1980) Cortisol production and metabolism in the human fetus and its reflection in the maternal urine. J Steroid Biochem 12:37

Naeye RL (1967) New observations in erythroblastosis fetalis. JAMA 200:281

Naeye RL, Harcke HT, Blanc WA (1971) Adrenal gland structure and the development of hyaline membrane disease. Pediatrics 47:650

Nagi AH (1970) Paraquat and adrenal cortical necrosis. Br Med J ii:669

Najjar SS, Slirin MS, Kublawi IS (1964) Cushing's syndrome due to bilateral adrenal hyperplasia in childhood (report of a case and review of the literature). J Med Liban 17:311

Nakamura J, Ohtani Y, Ohkawa T, Kanazawa M (1973) Massive adrenal hemorrhage in the newborn: 2 surviving cases by surgical treatment. J Urol 110:467

Nakanishi S, Inoue A, Kita T, Nakamura M, Chang ACY, Cohen SN, Nurma S (1979) Nucleotide sequence of cloned cDNA for bovine corticotropin-β-lipotropin precursor. Nature 278:423

Nelson DH (1980) The adrenal cortex: Physiological function and disease. Saunders, Philadelphia

Nelson DH, Meakin JW, Thorn GW (1960) ACTH-producing pituitary tumors following adrenalectomy for Cushing's syndrome. Ann Intern Med 52:560

Nerup J (1974a) Addison's disease – serological studies. Acta Endocrinol (Copenh) 76:142

Nerup J (1974b) Addison's disease – clinical studies. A report of 108 cases. Acta Endocrinol (Copenh) 76:127

Nerup J, Bendixen G (1969a) Anti-adrenal cellular hypersensitivity in Addison's disease. II. Correlation with clinical and serological findings. Clin Exp Immunol 5:341

Nerup J, Bendixen G (1969b) Anti-adrenal cellular hypersensitivity in Addison's disease. III. Species-specificity and subcellular localization of the antigen. Clin Exp Immunol 5:355

Neville AM (1978) The nodular adrenal. Invest Cell Pathol 1:99

Neville AM, Engel LL (1968). Steroid Δ-isomerase of the bovine adrenal gland: Kinetics, activation by NAD and attempted solubilization. Endocrinology 83:864

Neville AM, MacKay AM (1972) The structure of the human adrenal cortex in health and disease. Clin Endocrinol Metabol 1:361

Neville AM, O'Hare MJ (1978) Cell culture and histopathology of the human adrenal cortex in relation to hypercorticalism. In: James VHT, Serio M, Guisti G, Martini L (eds) The endocrine function of the human adrenal cortex. Academic Press, New York London, p 229

Neville AM, O'Hare MJ (1979) The human adrenal gland: Aspects of structure, function and pathology. In: James VHT (ed) The adrenal cortex. Raven, New York, p 1

Neville AM, Symington T (1966) Pathology of primary aldosteronism. Cancer 12:1854

Neville AM, Symington T (1967) The pathology of the adrenal gland in Cushing's syndrome. J Pathol 93:19

Neville AM, Symington T (1972) Bilateral adrenocortical hyperplasia in children with Cushing's syndrome. J Pathol 107:95

Neville AM, Webb JL (1965) The in vitro formation of 3-beta-hydroxyandrost-5-ene-7,17-dione by human adrenal glands. Steroids 6:421

Neville AM, Orr JC, Engel LL (1969a) The Δ^5-3β-hydroxysteroid dehydrogenase of bovine adrenal microsomes. J Endocrinol 43:599

Neville AM, Orr JC, Trofimow ND, Engel LL (1969b) A time study of the in vitro metabolism of 3β-hydroxyandrost-5-en-17-one by human adrenocortical tissue. Steroids 14:97

Neville AM, Webb JL, Symington T (1969c) The in vitro utilization of (4-^{14}C) dehydroisoandrosterone by human adrenocortical tumours associated with virilism. Steroids 13:821

Nevin NC, Dodge JA, Allen IV (1972) Two cases of trisomy D associated with adrenal tumours. J Med Genet 9:119

New MI (1970) Male pseudohemaphroditism due to 17α-hydroxylase deficiency. J Clin Invest 49:1930

New MI, Levine LS (1973) Congenital adrenal hyperplasia. In: Harris H, Hirschhorn K (eds) Adv human genetics. Plenum Press, New York, p 251

New MI, Peterson RE (1967) A new form of congenital adrenal hyperplasia. J Clin Endocrinol Metab 27:300

New MI, Miller B, Peterson RE (1966) Aldosterone excretion in normal children and in children with adrenal hyperplasia. J Clin Invest 45:412

New MI, Siegal EJ, Peterson RE (1973) Dexamethasone-suppressible hyperaldosteronism. J Clin Endocrinol Metab 37:93

New MI, Peterson RE, Saenger P, Levine LS (1976) Evidence for an unidentified ACTH-induced steroid hormone causing hypertension. J Clin Endocrinol Metab 43:1283

New MI, Levine LS, Biglieri EG, Pareira J, Ulick S (1977) Evidence for an unidentified steroid in a child with apparent mineralocorticoid hypertension. J Clin Endocrinol Metab 44:924

New MI, Lorenzen F, Pang S, Gunczler P, Dupont B, Levine LS (1979) 'Acquired' adrenal hyperplasia with 21-hydroxylase deficiency is not the same genetic disorder as congenital adrenal hyperplasia. J Clin Endocrinol Metab 48:356

New MI, Oberfield SE, Levine LS, Dupont B, Pollack M, Gill JR, Bartter FC (1980) Autosomal dominant transmission and absence of HLA linkage in dexamethasone suppressible hyperaldosteronism. Lancet I:550

Newell ME, Lippe BM, Ehrlich RM (1977) Testis tumors associated with congenital adrenal hyperplasia: A continuing diagnostic and therapeutic dilemma. J Urol 117:256

Newman PH, Silen W (1968) Myelolipoma of the adrenal gland. Arch Surg 97:637

Ney RL, Hammond W, Wright L, Davis WW, Acker J, Bartter FC (1966) Studies in a patient with an ectopic adrenocortical tumor. J Clin Endocrinol Metab 26:299

Nicolis GL, Babich AM, Mitty HA, Gabrilove LJ (1972) Observations on the cortisol content of human adrenal venous blood. J Clin Endocrinol Metab 38:638

Nichols J (1956) Studies of the adrenal glands of patients with low plasma sodium. Arch Pathol 62:419

Nichols J (1968) Adrenal cortex. In: Bloodworth JMB Jr (ed) 'Endocrine Pathology' Williams and Wilkins, Baltimore, p 224

Nichols J, Gourley W (1963) Adrenal weight-maintaining corticotropin in carcinoma of lung. JAMA 185:696

Nicholls MG, Espiner EA, Donald RA (1975a) Plasma aldosterone response to low dose ACTH stimulation. J Clin Endocrinol Metab 41:186

Nicholls MG, Espiner EA, Hughes H, Ross J, Stewart DT (1975b) Primary aldosteronism: A study in contrasts. Am J Med 59:334

Nishida S, Matsumura S, Horino M, Oyama H, Tenku A (1977) The variations of plasma corticosterone/cortisol ratios following ACTH stimulation or dexamethasone administration in normal men. J Clin Endocrinol Metab 45:585

Nishikawa T, Mikami K, Tamura Y, Yamamoto M, Kumagai A (1979) Comparative study of cyclic AMP-generation system, steroid biosynthesis and lipid metabolism in vitro in ACTH responsive and unresponsive adrenal tumors. Endocrinol Jpn 26:9

Nogeire C, Fukushima DK, Hellman L, Boyar RM (1977) Virilizing adrenal cortical carcinoma. Cancer 40:307

Nottelet E, Guillot E, Loiseau C, Philippe D, Barbet J (1976) Les corticosurrénalomas féminisants de l'enfant. Étude d'une observation et revue de la littérature. Sem Hop Paris 52:2369

Oberling C (1929) Les formations myelolipomateuses. Bull Assoc Fraç Canc 18:234

O'Bryan RM, Smith RW Jr, Fine G, Mellinger RC (1964) Congenital adrenocortical hyperplasia with Cushing's syndrome. JAMA 187:257

O'Connell TX, Aston SJ (1974) Acute adrenal hemorrhage complicating anticoagulant therapy. Surg Gynecol Obstet 139:355

O'Donnell WM (1950) Changing pathogenesis of Addison's disease, with special reference to amyloidosis. Arch Intern Med 86:266

O'Donohoe NV, Holland PDJ (1968) Familial congenital adrenal hypoplasia Arch Dis Child 43:717

Oelkers W, Brown JJ, Fraser R, Lever AF, Morton JJ, Robertson JIS (1974) Sensitization of the adrenal cortex to angiotensin II in sodium depleted man. Circ Res 34:69

Oelkers W, Schöneshöfer M, Schultze G, Brown JJ, Fraser R, Morton JJ, Lever AF, Robertson JIS (1975) Effect of prolonged low-dose angiotensin II infusion on the sensitivity of adrenal cortex in man. Circ Res Suppl 1 36–37:49

Ofuji N, Yasuhara T, Murakami M, Takahara J, Ofuji T (1977) A case of idiopathic Addison's disease with chronic thyroiditis and ovarian dysfunction. Jpn J Med Sci Biol 16:124

O'Hare MJ (1976) Monolayer cultures of normal adult rat adrenocortical cells: Steroidogenic responses to nucleotides, bacterial toxins and antimicrotubular agents. Experientia 32:251

O'Hare MJ, Hornsby PJ (1975) Absence of a circadian rhythm of corticosterone secretion in monolayer cultures of adult rat adrenocortical cells. Experientia 31:378

O'Hare MJ, Neville AM (1973a) Morphological responses to corticotrophin and cyclic AMP by adult rat adrenocortical cells in monolayer culture. J Endocrinol 56:529

O'Hare MJ, Neville AM (1973b) Steroid metabolism by adult rat adrenocortical cells in monolayer culture. J Endocrinol 58:447

O'Hare MJ, Neville AM (1973c) Effects of adrenocorticotrophin on steroidogenesis and proliferation by adult adrenal cells in monolayer culture. Biochem Soc Trans 1:1088

O'Hare MJ, Nice EC (1981) The analysis of steroid hormones in adrenal and testicular cells and tissues by high performance liquid chromatography. In: Kautsky M (ed) Steroid analysis by HPLC: Recent applications. Dekker, New York p 277

O'Hare MJ, Nice EC, Magee-Brown R, Bullman H (1976) High-pressure liquid chromatography of steroids secreted by cultured human adrenal and testis cells. J Chromatogr 125:357

O'Hare MJ, Ellison ML, Neville AM (1978) Tissue culture in endocrine research: Perspectives, pitfalls and potentials. Current Topics in Experimental Endocrinology 3:1

O'Hare MJ, Monaghan P, Neville AM (1979) The pathology of adrenocortical neoplasia: A correlated structural and functional approach to the diagnosis of malignancy. Hum Pathol 10:137

O'Hare MJ, Nice EC, Neville AM (1980a) The regulation of androgen secretion and sulfoconjugation in the adult human adrenal cortex: Studies with primary monolayer cell cultures. In: Genazzani AR, Thijssen JHH, Siiteri PK (eds) Adrenal androgens. Raven Press, New York, p 7

O'Hare MJ, Nice EC, Capp M (1980b) Reversed and normal-phase HPLC of 18-hydroxylated steroids and their derivatives: A comparison of selectivity, efficiency and recovery from biological samples. J Chromatogr 198:23

Olsson CA, Krane RJ, Klugo RC, Selikowitz SM (1973) Adrenal myelolipoma. Surgery 73:665

Omura T, Sato R, Cooper DY, Rosenthal O, Estabrook RW (1965) Function of cytochrome P-450 of microsomes Fed Proc 24:481

Oppenheimer EH (1964) Lesions in the adrenals of an infant following maternal corticosteroid therapy. Bull Johns Hopkins Hosp 114 14:146

Oppenheimer EH (1969) Cyst formation in the outer adrenal cortex. Arch Pathol 87:653

Oppenheimer EH (1970) Adrenal cytomegaly: studies by light and electron microscopy. Arch Pathol 90:57

Orme-Johnson NR, Light DR, White-Stevens RW, Orme-Johnson WH (1979) Steroid binding properties of beef adrenal cortical cytochrome P-450 which catalyzes the conversion of cholesterol into pregnenolone. J Biol Chem 254:2103

Orselli RC, Bassler TJ (1973) Theca granulosa cell tumor arising in adrenal. Cancer 31:474

Oshima H, Sarada T, Ochiai K, Tamaoki B-I (1969) A comparative study of steroid biosyntheses in vitro in clear cell adenoma and its adjacent tissue of human adrenal gland. Endocrinol Jpn 16:47

Øvlison B, Andersen JH (1966) Spontaneous remission in a case of Cushing's syndrome presumably due to adrenal tumor. J Clin Endocrinol Metab 26:294

Padfield PL, Allison MEM, Brown JJ, Ferriss JB, Fraser R, Lever AF, Luke RF, Robertson JIS (1975) Response of plasma aldosterone to fludrocortisone in primary hyperaldosteronism and other forms of hypertension. Clin Endocrinol (Oxf) 4:493

Padfield PL, Brown JJ, Davies D, Fraser R, Lever AF, Morton JJ, Robertson JIS (1981). The myth of idiopathic hyperaldosteronism. Lancet II:83

Pakravan P, Kenny FM, Depp R, Allen AC (1974) Familial congenital absence of adrenal glands. Evaluation of glucocorticoid, mineralocorticoid, and estrogen metabolism in the perinatal period. J Pediatr 84:74

Pang S, Levine LS, Cederqvist LL, Fuentes M, Riccardi VM, Holcombe JH, Nitowsky HM, Sachs G, Anderson CE, Duchon MA, Owens R, Merkatz I, New MI (1980) Amniotic fluid concentrations of Δ^5 and Δ^4 steroids in fetuses with congenital adrenal hyperplasia due to 21-hydroxylase deficiency and in anencephalic fetuses. J Clin Endocrinol Metab 51:223

Parker CR, Servy E, McDonough PG, Mahesh VB (1974) In vivo endocrine studies in adrenal rest tumor of ovary. Obstet Gynecol 44:327

Parker LN, Odell WD (1979) Evidence for existence of cortical androgen-stimulating hormone. Am J Physiol 236:616

Parker LN, Sack J, Fisher DA, Odell WD (1978) The adrenarche: Prolactin, gonadotropins, adrenal androgens, and cortisol. J Clin Endocrinol Metab 46:396

Parker L, Gral T, Perrigo V, Skowsky R (1981) Decreased adrenal androgen sensitivity to ACTH during aging. Metabolism 30:601

Parks GA, Bermudez JA, Anast CS, Bongiovanni AM, New MI (1971) Pubertal boy with the 3β-hydroxysteroid dehydrogenase defect. J Clin Endocrinol Metab 33:269

Parsons L, Thompson JE (1959) Symptomatic myelolipoma of the adrenal glands: Report of a case and review of literature. N Engl J Med 260:12

Pasqualini JR (1964) Conversion of tritiated 18-hydroxycorticosterone to aldosterone by slices of human cortico-adrenal gland and adrenal tumour. Nature 201:501

Pasqualini RQ, Gurevich N (1956) Spontaneous remission in a case of Cushing's syndrome. J Clin Endocrinol Metab 16:406

Pasqualini RQ, Wiqvist N, Diczfalusy E (1966) Biosynthesis of aldosterone by human foetuses perfused with corticosterone at mid-term. Biochim Biophys Acta 121:430

Pauerstein CJ, Solomon D (1968) LH and adrenal androgenesis. Obstet Gynecol 28:692

Pavlova EB, Pronina TS, Skebelskaya YB (1968) Histostructure of adenohypophysis of human fetuses and contents of somatotropic and adrenocorticotropic hormones. Gen Comp Endocrinol 10:269

Payan HM, Gilbert EF (1967) Micronodular phlebosclerosis. An aging change of venules of the kidney and adrenals. Angiology 18:384

Payan HM, Gilbert EF (1972) Interrupted eccentric longitudinal muscle fibers of the kidney and adrenal veins. Am Heart J 84:76

Payne AH, Jaffe RB (1972) Comparison of androgen synthesis in human fetal testis and adrenal: 3β-hydroxysteroid dehydrogenase-isomerase and 17β-steroid dehydrogenase activities. Biochim Biophys Acta 279:202

Peach MJ (1977) Renin–angiotensin system: Biochemistry and mechanisms of action. Physiol Rev 57:313

Pearson HA, Shanklin DR, Brodine CR (1965) Alpha-thalassemia as cause of nonimmunological hydrops. Am J Dis Child 109:168

Perchellet J-P, Sharma RK (1979) Mediatory role of calcium and guanosine 3′,5′-monophosphate in adrenocorticotropin-induced steroidogenesis by adrenal cells. Science 203:1259

Peretti E, Forest MG (1976) Unconjugated dehydroepiandrosterone plasma levels in normal subjects from birth to adolescence in human: The use of a sensitive radioimmunoassay. J Clin Endocrinol Metab 43:982

Peretti E, Forest MG (1978) Pattern of plasma dehydroepiandrosterone sulfate levels in human from birth to adulthood: Evidence for testicular production. J Clin Endocrinol Metab 47:572

Perlmutter M, Apfel AZ, Avin J, Hermann HB, Klein EA (1962) Cushing's syndrome in infancy: Report of a case. Metabolism 11:946

Peterman MG (1957) Suprarenal tumor (Cushing's syndrome). J Pediatr 50:59

Petersen KE, Tygstrup I, Thamdrup E (1977) Familial adrenocortical hypoplasia with early clinical and biochemical signs of mineralocorticoid deficiency (hypoaldosteronism). Acta Endocrinol (Copenh) 84:605

Petri M, Nerup J (1971) Addison's adrenalitis. Acta Pathol Microbiol Scand [A] 79:381

Peytremann A, Nicholson WE, Brown RD, Liddle GW, Hardman JG (1973) Comparative effects of angiotensin and ACTH on cyclic AMP and steroidogenesis in isolated bovine adrenal cells. J Clin Invest 52:835

Pinck RL, Constantacopoulos CG, Felice A, Ippolito J, Rubin B, Haller JO (1979) Adrenal hemorrhage in the newborn with evidence of bleeding while in utero. J Urol 122:813

Pirani CL (1952) Review: Relation of vitamin C to adrenocortical function and stress phenomena. Metabolism 1:197

Pitcock JA, Hartroft PM (1958) The juxtaglomerular cells in man and their relationship to the level of plasma sodium and to the zona glomerulosa of the adrenal cortex. Am J Pathol 34:863

Pittaway DE, Andersen RN, Givens JR (1973) In vitro studies on an HCG responsive, testosterone secreting adrenal cortical adenoma. Steroids 22:731

Plasse J-C, Lisboa BP (1973) Studies on the metabolism of steroids in the foetus. Metabolism of testosterone in the human foetal adrenals. Eur J Biochem 39:449

Plaut A (1958) Myelolipoma in the adrenal cortex (myeloadipose structures). Am J Pathol 34:487

Plotz CM, Knowlton AI, Ragan C (1952) Natural history of Cushing's syndrome Am J Med 13:597

Polansky S (1975) Luteinizing hormone, adrenal androgenesis and polycystic ovarian disease. Obstet Gynecol 45:451

Poortman J, Andriesse R, Agema A, Donker GH, Schwarz F, Thijssen JHH (1980) Adrenal androgen secretion and metabolism in postmenopausal women. In Genazzani AR, Thijssen JHH, Siiteri PK (eds) Adrenal androgens. Raven Press, New York 219

Popper H (1941) Histologic distribution of vitamin A in human organs under normal and under pathologic conditions. Arch Pathol 31:766

Porter B, Finzi M, Lieberman E, Mozes S (1977) The syndrome of congenital adrenal hyperplasia in Israel. Pediatrician 198:100

Powell LW Jr, Newman S, Hooker JW (1955) Cushing's syndrome: Report of a case in infant 12 weeks old. Am J Dis Child 90:417

Powell-Jackson JD, Calin A, Fraser R, Grahame R, Mason P, Missen GAK, Powell-Jackson PR, Wilson A (1974) Excessive deoxycorticosterone secretion from adrenocortical carcinoma. Br Med J ii:32

Powers JM, Schaumburg HH (1973) The adrenal cortex in adrenoleukodystrophy. Arch Pathol 96:305

Powers JM, Schaumburg HH (1974a) Adreno-leukodystrophy: Similar ultrastructural changes in adrenal cortical cells and Schwann cells. Arch Neurol 30:406

Powers JM, Schaumburg HH (1974b) Adreno-leukodystrophy (sex-linked Schilder's disease): A pathogenic hypothesis based on ultrastructural lesions in adrenal cortex, peripheral nerve and testis. Am J Pathol 76:481

Powers JM, Schaumburg HH (1981) The testis in adreno-leukodystrophy. Am J Pathol 102:90

Powers JM, Schaumburg HH, Johnson AB, Raine CS (1980) A correlative study of the adrenal cortex in adreno-leukodystrophy: Evidence for a fatal intoxication with very long chain saturated fatty acids. Enzyme histochemistry, fine structure, tissue culture, proposed molecular model and cellular pathogenesis. Invest Cell Pathol 3:353

Pozo E, Bigazzi M, Calaf J (1980) Induced human gestational hyperprolactinemia: Lack of action on fetal adrenal androgen synthesis. J Clin Endocrinol Metab 51:936

Prader A (1958) Die Häufigkeit des kongenitalen adrenogenitalen Syndroms. Helv Paediatr Acta 13:426

Prader A, Anders GJPA (1962) Zur Genetik der kongenitalen Lipoidhyperplasie der Nebennieren. Helv Paediatr Acta 17:285

Prader A, Gurtner HP (1955) Das Syndrom des Pseudohermaphroditismus masculinus bei Kongenitaler Nebennierenrinden-Hyperplasie ohne Androgenuberproduktion (adrenaler Pseudohermaphroditismus masculinus) Helv Paediatr Acta 10:397

Prader A, Anders GJPA, Habich H (1962) Zur Genetik des kongenitalen adrenogenitalen Syndroms. Helv Paediatr Acta 17:271

Prader A, Zachmann M, Illig R (1975) Luteinizing hormone deficiency in hereditary congenital adrenal hyperplasia. J Pediatr 86:421

Pratt JH, Luft FC (1979) The effect of extremely high sodium intake on plasma renin activity, plasma aldosterone concentration, and urinary excretion of aldosterone metabolites. J Lab Clin Med 93:724

Pratt JH, Sawin CT, Melby JC (1974) Remission of Cushing's disease after administration of adrenocorticotropin. Am J Med 57:949

Price WF, Farmer TA Jr (1969) Cushing's syndrome and adrenal medullary insufficiency with bilateral adrenal calcification. J Clin Endocrinol Metab 29:368

Purvis JL, Canick JA, Mason JI, Estabrook RW, McCarty JL (1973) Lifetime of adrenal cytochrome P-450 as influenced by ACTH. Ann NY Acad Sci 212:319

Putnam TI, Aceto T, Abbassi V, Kenny FM (1972) Cushing's disease with a spontaneous remission. Pediatrics 50:477

Quinan C, Berger AA (1933) Observations on human adrenals with especial reference to the relative weight of the normal medulla. Ann Intern Med 6:1180

Raafat F, Hashiemian MP, Abrishami MA (1973) Wolman's disease. Report of two new cases, with a review of the literature. Am J Clin Pathol 59:490

Race GJ, Wu HM (1961) Adrenal cortex functional zonation in the whale (Physeter catadon). Endocrinology 68:156

Radfar N, Kolins J, Bartter FC (1977) Evidence for cortisol secretion by testicular masses in congential adrenal hyperplasia. In: Lee PA, Plotnick LP, Kowarski AA, Migeon CJ (eds) Congenital adrenal hyperplasia. University Park Press, Baltimore London Tokyo p 331

Rae PA, Gutmann NS, Tsao J, Schimmer BP (1979) Mutations in cyclic AMP-dependent protein kinase and corticotropin (ACTH) – sensitive adenylate cyclase affect adrenal steroidogenesis. Proc Natl Acad Sci USA 76:1896

Raggatt PR, Engel LL, Symington T (1972) Fatty acid composition of the sterol ester fraction of human adrenal cortex in Cushing's syndrome and after treatment with aminoglutethimide. Lipids 7:474

Ramachandran J, Suyama AT (1975) Inhibition of replication of normal adrenocortical cells in culture by adrenocorticotropin. Proc Natl Acad Sci USA 72:113

Ramseyer J, Zala AP, Levy RP, Linton DS, Hirschmann H (1974) Secretion of 16α-hydroxyprogesterone and other steroids by the adult human adrenal. J Clin Endocrinol Metab 39:102

Rao AJ, Long JA, Ramachandran J (1978) Effects of antiserum to adrenocorticotropin on adrenal growth and function. Endocrinology 102:371

Rappaport R, Dray F, Legrand JC, Royer P (1968) Hypoaldostéronisme congénital familial par défaut de la 18-OH-déhydrogénase. Pediatr Res 2:456

Ratcliffe JG, Knight RA, Besser GM, Landon J, Stansfield AG (1972) Tumour and plasma ACTH concentrations in patients with and without the ectopic ACTH syndrome. Clin Endocrinol (Oxf) 1:27

Ratter SJ, Hogan P, Lowry PJ, Edwards CRW, Rees LH (1977). Comparison of plasma immunoreactive and bioactive corticotrophin. J Endocrinol 75:30P

Raux MC, Binoux M, Luton JP, Gourmelen M, Girard F (1975) Studies of ACTH secretion control in 116 cases of Cushing's syndrome. J Clin Endocrinol Metab 40:186

Rayfield EJ, Rose LI, Cain JP, Dluhy RG, Williams GH (1971) ACTH-responsive, dexamethasone-suppressible adrenocortical carcinoma. N Engl J Med 284:591

Re RN, Kourides IA, Weihl AC, Maloof F (1979) The relationship between endogenous hyper-prolactinaemia and plasma aldosterone. Clin Endocrinol (Oxf) 10:187

Reddy JK, Schimke RN, Chang CHJ, Svoboda DJ, Slaven J, Therou L (1972) Beckwith–Wiedemann syndrome. Arch Pathol 94:523

Rees LH, Ratcliffe JG (1974) Ectopic hormone production by non-endocrine tumours. Clin Endocrinol (Oxf) 3:263

Rees LH, Burke CW, Chard T, Evans SW, Letchworth AT (1975a) Possible placental origin of ACTH in normal human pregnancy. Nature 254:620

Rees LH, Grant DB, Wilson J (1957b) Plasma corticotrophin levels in Addison-Schilder's disease. Br Med J ii:201

Rees LH, Besser GM, Jeffcoate WJ, Goldie DJ, Marks V (1977) Alcohol-induced pseudo-Cushing's syndrome. Lancet I:726

Reichstein T (1936) Uber Cortin, das Hormon der Nebennierenrinde. Helv Chim Acta 19:29

Reidbord H, Fisher ER (1969) Aldosteronoma and nonfunctioning adrenal cortical adenoma. Comparative ultrastructural study. Arch Pathol 88:155

Reifenstein EC, Forbes AP, Albright F, Donaldson E, Carroll E (1945) The effect of methyl testosterone on urinary 17-ketosteroids of adrenal origin. J Clin Invest 24:416

Reiter EO, Fuldauer VG, Root AW (1977) Secretion of the adrenal androgen, dehydroepiandrosterone sulfate, during normal infancy, childhood, and adolescence, in sick infants, and in children with endocrinologic abnormalities. J Pediatr 90:766

Revach M, Shilo S, Cabili S, Rubenstein Z, Selzer G (1977) Hyperaldosteronism caused by adrenal cortical carcinoma. Isr J Med Sci 13:1123

Reyes FI, Boroditsky RS, Winter JSD, Faiman C (1974) Studies on human sexual development. II. Fetal and maternal serum gonadotropin and sex steroid concentrations. J Clin Endocrinol Metab 38:612

Riddick DH, Hammond CB (1975) Adrenal virilism due to 21-hydroxylase deficiency in the postmenarchial female. Obstet Gynecol 45:21

Riley C (1963) Lipids of human adrenals. Biochem J 87:500

Rimoin DL, Schimke RN (1971) Genetic disorders of the endocrine glands. Mosby, St Louis p 281

Riolan J (1629) Oeuvres anatomiques. Paris

Riou P, Evain D, Perrin F, Saez JM (1977) Adenosine 3′,5′-cyclic monophosphate dependent protein kinase in human adrenocortical tumors. J Clin Endocrinol Metab 44:413

Roberts G, Cawdery JE (1970) Congenital adrenal hypoplasia. J Obstet Gynaecol Br Cwlth 77:654

Roberts KD, Lieberman S (1970) The biochemistry of the 3β-hydroxy-Δ⁵-steroid sulfates. In: Bernstein S, Solomon S (eds) Chemical and biological aspects of steroid conjugation. Springer-Verlag, Berlin Heidelberg New York, p 219

Robinson MJ, Pardo V, Rywlin AM (1972) Pigmented nodules (black adenomas) of the adrenal. Hum Pathol 3:317

Rodin AE, Hsu L, Whorton EB (1976) Microcysts of the permanent adrenal cortex in perinates and infants. Arch Pathol 100:499

Roe TF, Kershnar AK, Weitzman JJ, Madrigal LS (1973) Beckwith's syndrome with extreme organ hyperplasia. Pediatrics 52:372

Rogoff JM, Stewart GN (1928) Studies on adrenal insufficiency in dogs. Am J Physiol 84:660

Romanoff LP, Baxter MN (1975) The secretion rates of deoxycorticosterone and corticosterone in young and elderly men. J Clin Endocrinol Metab 41:630

Rose LI, Williams GH, Emerson K, Villee DB (1969) Steroidal and gonadotropin evaluation of a patient with a feminizing tumor of the adrenal gland. In vivo and in vitro studies. J Clin Endocrinol Metab 29:1526

Rosenfeld RS, Rosenberg BJ, Fukushima DK, Hellman L (1975) 24-Hour secretory pattern of dehydroisoandrosterone and dehydroisoandrosterone sulfate. J Clin Endocrinol Metab 40:850

Rosenfield RL, Fang VS (1974) The effects of prolonged physiologic estradiol therapy on the maturation of hypogonadal teenagers. J Pediatr 85:830

Rosenfield RL, Root AW, Bongiovanni AM, Eberlein WR (1967) Idiopathic anterior hypopituitarism in one of monozygous twins. J Pediatr 70:114

Rosenfield RL, Rich BH, Wolfsdorf JI, Cassorla F, Parks JS, Bongiovanni AM, Wu CH, Shackleton CH (1980) Pubertal presentation of congenital Δ⁵-3β-hydroxysteroid dehydrogenase deficiency. J Clin Endocrinol Metab 51:345

Rösler A, Rabinowitz D, Theodor R, Ramirez LC, Ulick S (1977) The nature of the defect in a salt-wasting disorder of Jews in Iran. J Clin Endocrinol Metab 44:279

Ross EJ, Vant Hoff W, Crabbé J, Thorn GW (1960) Aldosterone excretion in hypopituitarism and after hypophysectomy in man. Am J Med 28:229

Rotter W (1949) Die Entwicklung der fetalen und kindlichen Nebennierenrinde. Virchows Arch 316:590

Rovner DR, Conn JW, Cohen EL, Berlinger FG, Kem DC, Gordon DL (1979) 17α-Hydroxylase deficiency. A combination of hydroxylation defect and reversible blockade in aldosterone synthesis. Acta Endocrinol (Copenh) 90:490

Rowntree LG, Greene CH, Swingle WW, Pfiffner JJ (1930) The treatment of patients with Addison's disease with the 'cortical hormone' of Swingle and Pfiffner. Science 72:482

Ruder HJ, Loriaux L, Lipsett MB (1972) Estrone sulfate: Production rate and metabolism in man. J Clin Invest 51:1020

Ruder HJ, Loriaux DL, Lipsett MB (1974) Severe osteopenia in young adults associated with Cushing's syndrome due to micronodular adrenal disease. J Clin Endocrinol Metab 39:1138

Ruiz-Palacios G, Pickering LK, vanEys J, Conklin R (1977) Disseminated herpes simplex with hepatoadrenal necrosis in a child with acute leukemia. J Pediatr 91:757

Russell MA, Opitz JM, Viseskul C, Gilbert EF, Bargman GJ (1977) Sudden infant death due to congenital adrenal hypoplasia. Arch Pathol 101:168

Russell P (1972) The adrenal glands in shock. Pathology 4:5

Russell RP, Masi AT (1973) Significant associations of adrenal cortical abnormalities with 'essential' hypertension. Am J Med 54:44

Russell RP, Masi AT, Richter ED (1972) Adrenal cortical adenomas and hypertension. Medicine 51:211

Saez JM, Rivarola MA, Migeon CJ (1967) Studies of androgens in patients with adrenocortical tumors. J Clin Endocrinol Metab 27:615

Saez JM, Loras B, Morera AM, Bertrand J (1971) Studies of androgens and their precursors in adrenocortical virilizing carcinoma. J. Clin Endocrinol Metab 32:462

Saez JM, Morera AM, Dazord A, Bertrand J (1972) Adrenal and testicular contribution to plasma oestrogens. J Endocrinol 55:41

Saez JM, Dazord A, Gallet D (1975) ACTH and prostaglandin receptors in human adrenocortical tumors. Apparent modification of a specific component of the ACTH-binding site. J Clin Invest 56:536

Saez JM, Morera AM, Gallet D (1977) Opposite effects of ACTH and glucocorticoids on adrenal DNA synthesis in vivo. Endocrinology 100:1268

Saez JM, Evain D, Gallet D (1978) Role of cyclic AMP and protein kinase on the steroidogenic action of ACTH, prostaglandin E$_1$ and dibutyryl cyclic AMP in normal adrenal cells and adrenal tumor cells from humans. J Cyclic Nucleotide Res 4:311

Sahagian-Edwards A, Holland JF (1954) Metastatic carcinoma to the adrenal glands with cortical hypofunction. Cancer 7:1242

Sakar SD, Cohen EL, Beierwaltes WH, Ice RD, Cooper R, Gold EN (1977) A new and superior adrenal imaging agent ^{131}I-6β-iodomethyl-19-norcholesterol (NP-59): Evaluation in humans. J Clin Endocrinol Metab 45:353

Salassa RM, Weeks RE, Northcutt RC, Carney JA (1974) Primary aldosteronism and malignant adrenocortical neoplasia. Trans Am Clin Climatol Assoc 86:163

Salassa RM, Laws ER, Carpenter PC, Northcutt RC (1978) Transsphenoidal removal of pituitary microadenoma in Cushing's disease. Mayo Clin Proc 53:24

Salomon MI, Tchertkoff V (1968) Incidence and role of adrenocortical tumors in hypertension. Geriatrics 23:179

Salti IS, Stiefel M, Ruse JL, Delarue NC, Laidlaw JC (1969) Non-tumorous 'primary' aldosteronism. I. Type relieved by glucocorticoid (glucocorticoid-remediable aldosteronism). Can Med Assoc J 101:1

Salyer WR, Moravec CL, Salyer DC, Guerin PF (1973) Adrenal involvement in cryptococcosis. Am J Clin Pathol 60:559

Samojlik E, Santen RJ, Wells SA (1977) Adrenal suppression with aminoglutethimide. II. Differential effects of aminoglutethimide in plasma androstenedione and estrogen levels. J Clin Endocrinol Metab 45:480

Samuels LT, Nelson DH (1975) Biosynthesis of corticosteroids. In: Greep RO, Astwood AB (eds) Handbook of physiology Vol VI. Adrenal gland. Am Physiol Soc, Washington, p 55

Sancho J, Re R, Burton J, Barger AC, Haber E (1976) The role of the renin angiotensin aldosterone system in cardiovascular homeostasis in normal human subjects. Circulation 53:400

Sandberg AA, Slaunwhite WR (1975) Adrenal corticosteroids (other than aldosterone) in the human: their secretion, determination, levels, and use in functional tests. In Dorfman RI (ed). 'Methods in investigative and diagnostic endocrinology' Vol 3 Steroid Hormones. North-Holland, Amsterdam p 121

Sandberg AA, Eik-Nes K, Migeon CJ, Samuels LT (1956) Metabolism of adrenal steroids in dying patients. J Clin Endocrinol Metab 16:1001

Sandor T, Fazekas AG, Robinson BH (1976) The biosynthesis of corticosteroids through the vertebrates. In: Chester Jones I, Henderson IW (eds) General, comparative and clinical endocrinology of the adrenal cortex Vol 1. Academic Press, New York p 25

Santander R, Gonzalez A, Suarez JA (1965) Case of probable mineralocorticoid excess without hypercortisolism due to a carcinoma of the adrenal cortex. J Clin Endocrinol Metab 25:1429

Sarason EL (1943) Adrenal cortex in systemic disease. Arch Intern Med 71:702

Sarett LH (1948) A new method for the preparation of 17(α)-hydroxy-20-keto pregnanes. J Am Chem Soc 70:1454

Sarosi GA, Voth DW, Dahl BA, Doto IL, Tosh FE (1971) Disseminated histoplasmosis: results of long-term follow-up. Ann Intern Med 75:511

Saruta T, Kaplan NM (1972) Adrenocortical steroidogenesis: the effects of prostaglandins. J Clin Invest 51:2246

Saruta T, Cook R, Kaplan NM (1972) Adrenocortical steroidogenesis: Studies on the mechanism of action of angiotensin and electrolytes. J Clin Invest 51:2239

Sayers G. White A, Long CNH (1943) Preparation of pituitary adrenotropic hormone. Proc Soc Exp Biol Med 52:199

Schambelan M, Slaton PE, Biglieri EG (1971) Mineralocorticoid production in hyperadrenocorticism: role in the pathogenesis of hypokalaemic alkalosis. Am J Med 51:299

Schaumburg HH, Richardson EP, Johnson PC, Cohen RB, Powers JM, Raine CS (1972) Schilder's disease. Sex-linked recessive transmission with specific adrenal changes. Arch Neurol 27:458

Schaumburg HH, Powers JM, Suzuki K, Raine CS (1974) Adreno-leukodystrophy (sex-linked Schilder disease). Ultrastructural demonstration of specific cytoplasmic inclusions in the central nervous system. Arch Neurol 31:210

Schaumburg HH, Powers JM, Raine CS, Suzuki K, Richardson EP (1975) Adrenoleukodystrophy. A clinical and pathological study of 17 cases. Arch Neurol 32:577

Schaumburg HH, Powers JM, Raine CS, Spencer PS, Griffin JW, Prineas JW, Boehme DM (1977) Adrenomyeloneuropathy: A probable variant of adrenoleukodystrophy. II. General pathologic, neuropathologic and biochemical aspects. Neurology 27:1114

Schimke RN (1978) Genetics and cancer in man. Churchill Livingstone, Edinburgh London New York, p 57

Schmidt MB (1926) Eine biglanduläre Erkrankung (Nebennieren und Schilddrüse) bein morbus Addisonii. Verh Dtsch Ges Pathol 21:212

Schneider G, Genel M, Bongiovanni AM, Goldman AS, Rosenfield RL (1975) Persistent testicular Δ^5-isomerase-3β-hydroxysteroid dehydrogenase (Δ^5—3β-HSD deficiency in the Δ^5-3βHSD form of congenital adrenal hyperplasia. J Clin Invest 55:681

Schöneshöfer M, Wagner GG (1977) Sex differences in corticosteroids in man. J Clin Endocrinol Metab 45:814

Schöneshöfer M, Schefzig B, Oelkers W (1979) Evidence of adrenal 18-hydroxylase inhibition by metyrapone in man. Horm Metab Res 11:306

Schor NA, Glick D (1970) Effect of vitamin A deficiency on 3β-hydroxysteroid dehydrogenase activity and corticosterone in the rat adrenal. Endocrinology 86:693

Schorr I, Hinshaw HT, Cooper MA, Mahaffee D, Ney RL (1972) Adenyl cyclase hormone responses of certain human endocrine tumors. J Clin Endocrinol Metab 34:447

Schteingart DE, Oberman HA, Friedman BA, Conn JW (1968) Adrenal cortical neoplasms producing Cushing's syndrome. A clinicopathologic study. Cancer 22:1005

Schteingart DE, Woodbury MC, Tsao HS, McKenzie AK (1979) Virilizing syndrome associated with an adrenal cortical adenoma secreting predominantly testosterone. Am J Med 67:140

Schweizer-Cagianut M, Froesch ER, Hedinger C (1980) Familial Cushing's syndrome with primary adrenocortical microadenomatosis (primary adrenocortical nodular dysplasia). Acta Endocrinol (Copenh) 94:529

Schwyzer R, Sieber P (1963) Total synthesis of adrenocorticotrophic hormone. Nature 199:172

Scott HW, Liddle GW, Mulherin JL, McKenna TJ, Stroup SL, Rhamy RK (1977) Surgical experience with Cushing's disease. Ann Surg 185:524

Scott RS, Espiner EA, Donald RA (1979) Intermittent Cushing's disease with spontaneous remission. Clin Endocrinol (Oxf) 11:561

Scully RE, Cohen RB (1961) Ganglioneuroma of adrenal medulla containing cells morphologically identical to hilus cells (extraparenchymal Leydig cells). Cancer 14:421

Scully RE, Galdabini JJ, McNeely BU (1979) Case records of the Massachusetts General Hospital. Case 23–1979. Presentation of case. N Engl J Med 300:1322

Seabold JE, Cohen EL, Beierwaltes WH, Hinerman DL, Nishiyama RH, Bookstein JJ, Ice RD, Balachandran S (1976) Adrenal imaging with [131]I-19-iodocholesterol in the diagnostic evaluation of patients with aldosteronism. J Clin Endocrinol Metab 42:41

Sekihara H, Sennett JA, Liddle GW, McKenna TJ, Yarbro LR (1976) Plasma 16β-hydroxy-dehydroepiandrosterone in normal and pathological conditions in man. J Clin Endocrinol Metab 43:1078

Sekihara H, Island DP, Liddle GW (1978) New mineralocorticoids: 5α-dihydroaldosterone and 5α-dihydro-11-deoxycorticosterone. Endocrinology 103:1450

Selye H (1946) The general adaptation syndrome and disease of adaptation. J Clin Endocrinol Metab 6:117

Selye H, Stone H (1950) Hormonally induced transformation of adrenal into myeloid tissue. Am J Pathol 26:211

Semple PF, Buckingham JC, Mason PA, Fraser R (1979) Suppression of plasma ACTH concentration by angiotensin II infusion in normal humans and in a subject with a steroid 17α-hydroxylase defect. Clin Endocrinol (Oxf) 10:137

Sen S, Shainoff JR, Bravo EL, Bumpus MF (1981) Isolation of aldosterone-stimulating factor (ASF) and its effect on rat adrenal glomerulosa cells in vitro. Hypertension 3:4

Serio M, Forti G, Giusti G, Bassi F, Giannotti P, Calabresi E, Mantero F, Armato U, Fiorelli G, Pinchera A (1980) In vivo and in vitro effects of prolactin on adrenal androgen secretion. In: Genazzani AR, Thijssen JHH, Siiteri PK (eds) Adrenal androgens. Raven Press, New York, p 71

Seron-Ferré M, Lawrence CC, Siiteri PK, Jaffe RB (1978) Steroid production by definitive and fetal zones of the human fetal adrenal gland. J Clin Endocrinol Metab 47:603

Serra GB, Perez-Palacios G, Jaffe RB (1971) Enhancement of 3β-hydroxysteroid dehydrogenase-isomerase in the human fetal adrenal by removal of the soluble cell fraction. Biochim Biophys Acta 244:186

Shackleton CDL, Honour JW, Dillon MJ, Chantler C, Jones RWA (1980) Hypertension in a four-year-old child: Gas chromatographic and mass spectrometric evidence of deficient hepatic metabolism of steroids. J Clin Endocrinol Metab 50:786

Shanklin DR, Richardson AP, Rothstein G (1963) Testicular hilar nodules in adrenogenital syndrome. Am J Dis Child 106:243

Shapiro B, Britton KE, Hawkins LA, Edwards CRW (1981). Clinical experience with ^{75}Se-selenomethylcholesterol adrenal imaging. Clin Endocrinol (Oxf) 15:19

Sheehan HL (1939) Simmond's disease due to post-partum necrosis of the anterior pituitary. Q J Med 8:277

Shirley IM, Cooke BA (1969) Metabolism of dehydroepiandrosterone by the separated zones of the human foetal and newborn adrenal cortex. J Endocrinol 44:411

Short RV (1960) The secretion of sex hormones by the adrenal gland. Biochem Soc Symp 18:59

Shrago SS, Waisman J, Cooper PH (1975) Spironolactone bodies in an adrenal adenoma. Arch Pathol 99:416

Siegler RL, Rallison ML (1978) Hypertension with virilizing adrenal tumor. Pediatrics 61:925

Siemerling E, Creuzfeldt HG (1923) Bronzkrankheit und sklerosierende Encephalomyelitis. Arch Psychiatr Nervenkr 68:217

Sikl H (1948) Addison's disease due to congenital hypoplasia of the adrenals in an infant aged 33 days. J Pathol Bacteriol 60:323

Silman RE, Chard T, Lowry PJ, Smith I, Young IM (1976) Human foetal pituitary peptides and parturition. Nature 260:716

Silman RE, Chard T, Lowry PJ, Mullen PE, Smith I, Young IM (1977) Human fetal corticotrophin and related pituitary peptides. J Steroid Biochem 8:553

Silman RE, Holland D, Chard T, Lowry PJ, Hope J, Robinson JS, Thorburn GD (1978) The ACTH 'family tree' of the rhesus monkey changes with development. Nature 276:526

Simmonds M (1919) Zwergwuchs bei Atrophie des Hypophysisvorderlappens. Dtsch Med Wochenschr 45:487

Simonian MH, Gill GN (1981) Regulation of the fetal human adrenal cortex: Effects of adrenocorticotropin on growth and function of monolayer cultures of fetal and definitive zone cells. Endocrinology 108:1769

Simonian MH, Hornsby PJ, Ill CR, O'Hare MJ, Gill GN (1979) Characterisation of cultured bovine adrenocortical cells and derived clonal lines: Regulation of steroidogenesis and culture life span. Endocrinology 105:99

Simpson ER, Mason JI (1976) Molecular aspects of the biosynthesis of adrenal steroids. Pharmacol Ther B 2:339

Simpson ER, McCarthy JL, Peterson JA (1978) Evidence that the cycloheximide-sensitive site of adrenocorticotropic hormone action is in the mitochondrion. J Biol Chem 253:3135

Simpson SA, Tait JF, Bush IE (1952) Secretion of a salt-retaining hormone by the mammalian adrenal cortex. Lancet II:226

Simpson SA, Tait JF, Wettstein A, Neher R, von Euw J, Schindler O, Reichstein T (1954) Konstitution des Aldosterons, des neuen Mineralocorticoids. Experientia 10:132

Sinclair-Smith C, Kahn LB, Cywes S (1975) Malacoplakia in childhood. Arch Pathol 99:198

Sinterhauf K, Herzog P, Diedrichsen G, Lommer D (1974a) In vitro Corticosteroidbiosynthese in menschlichen Nebennieren. II. Vergleich zwischen normalen und hyperplastischen (Cushing) Nebennieren. Klin Wocheschr 52:1103

Sinterhauf K, Herzog P, Diedrichsen G, Lommer D (1974b) In vitro Corticosteroidbiosynthese in menschlichen Nebennieren. I. Inkubation von Schnitten und Homogenaten frischen und tiefgefroren gelagerten Gewebes. Klin Wochenschr 52:816

Six R, Leclercq R, Noeninckx F (1972) Hypermineralocorticoidism: The sole clinical manifestation of an adrenal cortical carcinoma. Acta Clin Belg 27:426

Sizonenko PC (1975) Endocrine laboratory findings in pubertal disturbances. Clin Endocrinol Metab 4:173

Sklar CA, Kaplan SL, Grumbach MM (1980) Evidence for dissociation between adrenarche and gonadarche: Studies in patients with idiopathic precocious puberty, gonadal dysgenesis, isolated gonadotropin deficiency, and constitutionally delayed growth and adolescence. J Clin Endocrinol Metab 51:548

Slaton PE, Schambelan M, Biglieri EG (1969) Stimulation and suppression of aldosterone secretion in patients with an aldosterone-producing adenoma. J Clin Endocrinol Metab 29:239

Sloper JC (1955) The pathology of the adrenals, thymus and certain other endocrine glands in Addison's disease: An analysis of 37 necropsies. Proc R Soc Med 48:625

Smith HC, Posen S, Clifton-Bligh P, Casey J (1978) A testosterone-secreting adrenal cortical adenoma. Aust NZ J Med 8:171

Smith JA Jr, Middleton RG (1979) Neonatal adrenal hemorrhage. J Urol 122:674

Smith JM, Keane FB, O'Flynn JD, Collins PG (1979) Primary nonfunctioning carcinoma of adrenal cortex. Urology 13:253

Smith PE (1930) Hypophysectomy and a replacement therapy in the rat. Am J Anat 45:205

Snaith AH (1958) A case of feminizing adrenal tumor in a girl. J Clin Endocrinol Metab 18:318

Snearly RG, Ram MD (1978) Myelolipoma of adrenal. Urology 11:411

Sober I, Hirsch M (1965) Unilateral massive adrenal hemorrhage in newborn infant. J Urol 93:430

Sobrinho LG, Kase NG (1970) Adrenal rest cell tumor of the ovary. Obstet Gynecol 36:895

Sobrinho LG, Kase NG, Grunt JA (1971) Changes in adrenocortical function of patients with gonadal dysgenesis after treatment with estrogen. J Clin Endocrinol Metab 33:110

Soffer LJ, Geller J, Gabrilove JL (1957) Response of the plasma 17-hydroxycorticosteroid level to gel-ACTH in tumorous and non-tumorous Cushing's syndrome. J Clin Endocrinol Metab 17:878

Soffer LJ, Dorfman RI, Gabrilove JL (1961a) The human adrenal gland. Lea and Febiger, Philadelphia

Soffer LJ, Iannaccone A, Gabrilove JL (1961b) Cushing's syndrome: A study of fifty patients. Am J Med 30:129

Solomon IL, Schoen EJ (1975) Blood testosterone values in patients with congenital virilizing adrenal hyperplasia. J Clin Endocrinol Metab 40:355

Solomon S, Bird CE, Ling W, Iwamiya M, Young PCM (1967) Formation and metabolism of steroids in the fetus and placenta. Recent Prog Horm Res 23:297

Solomon SS, Swersie JP, Paulsen CA, Biglieri EG (1968) Feminizing adrenocortical carcinoma with hypertension. J Clin Endocrinol Metab 28:608

Sommers SC, Carter ME (1975) Adrenocortical postirradiation fibrosis. Arch Pathol 99:421

Sommers SC, Terzakis JA (1970) Ultrastructural study of aldosterone-secreting cells of the adrenal cortex. Am J Clin Pathol 54:303

Sommerschild HC (1970) Haematoma of the adrenal gland in newborns presenting as an asymptomatic abdominal mass. Z Kinderchir 8:84

Sonino N, Levine LS, Vecsei P, New MI (1980) Parallelism of 11β- and 18-hydroxlation demonstrated by urinary free hormones in man. J Clin Endocrinol Metab 51:557

Sorkin SZ (1957) The adrenals before Addison. J Mt Sinai Hosp 24:1238

Southren AL, Weisenfeld S, Laufer A, Goldner MG (1961) Effect of o,p'-DDD in a patient with Cushing's syndrome. J Clin Endocrinol Metab 21:201

Spark RF, Etzkorn JR (1977) Absent aldosterone response to ACTH in familial glucocorticoid deficiency. N Engl J Med 297:917

Spark RF, Gordon SJ, Dale SL, Melby JC (1968) Aldosterone production after suppression of corticotropin secretory activity. Arch Intern Med 122:394

Spaulding SW, Masuda T, Osawa Y (1980) Increased 17β-hydroxysteroid dehydrogenase activity in a masculinizing adrenal adenoma in a patient with isolated testosterone overproduction. J Clin Endocrinol Metab 50:537

Sperling MA, Wolfsen AR, Fisher DA (1973) Congenital adrenal hypoplasia: An isolated defect of organogenesis. J Pediatr 82:444

Spinner MW, Blizzard PM, Childs B (1968) Clinical and genetic heterogeneity in idiopathic Addison's disease and hypoparathyroidism. J Clin Endocrinol Metab 28:795

Sprague RG, Randall RV, Salassa RM, Scholtz DA, Priestly JT, Halters N, Bulbulian AH (1955) In: American med assoc sci exhibits. Grune & Stratton, New York. p 315

Starkel S, Wegrzynowski J (1910) Beitrag zur Histologie der Nebenniere bei Feten und Kindern. Arch Anat Entwicklungsgesch 34:214

Stewart DR, Morris-Jones PM, Jolleys A (1974) Carcinoma of the adrenal gland in children. J Pediatr Surg 9:59

Stirling GA, Keating VJ (1958) The size of the adrenals in Jamaicans. Br Med J iii:1016

Stoerk O (1908) Zur Histogenese der Grawitz'schen Neirengeschwülste. Beitre Pathol Anat 43:393

Strecker JR, Lauritzen C, Dahlén H, Jonatha W, Gossler W, Tettenborn U (1977) Injections of ACTH and HCG into the fetus during mid-pregnancy legal abortion performed by intra-amniotic instillation of prostaglandin. Influence on maternal plasma oestrogens and testosterone. Horm Metab Res 9:409

Studzinski GP, Symington T, Grant JK (1962) Triphosphopyridine nucleotide-linked dehydrogenases in the adrenal cortex in man: The effect of corticotrophin and the distribution of enzymes. Acta Endocrinol (Copenh) 40:232

Studzinski GP, Hay DCF, Symington T (1963) Observations on the weight of the human adrenal gland and the effect of preparations of corticotropin of different purity on the weight and morphology of the human adrenal gland. J Clin Endocrinol Metab 23:248

Sutherland DJA, Ruse JL, Laidlaw JC (1966) Hypertension, increased aldosterone secretion and low plasma renin activity relieved by dexamethasone. Can Med Assoc J 95:1109

Suzuki S (1976) ACTH secretion and adrenocortical responsiveness in Cushing's syndrome due to adrenocortical hyperplasia. Folia Endocrinol Jpn 52:828

Swann HG (1940) The pituitary-adrenocortical relationship. Physiol Rev 20:493

Swingle WW, Pfiffner JJ (1930) An aqueous extract of the suprarenal cortex which maintains the life of bilaterally adrenalectomized cats. Science 71:321

Symington T (1962) The morphology and zoning of the human adrenal cortex. In: Currie AR, Symington T, Grant JK (eds) The human adrenal cortex. Livingstone, Edinburgh London, p 3

Symington T (1969) Functional pathology of the human adrenal gland. Livingstone, Edinburgh

Symington T, Currie AR, Curran RC, Davidson JN (1955) Reactions of the adrenal cortex in conditions of stress. In: The human adrenal cortex. Ciba Fdn Colloq Endocrinol 8:70

Symington T, Duguid WP, Davidson JN (1956) Effect of exogenous corticotropin on the histochemical pattern of the human adrenal cortex and a comparison with the changes during stress. J Clin Endocrinol Metab 16:580

Symonds DA, Driscoll SG (1973) An adrenal cortical rest within the fetal ovary: Report of a case. Am J Clin Pathol 60:562

Szabo D, Gyevai A, Glaz E, Stark E, Peteri M, Alant O (1975) Changes in the fine structure and function of a hormone-secreting adrenocortical tumour investigated in tissue culture. Virchows Arch [Pathol Anat] 367:273

Szabo S, Huttner I, Kovacs K, Horvath E, Szabo D, Horner HC (1980) Pathogenesis of experimental adrenal hemorrhagic necrosis ('apoplexy'). Ultrastructural, biochemical, neuropharmacologic, and blood coagulation studies with acrylonitrile in the rat. Lab Invest 42:533

Szent-Györgi A (1928) Observations on the function of peroxidase systems and the chemistry of the adrenal cortex. Biochem J 22:1387

Tähkä H (1951) On the weight and structure of the adrenal glands and the factors affecting them in children of 0–2 years. Acta Paediatr Scand [Suppl] 81:1

Tait JF, Tait SAS (1978) A short history of aldosterone. Trends Biochem Sci 4:273

Takayasu K, Okuda K, Yoshikawa I (1970) Fatty acid composition of human and rat adrenal lipids: Occurrence of ω6-docosatrienoic acid in human adrenal cholesterol ester. Lipids 5:743

Tan SY, Mulrow PJ (1975) The contribution of the zona fasciculata and glomerulosa to plasma 11-deoxycorticosterone levels in man. J Clin Endocrinol Metab 41:126

Tan SY, Genel M, Forman BH, Mulrow PJ (1977) Steroid profile in a case of adrenal carcinoma with severe hypertension. Am J Clin Pathol 67:591

Tang CK, Grey GF (1975) Adrenocortical neoplasms, prognosis and morphology. Urology 5:691

Tang C-K, Harriman BB, Toker C (1979) Myxoid adrenal cortical carcinoma. A light and electron microscopic study. Arch Pathol 103:635

Tanimura T, Nelson T, Hollingsworth RR, Shepard TH (1971) Weight standards for organs from early human fetuses. Anat Rec 171:227

Tannenbaum M (1973) Ultrastructural pathology of the adrenal cortex. In: Sommers SC (ed) Pathology annual vol 8. Appleton Century Crofts, New York, p 109

Taylor T, Hamilton W (1973) Human foetal adrenal 4-ene-3-oxosteroid synthesis: An investigation of (4-^{14}C) pregnenolone and (4-^{14}C)dehydroepiandrosterone metabolism using new techniques. J Endocrinol 56:387

Tchertkoff V, Salomon MI, Garret R (1979) Adrenal cortical nodules. Arch Pathol 103:100

Telegdy G, Weeks JW, Archer DF, Wiqvist N, Diczfalusy E (1970) Acetate and cholesterol metabolism in the human foeto-placental unit at mid-gestation. 3. Steroids synthesised and secreted by the foetus. Acta Endocrinol (Copenh) 63:119

Thiele J (1974) Feinstruktutrelle Untersuchungen an einem endokrin aktiven Carcinom der Nebennierenrinde. Virchows Arch [Cell Pathol] 17:51

Thistlethwaite D, Darling JAB, Fraser R, Mason PA, Rees LH, Harkness RA (1975) Familial glucocorticoid deficiency. Studies of diagnosis and pathogenesis. Arch Dis Child 50:291

Thomas H (1911) Ueber die Nebenniere des Kindes und ihre Veränderungen bei Infektionskrankheit. Beitr Pathol Anat 50:495

Thomsen M, Platz P, Andersen OO, Christy M, Lynsgoe J, Nerup J, Rasmussen K, Ryder LP, Staub Neilsen L, Svejgaard A (1975) MLC typing in juvenile diabetes mellitus and idiopathic Addison's disease. Transplant Rev 22:122

Thorburn MJ, Wright ES, Miller CG, Smith-Read EH (1970) Exomphalo-macroglossia-gigantism syndrome in Jamaican infants. Am J Dis Child 119:316

Thorn GW, Dorrance SS, Day E (1942) Addison's disease: Evaluation of synthetic deoxycorticosterone acetate therapy in 158 patients. Ann Intern Med 16:1053

Tipton RH, Pennington GW, Lunt RL, Clarke RG (1971) Androgen-secreting tumour of the adrenal cortex without masculinization. Br Med J ii:744

Tobian L (1960) Interrelationship of electrolytes, juxtaglomerular cells and hypertension. Physiol Rev 40:280

Todesco S, Terribile V, Borsatti A, Mantero F (1975) Primary aldosteronism due to a malignant ovarian tumor. J Clin Endocrinol Metab 41:809

Touchstone JC, Kasparow M (1970) Isolation of 20-hydroxycorticoids from incubated human adrenal tissue. Steroids 15:227

Touchstone JC, Kasparow M, Blakemore WS (1965) Production of 11β, 17,20α,21-tetrahydroxypregn-4-en-3-one and the 20β-epimer by human adrenal tissue. J Clin Endocrinol Metab 25:1463

Touitou Y, Bogdan A, Luton JP (1978) Changes in corticosteroid synthesis of the human adrenal cortex in vitro, induced by treatment with o,p'-DDD for Cushing's syndrome: evidence for the sites of action of the drug. J Steroid Biochem 9:1217

Treager HS, Gabuzda GJ, Zamchek N, Davidson CS (1950) Response to adrenocorticotrophic hormone in clinical scurvy. Proc Soc Exp Biol Med 75:517

Trygstad CW, Mangos JA, Bloodworth JMB, Lobeck CC (1969) A sibship with Bartter's syndrome: Failure of total adrenalectomy to correct the potassium wasting. Pediatrics 44:234

Tsutsui Y, Hirabayashi N, Ito G (1970) An autopsy case of congenital lipoid hyperlasia of the adrenal cortex. Acta Pathol Jpn 20:227

Tucci JR, Espiner EA, Jagger P, Pauk GL, Lauler DP (1967) ACTH stimulation of aldosterone secretion in normal subjects and in patients with chronic adrenocortical insufficiency. J Clin Endocrinol Metab 27:568

Tuck ML, Chandler DW, Mayes DM (1977) The influences of ACTH, dietary sodium, upright posture and angiotensin II on plasma 18-hydroxy-11-deoxycorticosterone levels in normal subjects. J Clin Endocrinol Metab 45:893

Tulcinsky DB, Deutsch V, Bubis JJ (1970) Myelolipoma of the adrenal gland Br J Surg 57:465

Twersky J, Levin DC (1975) Metastatic melanoma of the adrenal: An unusual case of adrenal calcification. Radiology 116:627

Tyrell JB, Brooks RM, Fitzgerald PA, Cofoid PB, Forsham PH, Wilson CB (1978) Cushing's disease. Selective trans-sphenoidal resection of pituitary microadenomas. N Engl J Med 298:753

Ulick S (1976a) Adrenocortical factors in hypertension. I. Significance of 18-hydroxy-11-deoxy-corticosterone. Am J Cardiol 38:814

Ulick S (1976b) Diagnosis and nomenclature of the disorders of the terminal portion of the aldosterone biosynthetic pathway. J Clin Endocrinol Metab 43:92

Ulick S, Gautier E, Vetter KK, Markello JR, Yaffe S, Lowe CU (1964) An aldosterone biosynthetic defect in a salt-losing disorder. J Clin Endocrinol Metab 24:669

Ulick S, Ramirez LC, New MI (1977) An abnormality in steroid reductive metabolism in a hypertensive syndrome. J Clin Endocrinol Metab 44:799

Ulick S, Eberlein WR, Bliffeld AR, Chu MD, Bongiovanni AM (1980) Evidence for an aldosterone biosynthetic defect in congenital adrenal hyperplasia. J Clin Endocrinol Metab 51:1346

Unsicker K (1971) On the innervation of the rat and pig adrenal cortex. Z Zellforsch 116:151

Uotila UU (1940) The early embryological development of the fetal and permanent adrenal cortex in man. Anat Rec 76:183

Uras A, Budak D, Ariogul O, Görpe A, Tahsinoglu M (1978) A functioning black adenoma of the adrenal gland. Clin Oncol 4:181

Urban MD, Lee PA, Gutai JP, Migeon CJ (1980) Androgens in pubertal males with Addison's disease. J Clin Endocrinol Metab 51:925

Uretsky G, Freund H, Charuzi I, Luttwak EM (1978) Cysts of the adrenal gland. Eur Urol 4:97

Urushibata K (1971) Fine structure of adrenocortical cell in Cushing's syndrome. Nagoya J Med Sci 34:27

Uttley WS (1968) Familial congenital adrenal hypoplasia. Arch Dis Child 43:724

Vagnucci AH (1969) Selective aldosterone deficiency. J Clin Endocrinol Metab 29:279

Valente M, Pennelli N, Segato P, Bevilacqua L, Thiene G (1978) Androgen producing adrenocortical carcinoma. A histological and ultrastructural study of two cases. Virchows Arch [Pathol Anat] 378:91

Van der Water JM, Fonkalsrud EW (1966) Adrenal cysts in infancy. Surgery 60:1267

Van Hale HM, Turkel SB (1979) Neuroblastoma and adrenal morphologic features in anencephalic infants. Arch Pathol 103:119

Van Seters AP, Van Aalderen W, Moolenaar AJ, Gorsiro MCB, Van Roon F, Backer ET (1981) Adrenocortical tumour in untreated congenital adrenocortical hyperplasia associated with inadequate ACTH suppressibility. Clin Endocrinol (Oxf) 14:325

Varma MM, Huseman CA, Johanson AJ, Blizzard RM (1977) Effect of prolactin on adrenocortical and gonadal function in normal men. J Clin Endocrinol Metab 44:760

Vecsei P, Purjesz I, Wolff HP (1969) Studies on the biosynthesis of aldosterone in solitary adenoma and in nodular hyperplasia of the adrenal cortex in patients exhibiting Conn's syndrome. Acta Endocrinol (Copenh) 62:391

Veldhuis JD, Kulin HE, Santen RJ, Wilson TE, Melby JC (1980) Inborn error in the terminal step of aldosterone biosynthesis: Corticosterone methyl oxidase type II deficiency in a North American pedigree. N Engl J Med 303:117

Velican C (1948) Embryogenèse de la surrénale humaine. Arch Anat Microsc Morphol Exp 37:73

Verberckmoes R, VanDamme B, Clement J (1976) Bartter's syndrome with hyperplasia of renomedullary interstitial cells. Successful treatment with indomethacin. Kidney Int 9:302

Vermeulen A, Ando S (1978) Prolactin and adrenal androgen secretion. Clin Endocrinol (Oxf) 8:295

Vermeulen A, Rubens R (1979) Adrenal virilism. In: James VHT (ed) The adrenal gland. Raven Press, New York, p 259

Vermeulen A. Verdonck L (1976) Radioimmunoassay of 17β-hydroxy-5α-androstan-3-one, 4-androstene-3,17-dione, dehydroepiandrosterone, 17-hydroxyprogesterone and progesterone and its application to human male plasma. J Steroid Biochem 7:1

Vermeulen A, Suy E, Rubens R (1977) Effect of prolactin on plasma DHEA(S) levels. J Clin Endocrinol Metab 44:1222

Vihko R, Ruokonen A (1975) Steroid sulphates in human adult testicular steroid synthesis. J Steroid Biochem 6:353

Vilar O, Tullner WW (1959) Effects of o,p′-DDD on histology and 17-hydroxycorticosteroid output of the dog adrenal cortex. Endocrinology 65:80

Villee CA, Loring JM (1965) Synthesis of steroids in the newborn human adrenal in vitro. J Clin Endocrinol Metab 25:307

Villee CA, Loring JM (1969) The synthesis and cleavage of steroid sulphates in the human fetus and placenta. In: Pecile A, Finzi C (eds) The foeto-placental unit. Excerpta Med Found, Amsterdam, p 182

Villee DB, Engel LL, Villee CA (1959) Steroid hydroxylation in human fetal adrenals. Endocrinology 65:465

Villee DB, Engel LL, Loring JM, Villee CA (1961) Steroid hydroxylation in human fetal adrenals: formation of 16α-hydroxyprogesterone, 17-hydroxyprogesterone and deoxycorticosterone. Endocrinology 69:354

Vinson GP, Whitehouse BJ (1976) In vitro modification of rat adrenal zona fasciculata/reticularis function by the zona glomerulosa. Acta Endocrinol (Copenh) 81:340

Vinson GP, Whitehouse BJ, Dell A, Etienne T, Morris HR (1980) Characterisation of an adrenal zona glomerulosa-stimulating component of posterior pituitary extracts as α-MSH. Nature 284:464

Visser HKA, Cost WS (1964) A new hereditary defect in the biosynthesis of aldosterone: Urinary C_{21}-corticosteroid pattern in three related patients with a salt-losing syndrome, suggesting an 18-oxidation defect. Acta Endocrinol (Copenh) 47:589

Visser JW, Boeijinga JK, Meer CD (1974) A functioning black adenoma of the adrenal cortex: A clinico-pathological entity. J Clin Pathol 27:955

Voigt KH, Fehm HL, Pfeiffer EF (1975) Dissociation of in vivo and in vitro 'autonomy' in a human adrenocortical tumour. Acta Endocrinol (Copenh) 78:302

Völpel M (1971) Hiluszellwucherungen im Ovar bei connatalem adrenogenitalem Syndrom. Virchows Arch [Pathol Anat] 352:43

Voutilainen R, Kahri AI, Salmenperä M (1979) The effects of progesterone, pregnenolone, estriol, ACTH and hCG on steroid secretion of cultured human fetal adrenals. J Steroid Biochem 10:695

Wahl HR (1951) Adrenal cysts. Am J Pathol 27:758

Wajchenberg BL, Goldman J, Kyan TS, Achando SS, Thomsen YL, Lima SS (1980) Oestrogen dynamics in adrenal venous effluents in congenital virilizing adrenal hyperplasia. Clin Endocrinol (Oxf) 13:401

Waldhäusl W, Herkner K, Nowotny P, Bratusche-Marrain P (1978) Combined 17α- and 18-hydroxylase deficiency associated with complete male pseudohermaphroditism and hypoaldosteronism. J Clin Endocrinol Metab 46:236

Wallach S, Brown H, Englert E, Eik-Nes K (1957) Adrenocortical carcinoma with gynecomastia: A case report and review of the literature. J Clin Endocrinol Metab 17:945

Ward TJ, Grant JK (1963) The metabolism of progesterone by adrenocortical tissues from patients with Cushing's syndrome. J Endocrinol 26:139

Warkany J (1971) Congenital malformations. Year Book Medical Publishers Inc, Chicago, p 427

Warne GL, Carter JN, Faiman C, Reyes FI, Winter JSD (1978) Hormonal changes in girls with precocious adrenarche: A possible role for estradiol or prolactin. J Pediatr 92:743

Waterhouse R (1911) A case of suprarenal apoplexy. Lancet I:577

Wegienka LC, Wuepper KD, Komarmy LE, Forsham PH (1966) Cushing's syndrome with adrenal medullary insufficiency and adrenal autoantibodies. Lancet I:741

Weinberger MH, Kem DC, Gomez-Sanchez C, Kramer NJ, Martin BT, Nugent CA (1975) The effect of dexamethasone on the control of plasma aldosterone concentration in normal recumbent man. J Lab Clin Med 85:957

Weinberger MH, Grim CE, Hollifield JW, Kem DC, Ganguly A, Kramer NJ, Yune HY, Wellman H, Donohue JP (1979) Primary aldosteronism: Diagnosis, localization and treatment. Ann Intern Med 90:386

Weiner N (1975) Control of the biosynthesis of adrenal catecholamines by the adrenal medulla. In: Greep RO, Astwood EB (eds) Handbook of physiology vol VI, Adrenal gland. American Physiological Society, Washington p 357

Weinstein RL, Kliman B, Neeman J, Cohen RB (1970) Deficient 17-hydroxylation in a corticosterone producing adrenal tumor from an infant with hemihypertrophy and visceromegaly. J Clin Endocrinol Metab 30:457

Weiss L, Mellinger RC (1970) Congenital adrenal hypoplasia – An X-linked disease. J Med Genet 7:27

Welbourn RB, Montgomery DAD, Kennedy TL (1971) The natural history of treated Cushing's syndrome. Br J Surg 58:1

Weliky I, Engel LL (1963) Metabolism of progesterone-4-C^{14} and pregnenolone-7-H^3 by human adrenal tissue. J Biol Chem 238:1302

Wells HG (1930) Addison's disease with selective destruction of the suprarenal cortex. Arch Pathol 10:499

Werk EE, Sholiton LE, Kalejs L (1973) Testosterone-secreting adrenal adenoma under gonadotropin control. N Eng J Med 289:767

West CD, Meikle AW (1980) Laboratory tests for the diagnosis of Cushing's syndrome and adrenal insufficiency and factors effecting those tests. In: deGroot LJ et al. (eds) Endocrinology vol 2. Grune & Stratton, New York, p 1157

West CD, Damast B, Pearson OH (1958) Adrenal estrogens in patients with metastatic breast cancer. J Clin Invest 37:341

West CD, Kumagai LF, Simons EL, Dominguez OV, Berliner DL (1964) Adrenocortical carcinoma with feminization and hypertension associated with a defect in 11β-hydroxylation. J Clin Endocrinol Metab 24:567

West CD, Atcheson JB, Stanchfield JB, Rallison ML, Chavre VJ, Tyler FH (1979) Multiple or single 21-hydroxylases in congenital adrenal hyperplasia. J Steroid Biochem 11:1413

Westphal U (1971) Steroid-protein interactions. Monographs on Endocrinology Vol 4. Springer Verlag, Berlin

Wheeler TD, Vincent S (1917) The question as to the relative importance to life of cortex and medulla of the adrenal bodies. Trans R Soc Can 11:125

Whitehouse BJ, Vinson GP (1968) Corticosteroid biosynthesis from pregnenolone and progesterone by human adrenal tissue in vitro. A kinetic study. Steroids 11:245

Whittaker LD (1968) Myelolipoma of the adrenal gland. Arch Surg 97:628

Wilbur OM, Rich AR (1953) A study of the role of adrenocorticotropic hormone (ACTH) in the pathogenesis of tubular degeneration of the adrenals. Bull Johns Hopkins Hosp 93:321

Wilkins L, Ravitch MM (1952) Adrenocortical tumor arising in the liver of a 3-year-old boy with signs of virilism and Cushing's syndrome. Report of a case with cure after partial resection of the right lobe of liver. Pediatrics 9:671

Williams GH, Braley LM (1977) Effects of dietary sodium and potassium intake and acute stimulation on aldosterone output by isolated human adrenal cells. J Clin Endocrinol Metab 45:55

Williams GH, Braley LM, Underwood RH (1976) The regulation of plasma 18-hydroxy-11-deoxycorticosterone in man. J Clin Invest 58:221

Williams GH, Dluhy RG (1972) Aldosterone biosynthesis: Interrelationship of regulatory factors Am J Med 53:595

Williams GH, Hollenberg NK, Brown C, Mersey JH (1978) Adrenal responses to pharmacological interruption of the renin-angiotensin system in sodium-restricted normal man. J Clin Endocrinol Metab 47:725

Williams GH, Rose LI, Dluhy RG, Dingman JF, Lauler DP (1971) Aldosterone response to sodium restriction and ACTH stimulation in panhypopituitarism. J Clin Endocrinol Metab 32:27

Williams GH, Tuck ML, Rose LI, Dluhy RG, Underwood RH (1972) Studies of the control of plasma aldosterone concentration in normal man. III. Response to sodium chloride infusion. J Clin Invest 51:2645

Wilms G, Baert A, Marchal G, Goddeeris P (1979) Computed tomography of the normal adrenal glands: correlative study with autopsy specimens. J Comput Assist Tomogr 3:467

Winter JSD, Fujieda K, Faiman C, Reyes FI, Thliveris J (1980) Control of steroidogenesis by human fetal adrenal cells in tissue culture. In:Genazzani AR, Thijssen JHH, Siiteri P (eds) Adrenal androgens. Raven Press, New York, p 55

Winters AJ, Oliver C, Colston C, MacDonald PC, Porter JC (1974) Plasma ACTH levels in the human fetus and neonate as related to age and parturition. J Clin Endocrinol Metab 39:269

Winters AJ, Colston C, MacDonald PC, Porter JC (1975) Fetal plasma prolactin levels. J Clin Endocrinol Metab 41:626

Wintersteiner O, Pfiffner JJ (1935) Chemical studies on the adrenal cortex. II. Isolation of several physiologically inactive crystalline compounds from active extracts. J Biol Chem 111:599

Wohltmann H, Mathur RS, Williamson HO (1980) Sexual precocity in a female infant due to feminizing adrenal carcinoma. J Clin Endocrinol Metab 50:186

Wolman M, Sterk VV, Gratl S, Frenkel M (1961) Primary familial xanthomatosis with involvement and calcification of adrenal. Pediatrics 28:742

Wong T-W, Warner NE (1971) Ovarian thecal metaplasia in the adrenal gland. Arch Pathol 92:319

Woolley PG (1903) Adrenal tumours. Am J Med Sci 125:33

Wright RD (1963) Blood flow through the adrenal gland. Endocrinology 72:418

Wüchner U, Mieler W (1977) Zwillinge mit beidseitiger Nebennierenagenesie. Kinderaerztl Prax 9:405

Wuepper KD, Wegienka LC, Fudenberg HH (1969) Immunologic aspects of adrenocortical insufficiency. Am J Med 46:206

Xarli VP, Steele AA, Davis PJ, Buescher ES, Rios CN, Garcia-Bunuel R (1978) Adrenal hemorrhage in the adult. Medicine 57:211

Yalow RS, Berson S (1971) The heterogeneity of immunoreactive human ACTH in plasma and in extracts of ACTH-producing thymoma. Biochem Biophys Res Commun 44:439

Yalow RS, Berson S (1973) Characteristics of 'big ACTH' in human plasma and pituitary extracts. J Clin Endocrinol Metab 36:415

Yamaji T, Ishibashi M, Katayama S, Kosaka K (1980) Serum 16β-hydroxydehydroepiandrosterone sulfate in man. J Clin Endocrinol Metab 50:955

Yamasaki H, Shimuzu K (1973) Intracellular distribution and substrate specificity of the 16α-hydroxylase in the adrenal of human fetus. Steroids 22:637

Yates J, Deshpande N (1975) Evidence for the existence of a single 3β-hydroxysteroid dehydrogenase/$\Delta^{5,4}$-3-oxosteroid isomerase complex in the human adrenal cortex. J Endocrinol 64:195

Yotsumoto S, Aizawa T, Kotani M, Yamada T (1979) Virilizing adrenal adenoma stimulated by dexamethasone in a middle-aged woman. J Clin Endocrinol Metab 48:660

Zachmann M, Prader A (1975) Gynecomastia with congenital virilizing adrenal hyperplasia (11β-hydroxylase deficiency). J Pediatr 87:839

Zachmann M, Völlmin JA, New MI, Curtius H-C, Prader A (1971) Congenital adrenal hyperplasia due to deficiency of 11β-hydroxylation of 17α-hydroxylated steroids. J Clin Endocrinol Metab 33:501

Zager PG, Hsueh WA, Luetscher JA, Biglieri EG, Dowdy AJ (1980) Effect of des-Asp[1]-angiotensin II on secretion and metabolism of aldosterone. J Clin Endocrinol Metab 50:874

Zipser RD, Rude RK, Zia PK, Fichman MP (1979) Regulation of urinary prostaglandins in Bartter's syndrome. Am J Med 67:263

Zumoff B, Fukushima DK, Weitzmann ED, Kream J, Hellman L (1974) The sex difference in plasma cortisol concentration in man. J Clin Endocrinol Metab 39:805

Zwierzina WD (1979) Ultrastruktur der normalen menschlichen Nebennierenrinde. Acta Anat (Basel) 103:409

Subject Index